Modelling and Computational Approaches for Multi-Scale Phenomena in Cancer Research

From Cancer Evolution to Cancer Treatment

Modelling and Computational Approaches for Multi-Scale Phenomena in Cancer Research

From Cancer Evolution to Cancer Treatment

editors

Raluca Eftimie
University of Franche-Comté, France

Dumitru Trucu
University of Dundee, UK

World Scientific

NEW JERSEY · LONDON · SINGAPORE · BEIJING · SHANGHAI · HONG KONG · TAIPEI · CHENNAI · TOKYO

Published by

World Scientific Publishing Europe Ltd.

57 Shelton Street, Covent Garden, London WC2H 9HE

Head office: 5 Toh Tuck Link, Singapore 596224

USA office: 27 Warren Street, Suite 401-402, Hackensack, NJ 07601

Library of Congress Cataloging-in-Publication Data
Names: Eftimie, Raluca, editor. | Trucu, Dumitru, editor.
Title: Modelling and computational approaches for multi-scale phenomena in cancer research :
    from cancer evolution to cancer treatment / editors, Raluca Eftimie,
    University of Franche-Comté, France, Dumitru Trucu, University of Dundee, UK.
Description: New Jersey : World Scientific, [2025] | Includes bibliographical references and index.
Identifiers: LCCN 2023057790 | ISBN 9781800614376 (hardcover) |
    ISBN 9781800614383 (ebook) | ISBN 9781800614390 (ebook other)
Subjects: LCSH: Cancer--Mathematical models. | Cancer--Computer simulation. |
    Cancer--Research. | Multiscale modeling. | Biological models.
Classification: LCC RC267 .M636 2025 | DDC 616.99/40072--dc23/eng/20240325
LC record available at https://lccn.loc.gov/2023057790

British Library Cataloguing-in-Publication Data
A catalogue record for this book is available from the British Library.

For any available supplementary material, please visit
https://www.worldscientific.com/worldscibooks/10.1142/Q0424#t=suppl

Desk Editors: Balasubramanian Shanmugam/Rosie Williamson/Shi Ying Koe

Typeset by Stallion Press
Email: enquiries@stallionpress.com

Preface

Despite the progress recorded over the past few decades, the understanding of the basic mechanisms behind the solid tumours development and invasion is far from being complete. The wide complexity of intertwined processes involved in cancer growth and spread pose tremendous challenges in the current endeavours for deciphering the overall solid tumour dynamics as well for identifying effective avenues of invasion control and treatment. Nevertheless, horizons of hope are definitely there, and these arise from the many increasing interdisciplinary approaches that were advanced over the past three decades, where clinical *in vivo* investigations were not only complemented with wet-lab *in vitro* analysis but also by increasingly sophisticated mathematical modelling and computational simulations that were able to replicate *in silico* key aspects involved in cancer development and spread. Moreover, mathematical and computational modelling offers unparalleled opportunity for scrutinising existing biological perspectives and clinical approaches as well as for advancing new hypothesis for experimental investigations.

Starting with an overview of clinical challenges in treating grade 4 brain tumours (glioblastomas), this book aims to give a perspective over several significant current mathematical modelling approaches and computational simulation advances for key processes in solid tumour development, detection, and treatment. These include both single-scale and multi-scale modelling, involving a series of approaches that local and non-local techniques at each scale considered (whether tissue- or cell-scales) as well as for the cross-talk between the dynamics at tissue- and cell- scales when the integrated two-scale tumour dynamics is considered.

This book is aimed at both young researchers and senior investigators in the area of mathematical modelling for solid tumour growth, with the ultimate hope to inspire and stimulate fresh perspectives in this highly active mathematical and computational research direction. While mindful that this book is not an exhaustive recap and rather just a projection within the wide range of modelling and analysis methodologies that are currently being developed for addressing cancer progression, it is hoped that the works selected and the topics addressed here will act as a catalyst for generating new ideas in mathematical modelling, analysis, and computational approaches, both for advancing the understanding of solid tumour dynamics beyond the current state and by taking forward the frontiers of mathematics with novel concepts that will be necessary for expressing the newly acquired knowledge.

Raluca Eftimie
Dumitru Trucu

About the Editors

Raluca Eftimie is a Professor in Mathematics at the University of Franche-Comté, France (and honorary professor at the University of Dundee, UK), interested in single-scale and multi-scale modelling of various phenomena in biology and medicine. She is on the Editorial Boards of multiple journals in Applied Mathematics/Mathematical Biology. She has previously published a research monograph on *Hyperbolic and Kinetic Models for Self-Organised Biological Aggregations: A Modelling and Pattern Formation Approach* (Springer, 2018).

Dumitru Trucu is a Reader in Mathematics at the University of Dundee, UK. His research interest is in the area of computational multi-scale moving boundary modelling and analysis for multi-scale structured processes involved with solid tumours growth and spread in fibrous tissue environments. He has previously co-authored a research monograph on *Mathematical Models and Methods for Living Systems*: Levico Terme, Italy 2014 — Lecture Notes in Mathematics 2167 — CIME Foundation Subseries (Springer, 1st ed., 2016).

Contents

Chapter 1

Introduction: Brief Review of Multi-Scale Aspects in Cancer

Raluca Eftimie[*]

Laboratoire de mathématiques de Besançon,
Université de Franche-Comté,
Besançon, France
raluca.eftimie@univ-fcomte.fr

Experimental and clinical studies published over the last few decades have emphasised the complex biological processes that take place inside the tumour microenvironment during the evolution of primary tumours as well as secondary tumours (i.e., metastases). These processes occur at multiple scales (molecular, cellular, and tissue scales) and their complex interlinking and continuous evolution have significant impacts on the success of anti-tumour therapies. In this introductory chapter, we discuss some multi-scale biological aspects related to tumour progression that are discussed in more detail in the rest of the chapters. The goal of this chapter is also to draw a link between the various other chapters of this book.

---

[*]The author is also an Honorary Professor at School of Science and Engineering, University of Dundee, Dundee, UK. Email address: r.a.eftimie@dundee.ac.uk.

1. Introduction to Multi-Scale Aspects in Cancer

The complexity and diversity of neoplastic diseases, that generated a huge scientific literature over the last century but for which no general treatment was found yet, were captured in the six hallmarks of cancer proposed in the seminal paper by Hanahan and Weinberg (2000) [1]: self-sufficiency in growth signals, insensitivity to anti-growth signals, tissue invasion and metastasis, limitless replicative potential, sustained angiogenesis, and evading apoptosis. A decade later, these six hallmarks were then completed with two more hallmarks [2], namely deregulation in cellular energetics and avoidance of immune destruction, and two enabling characteristics (genome instability and mutation and tumour-promoting inflammation). These eight hallmarks, which are shared by all known cancers [1], emphasise the multi-scale aspect of cancers: they are regulated by various intracellular signalling pathways (some of which being redundant) [2], to allow tumour cells to interact with each other and with the environment (i.e., stroma and immune cells) in a dynamic manner during the multiple stages of tumour development.

These dynamic interactions also lead to tumour heterogeneity [3] and immunological heterogeneity [4] inside the tumour-immune microenvironment, which is another aspect of the multi-scale characteristics of neoplastic diseases. Tumour heterogeneity refers to the existence of sub-populations of cells inside the various spatial regions of primary and/or secondary (i.e., metastasis) tumour aggregations, with different genotypes and phenotypes, which display different biological behaviours [3]. Immunological heterogeneity refers to the diversity of immune cells infiltrating tumours, the diversity of cytokine/chemokine environment inside tumours, the diversity in the cytotoxic anti-tumour activity of different immune cells, and the diversity of immunosuppressive aspects of tumours [4]. For both tumour and immune cells, there are two types of heterogeneity: spatial heterogeneity, characterised by uneven localisation of tumour and immune cells within spatial regions of the tumour microenvironment [4], and temporal heterogeneity characterised by a dynamical evolution of tumour cells and immune responses during the course of tumour progression or following treatment [4]. All these heterogeneity aspects observed at tissue level are the result of heterogeneity at molecular and cell levels in both tumour and immune cells.

Moreover, there is a correlation between the heterogeneity of tumour cells and the heterogeneity of immune cells, suggesting a co-evolution of the tumour and immune cells that reinforces the temporal heterogeneity. In addition, histopathologists have known for a long time that there are not only (i) morphological differences between different regions of a tumour tissue or between different tumours inside a single patient but also (ii) differences in tumour behaviour between different patients that have the same type of tumour [3]. To address heterogeneity issue (i), histopathologists routinely examine different sections of the same tumour to grade the cancers and make predictions about their evolution and the survival of the patient. More recently, to improve detection accuracy and reduce time, the clinical-pathological examinations of tumour tissues by trained pathologists have started to be helped by the use of machine learning algorithms, as is discussed in the following. In regard to heterogeneity issue (ii), this is mainly manifested as differential or mixed responses of patients to anti-tumour therapies [3]. These mixed responses are the result of dynamic interactions between the tumour and immune components of the tumour-immune microenvironment. It should be mentioned that such mixed responses could be also observed inside the same patient, where anti-tumour drugs can eliminate some tumours but not all, following the accumulation of new molecular aberrations as a consequence of tumour progression [5].

Understanding these dynamic changes, which are the result of multiple interactions between the various components of the tumour microenvironment at molecular, cellular, and tissue scales, is crucial for the development of new successful anti-cancer therapies [2]. Unfortunately, the complexity of these interactions that can be local or nonlocal, uni-directional or multi-directional, temporal or spatio-temporal, makes it very difficult for the human mind to understand them. In the most recent review in these series of hallmarks of cancer, Hanahan [6] emphasised the continuous discovery of new facets of the disease as a result of more powerful experimental and computational tools and technologies.

Computational and mathematical models are often used to analyse available data, to qualitatively and/or quantitatively reproduce stationary and dynamic patterns observed in the data, or to investigate the range of outcomes when certain hypotheses are made about a biological system (hypotheses which cannot be tested experimentally due to financial or technical/methodological constraints) [7]. In the context of cancer research, the past few decades have focussed mainly on mathematical models for single-scale data. However, advances in experimental approaches have emphasised the importance of cell–cell and cell–environment interactions across multiple scales (molecular, cellular, and tissue scales) on the overall evolution of the tumour and the need for new mathematical modelling and computational approaches to understand these multi-scale interactions by connecting back to the data [8]. Also, recent advances in artificial intelligence have led to the development of various computational approaches (e.g., based on image preprocessing and image segmentation algorithms) for the automatic detection of cancer cells inside tissues (i.e., macroscale level) [9], while taking into consideration various information about the cellular and molecular structure of these tissues. In addition, machine learning (ML) computational approaches have been used, for example, to predict patient survival for multiple cancer types [10] and to predict therapeutic responses for different anticancer therapies [11]. While the future of the mathematical oncology field will see the integration of ML approaches with deterministic and stochastic mathematical models towards the development of "digital twins" [12] (i.e., digital replica of cells, tissues, organs, and even patients) to be used for personalised cancer therapies, we acknowledge that we are not there yet and we still need to develop new mathematical models, to understand if such models can reproduce the observed cancer dynamics, and to understand the power and limitations of these mathematical models.

The goal of this book is to review a few state-of-the-art approaches in the mathematical and computational modelling of cancer development and evolution as a result of single-scale and multi-scale interactions between cancer cells and their environment, in the mathematical modelling of various cancer therapies, in the development of new mathematical and computational tools for parametrisation of these models with various single-scale and multi-scale data, while emphasising current open problems in the field.

In the following, we summarise briefly the chapters in this book, some of which are more biological while others are more mathematical. However, altogether all these chapters tell a story about our current understanding of the complexity of the cancer problem (and the heterogeneity of the tumour-immune microenvironment) and the need to develop new modelling, analytical, and computational tools to integrate cancer data across different spatial and spatio-temporal scales. In fact, all these chapters focus one way or another on data: available data, unavailable data, use of multi-scale data, and/or some experimental knowledge to inform the development of complex mathematical models, methods to parametrise the mathematical models using such data. Also, most of the chapters end with a short discussion of some open problems related to the respective topics.

2. Mathematical and Biophysical Models for Cancer

To ensure a logical flow in the presentation of the problem, this book starts with presentations of various biological and biomechanical aspects related to molecular/cellular/tissue dynamics of tumour cells as well as other cells in the tumour microenvironment, such as immune cells. These biological presentations are followed by presentations of mathematical models as well as computational and analytical approaches used to investigate these models and to connect with the available data. Hence, Chapters 2–4 have strong biological/ immunological/biomechanical components followed by discussions of various modelling approaches; Chapters 5–7 have strong modelling components combined with detailed computational investigations of the behaviours of the multi-scale models presented in each of those studies; Chapters 8 and 9 focus on computational and analytical approaches aimed at identifying model parameters from real/synthetic datasets. To highlight the results in this book, in the following, we summarise briefly the various chapters while emphasising the connecting ideas presented throughout these chapters.

Chapter 2 focusses on glioblastoma (GBM), as a case study for a highly aggressive (and also a very common) tumour and for the use of mathematical models for the development of cancer precision medicines. The chapter starts with a clinical presentation and management of GBM, after which the authors discuss various factors that lead to the very poor prognosis of GBM, the hystopathogenesis of GBM, and then the hallmarks of cancer relevant to the maintenance and progression of GBM. After this discussion focussed mostly on microscale aspects of GBM, the authors talk about the macroscopic growth patterns and morphology of GBM. This chapter concludes with a summary of a few types of mathematical models derived over the past years to address some of the clinical challenges associated with GBM, followed by a discussion of possible future directions and scope of single-sale and multi-scale mathematical models of GBM and their integration with data. Overall, this chapter summarises the complex interplay of various factors at genetic, molecular, microscopic, and macroscopic levels behind this most common and most aggressive brain tumour and sets the stage for all other chapters in this book (some also focussed on brain tumours).

Chapter 3 focusses on general biological and modelling aspects related to immune responses to cancers. It starts with a brief review of some immune cells involved in the fight against cancers, as well as some current immunotherapies targeting immune–tumour interactions at molecular level. These biological aspects then form the basis for the discussion of some classes of continuum multi-scale mathematical models for cancer-immune interactions and the impact of different immunotherapies. The chapter ends with a brief discussion of some open problems related to the parameterisation of these models with single-scale and multi-scale data.

Chapter 4 focusses on biophysical modelling of tumour viscoelasticity and surface tension in the context of breast cancer spheroids. The authors start with a biological and biophysical review of some main parameters that influence the rearrangement of cell spheroids as a result of their collective motion: tissue surface tension and solid stress accumulation (both normal and shear stress). Then, they review in detail two multi-scale models for the fusion of cell spheroids: (i) a model for the constitutive behaviour of two epithelial spheroids: the Zener model, characterised by dominant viscous behaviour occurring on a short time scale and an elastic behaviour occurring on a long time scale, and (ii) a model for the constitutive behaviour of two cancer spheroids: the Maxwell model, characterised by a dominant elastic behaviour on a short time scale and a viscous behaviour on a long time scale.

Chapter 5 focusses on kinetic transport models for cell migration in response to different superposing stimuli. The authors start by reviewing the general form of a kinetic transport equation for the movement of cells characterised by a certain speed and polarisation direction as internal states. Then they show the derivation of such kinetic models from microscopic stochastic processes and present approaches to recover some of the main statistical properties of the cell populations from the kinetic equations. The chapter ends with the presentation and numerical investigation of three case studies for different non-local cell sensing of environmental stimuli: (i) chemotaxis and physical limits of migration on the extracellular matrix (ECM), (ii) contact guidance and steric hindrance in the context of breast cancer migration on the ECM, and (iii) contact guidance and chemotaxis.

Chapter 6 focusses on a multi-scale moving-boundary mathematical model for the use of combination chemo-viro-therapy in cancer treatments. This therapy combines a classical chemotherapy approach with a therapy using oncolytic viruses (i.e., viruses that selectively replicate inside and destroy cancer cells). The microscale sub-model considers the dynamics of the matrix degrading enzymes in small microdomains on tumour boundary. The macroscale sub-model considers the spatio-temporal changes in the densities of infected and uninfected tumour cells, extracellular matrix (ECM), oncolytic viruses, and the concentration of the chemotherapy drug. The two sub-models are connected through the following: (a) the production of microscale matrix-degrading enzymes by the infected and uninfected cancer cells and (b) the degradation of the ECM by these enzymes, which changes the boundaries of the tumour at the macroscale. Numerical simulations are used to investigate different case studies: (i) virotherapy as a monotherapy; (ii) chemotherapy as a monotherapy; (iii) sequential combination therapy: first oncolytic virus and then chemotherapy; (iv) sequential combination therapy: chemotherapy first and then viral therapy; (v) simultaneous chemotherapy and virotherapy with constant influx of therapies or temporal-pulsed injections or spatio-temporal pulsed injections (i.e, viral injection at different positions in space). The simulations identified the best treatment scenario (for the parameter values considered in the study): injection of both OV and the chemotherapy drug with five initial doses at different spatial locations inside/outside tumour.

Chapter 7 focusses on a multi-scale mathematical model for the impact of interferon (IFN) response on oncolytic virus (OV) therapies against cancers. To investigate the complex role of IFN on cancer therapies, which has an impact on the spatio-structural heterogeneity of cells inside solid tumours, the three variables in this model (cancer cell population, molecular IFN population, and oncolytic viruses population) are structured by space, internal viral load, and surface–ligand binding of IFN. Numerical simulations, performed with some arbitrary parameter values, investigate the evolution of cancer population under OV treatment in the absence and in the presence of an IFN immune response. The results show time-variation in the cancer cells across the physical space and the space of the structural variables (i.e., viral load and surface–ligand binding of IFN). Overall, this study emphasises the ability of mathematical models to capture simultaneously spatial and biochemical heterogeneity within the framework of temporal dynamics of various populations inside the tumour microenvironment.

Chapter 8 focusses on a data-driven growth model for the formation of astrocytoma tumours that incorporates a mechano-biological triggering hypothesis for the malignant transformation from grade 2 to grade 3 astrocytomas. The authors start with a discussion of the classification and the grading system of brain cancers, followed by a presentation various aspects related to malignant transformations of these cancers across the different evolution stages. Next, they present imaging techniques used for the diagnosis of low grade gliomas, followed by a detailed discussion of available data and the description of the model equations. The numerical outputs of the model are calibrated against patient data 69 days after the initial detection data. Finally, the model is evaluated on its prediction of a malignant transformation observed in the patient data more than 600 days after the initial detection.

Chapter 9 focusses on an inverse problem that aims to estimate the original tumour size based on the size of the tumour at a final time, to generate further insight into tumour growth and its origin. To this end, the authors investigate the backward evolution of a reaction-diffusion mathematical model describing a brain tumour. The inverse problem is formulated as a minimisation of a cost functional that compares the solution of the mathematical model and the data, with the initial tumour density as the control parameter. For numerical simulations, the authors used Magnetic Resonance Tomography images from the BraTS'20 dataset (i.e., real brain images of two patients), on which they first simulated the growth of an initial tumour until a final state (by solving forward in time the reaction-diffusion model). Then, they used two approaches, namely Nonlinear

Conjugate Gradient (NCG) method and the Landweber method, to reconstruct the initial tumour data. The results showed that the error between the original tumour and the numerically reconstructed tumour is small, and the computational approaches are capable to reconstruct past tumour cells distributions.

In summary, all chapters in this book emphasise the power of mathematical and computational modelling for complementing experimental and clinical studies to understand the evolution of solid tumours as a results of single-scale and multi-scale interactions between the various components of the tumour-immune microenvironment and to understand and predict the success of different anti-tumour therapies. Although prediction depends on available relevant data, which is sometimes lacking at this moment [8], the mathematical and computational approaches presented here emphasise the path towards precision medicine that will dominate the oncological and mathematical-oncology research in the upcoming years. They also emphasise the fact that before we arrive at incorporating data into these models to completely parametrise them, we need to explore the power and limitations of such models to reproduce the experimentally observed and clinically observed behaviours and to investigate the mathematical and computational challenges that prevent the straightforward parametrisation of such multi-scale models.

References

[1]   D. Hanahan and R. Weinberg, The hallmarks of cancer, *Cell.* **100**, 57–70 (2000).

[2]   D. Hanahan and R. Weinberg, Hallmarks of cancer: The next generation, *Cell.* **144**, 646–674 (2011).

[3]   R. Fisher, L. Pusztai, and C. Swanton, Cancer heterogeneity: Implications for targeted therapeutics, *British Journal of Cancer.* **108**(3), 479–485 (2013).

[4]   Q. Jia, A. Wang, Y. Yuan, B. Zhu, and H. Long, Heterogeneity of the tumour immune microenvironment and its clinical relevance, *Experimental Hematology & Oncology.* **11**, 24 (2022).

[5]   F. Janku, Tumour heterogeneity in the clinic: Is it a real problem? *Therapeutic Advances in Medical Oncology.* **6**(2), 43–51 (2014).

[6]   D. Hanahan, Hallmarks of cancer: New dimensions, *Cancer Discovery.* **22**(1), 31–46 (2022).

[7]   R. Eftimie, J. Gillard, and D. Cantrell, Mathematical models for immunology: Current state of the art and future research directions, *Bulletin of Mathematical Biology.* **78**, 2091–2134 (2016).

[8]   R. Eftimie, Grand challenges in mathematical biology: Integrating multi-scale modelling and data, *Frontiers in Applied Mathematics and Statistics.* **8**, 1010622 (2022).

[9]   W. He, T. Liu, Y. Han, W. Ming, J. Du, Y. Liu, *et al.*, A review: The detection of cancer cells in histopathology based on machine vision, *Computers in Biology and Medicine.* **146**, 105636 (2022).

[10]   E. Wulczyn, D. Steiner, Z. Xu, A. Sadwani, H. Wang, I. Flament-Auvigne, *et al.*, Deep learning-based survival prediction for multiple cancer types using histopathology images, *PLoS One.* **15**(6), e0233678 (2020).

[11]   R. Rafique, S. Islam, and J. Kazi, Machine learning in the prediction of cancer therapy, *Computational and Structural Biotechnology Journal.* **19**, 4003–4017 (2021).

[12]   R. Eftimie, A. Mavrodin, and S. Bordas, From digital control to digital twins in medicine: A brief review and future perspectives, *Advances in Applied Mechanics.* **56**, 323–368 (2023).

Chapter 2

Using Mathematical Models to Predict Glioblastoma Growth and Response to Treatment in a Patient-Specific Manner

Dana L. Hutton* and **Kismet Hossain-Ibrahim**[*,†,‡]

*School of Medicine, University of Dundee,
Dundee, UK
†Department of Neurosurgery,
Ninewells Hospital and Medical School,
NHS Tayside, Dundee, UK
‡k.z.hossainibrahim@dundee.ac.uk

Mathematical neuro-oncology is a growing field in brain tumour treatment, being used to model the effect of treatment on glioblastoma (GBM), the most malignant primary brain tumour. GBM is particularly heterogeneous, with highly variable patient response to current standard of care: surgery, radiotherapy, and chemotherapy. Median survival despite treatment is only 14–15 months, so novel treatments are needed. Researchers are using machine learning to predict growth patterns of GBM after surgery. Linking these models with individual patient (MRI imaging) data, we hope this chapter assists mathematicians and clinicians to work together and predict individual patient responses to existing and novel chemotherapy, radiotherapy, and experimental regimes (e.g., immunotherapy, oncolytic viral therapy, interstitial laser, and focused ultrasound). We summarise the complex interplay involved in glioma growth at a genetic, molecular, microscopic, and macroscopic level, which needs to be integrated into future *in silico* models in order to accurately predict patient response to treatment. Predictive modelling is safer than testing potentially toxic novel treatments directly on patients (i.e., can be used prior to clinical trials), can model dosing and timing regimes, and is individualised. This may enable us to apply precision medicine to GBM treatment and allow clinicians to ultimately improve patient outcome.

1. Introduction

Glioblastoma multiforme (GBM) is an aggressive primary brain tumour which, despite recent efforts, with almost all patients dying within 2 years of diagnosis [1]. Thus, finding strategies to improve the outcomes for patients with GBM remain at the frontier of neuro-oncology-based research.

Mathematical neuro-oncology (MNO), a termed coined by *Rockne and Baldock* [2], requires the use of mathematical expertise in computer modelling to 'map' the growth of GBMs, in order to predict subsequent GBM tumour behaviour *in silico*. New MNO techniques take into account both the biological process that take place on a *microscopic* level (based on histopathological analysis of tumours) and the *macroscopic* level, analysing the growth patterns of large groups of cells (visualised through techniques which take serial images of the tumour over time, such as magnetic resonance imaging (MRI) of patients' tumours).

A form of artificial intelligence known as *machine learning* can be utilised for MNO models. It is patient-specific, as it incorporates MRI data into the model being utilised. Machine learning starts with the size and shape of a tumour demonstrated by the MRI scan at diagnosis. From this, an MNO model is used to predict tumour growth, and this prediction is compared to the growth observed in later MRI scans. If the model and the scan do not match, the model is adjusted until it predicts something that more closely represents what is seen in subsequent scans. By repeating this process on several different patient datasets, the computer 'learns' to improve its accuracy in predicting how the tumour will grow. MNO models now incorporate data detailing patient interventions, such as radiotherapy and chemotherapy, with the aim of predicting how an individual patient's tumour will respond to different treatments.

Individualised mathematical models of GBM growth patterns may enable us to apply precision-medicine to GBM treatment, and also to guide the delicate equipoise involved in the management of these patients. There are a few ways in which we can achieve this in the future: (1) treatments are selected on an individual basis by being based on the best computer-modelled outcome for them; (2) computerised mathematical models can be used as a safe alternative to test novel treatments, instead of trying them out on patients; (3) models' predictive of individual patient response to treatment can enable the early implementation of more or less aggressive treatment regimens of an appropriate time scale (e.g., redo surgery or second line chemotherapy).

Different mathematical research groups have modelled different aspects of the complex interplay involved in glioma growth at a genetic, molecular, microscopic and, macroscopic level. The future of the MNO field will not only rely on the integration of such models to predict tumour growth as accurately as possible, incorporating new discoveries as they arise, but also to do so in a way that assists clinicians in dealing with the challenges faced in the management of patients with GBM. However, before discussing the needs of new models that could predict the infiltrative behaviour of tumours, first we must further our understanding of the biological mechanisms which underpin malignant tumours at the microscopic level, as well as the diffuse, infiltrative macroscopic patterns of tumour growth observed with clinical imaging, both of which are discussed in this chapter, using GBM as an example. We then summarise different models of MNO that take into account these biological mechanisms before discussing potential future directions of mathematical modelling research that can ultimately be used to aid clinical management of GBM.

2. Introduction to Glioblastoma (GBM)

2.1. *Clinical presentation and management of GBM*

Glioblastoma (GBM) is the most common primary brain tumour (1). Under the World Health Organisation grading of central nervous system (CNS) tumours, GBM is classified under WHO grade IV — the most aggressive grade (Table 1). The median overall survival

Table 1.   World Health Organisation (WHO) grading of glioma.

WHO Grade	Features
I	*Pilocytic astrocytoma* • Circumscribed, benign tumours • Low proliferative potential • May occur during childhood and in young adults
II	*Low-grade glioma* • Diffusely infiltrative • Increased cellular abnormalities
III	*Low-grade glioma* • Diffusely infiltrative • Increased cellular abnormalities • De-differentiation and mitotic cell activity
IV	*Glioblastoma multiforme* • Diffusely infiltrative • Increased cellular abnormalities • De-differentiation and mitotic cell activity • Pathological proliferation of small blood vessels (neovascularisation) and/or necrosis

(OS) of GBM in the UK (2007–2011 data) was 6.1 months (rising to 14.9 months if <69 years and maximally treated); overall 1-, 2-, and 5-year survival rates were 28.4%, 11.5%, and 3.4%, respectively [3].

GBM incidence increases with age and is more common in males than females. Age-stratified median survival in the UK was found to decrease significantly ($p < 0.0001$) with increasing age at diagnosis, from 16.2 months for the youngest group (20–44 years) to just 3.2 months for the eldest group (70+ years) [3]. The majority of GBMs arise spontaneously. However, one known risk factor for GBM is previous exposure to ionising radiation. Other factors such as smoking and viral infection are still inconclusive. Approximately 5% of all GBMs are associated with a hereditary predisposition to cancer development, featuring genetic disorders (e.g., *NF1, NF2, tuberous sclerosis, Von Hippel Lindau, and Li-Fraumeni syndrome*) [4]. Not all gliomas are malignant, with previous classification being based on histopathological features summarised in Table 1, with Grade III and IV gliomas being malignant, but note that all Grade II tumours eventually transform to a higher malignant grade. However, as discussed in the following, this has been superseded by a more recent WHO classification incorporating molecular markers that better predict tumour prognosis.

Patients tend to present with intractable headaches, as well as seizures occurring in up to 25%. The nature of any other progressive neurological deficit which a patient may present with depends on the tumour's anatomical site. A key feature of GBM is peritumoral vasogenic oedema, which is often the underlying cause of clinical signs and symptoms secondary to raised intracranial pressure (e.g., headaches and, eventually, drowsiness). Symptomatic patients are initially treated with corticosteroids (preferably dexamethasone) to reduce this vasogenic oedema [6]. Following the work of Stupp *et al.*, the standard of care for newly diagnosed GBM features maximally safe neurosurgical resection, followed by concurrent radiation and the oral DNA-alkylating agent, temozolomide (TMZ). This is known as the 'Stupp Protocol' [7]. Although maximal combination therapy has shown to prolong the median survival for newly diagnosed patients (aged 69 years and younger) to 14.9 months, this prognosis for GBM patients is still far from ideal [3]. Other, novel options for GBM include gene therapy, targeted therapies (e.g., anti-angiogenics), immunotherapy, and therapeutic vaccines [4], but none have significantly and consistently improved survival.

Almost all patient's tumours will progress (termed recurrent GBM) despite maximal combination therapy. There is, as yet, no established standard of care for progressive (recurrent) GBM, with little evidence for first-line interventions to prolong OS. Options include further resection, reirradiation, and novel chemotherapeutics, with second-line experimental therapy including tumour-treating fields (in the US), immunotherapy, and combined approaches [1, 6]. However, many patients may not be suitable for any therapy at tumour recurrence and may receive supportive care alone (palliation).

Since the Stupp protocol was introduced in 2005, the only Phase 3 clinical trial intervention to show significant (albeit small) improvement in survival is tumour-treating field (TTF), which is an emerging non-invasive anti-cancer treatment. TTF involves the transcutaneous delivery of low-intensity alternating electric fields via cutaneous transducer arrays configured to provide optimal tumour site coverage. The use of TTF with other chemotherapy may be considered when treating patients with progressive GBM. However, the AANS CNS guidelines state that there is insufficient evidence to recommend TTF to increase OS in progressive GBM patients [8]. Additionally, factors which are now being regarded to a higher extent are patient quality of life (acceptability of the novel treatment) and cost, with TTF therapy being deemed too expensive to be endorsed by many healthcare systems and has poor patient compliance — as patients are required to regularly shave their hair as well as wearing and carrying the device around, with skin irritation a common side effect [9].

2.2. *Why is the prognosis of GBM so poor?*

The reason behind the adverse outcomes for GBM patients is multifactorial. However, a key factor that contributes to long-term survival is the extent of neurosurgical resection [1, 4]. Gross total resection is associated with improved outcome in both newly diagnosed [10] and recurrent GBM [11,12] but only if surgery is combined with chemoradiotherapy [13]. Difficulties in achieving substantial *safe* resection include tumour location (e.g., near eloquent areas of the brain) and the highly invasive nature of the tumour itself. Another obstacle to the treatment of GBM is the presence of the blood–brain barrier (BBB), a physiological barrier coordinated by a series of physical, transport, and metabolic properties possessed by the endothelial cells that line blood vessels within the CNS. The BBB tightly regulates CNS homeostasis by allowing the movement and delivery of ions, molecules, and cells that facilitate optimal neuronal function while 'blocking' the entry of toxins and pathogens that are damaging to the brain [14]. It is also a barrier for many therapeutic agents (including TMZ), hindering their penetration into CNS from the peripheral circulation.

Heterogeneity is a morphological hallmark of GBM, hence the term 'multiforme' (i.e., can arise as multiple distinct entities), and is most often the underlying reason GBMs will progress/recur despite maximal combination therapy. Genotypic and phenotypic variations exist among gliomas cells within a single tumour (intra-tumoral heterogeneity) and between patients (intertumoral heterogeneity) [5]. In recent years, a pivotal movement in GBM research was achieved following the demonstration of different prognostic relevant sub-types that highlight *inter* tumoral heterogeneity. Many researchers have attempted to refine the classification of primary and secondary GBM into several different sub-types. A recent example includes the proposal of four molecular sub-types, based on characteristic somatic alterations and gene expression signatures of different tissue types: (1) neuro-progenitor cells (**Pro-neural**), (2) neurons (**Neural**), (3) mesenchymal tissue (**Mesenchymal (MES)**), or (4) proliferating cells with receptor tyrosine kinase activation (**Classical (CL)**) [3]. This may be useful in mathematical models trying to link such biomarkers to prognosis. However, this sub-classification neglects *intra*-tumoral heterogeneity [15].

Intra-tumoral heterogeneity arises either from a self-renewing cancer stem cell population or due to clonal expansion of glioma cells harbouring specific genetic and epigenetic alterations that promote cancer cell migration and invasion. In addition to *genetic* heterogeneity, interactions between glioma cells and the surrounding normal parenchyma and immune cells (tumour microenvironment) lead to phenotypic diversity. Supporting the theory of GBM intra-tumoral heterogeneity, Sottorvia *et al.* presented an integrated genomic analysis that illustrated most patients display more than one molecular sub-type within a single tumour (e.g., *both pro-neural and mesenchymal*). The group were also able to 'map' oncogenic genetic changes in both time and space to further expand on the features of the different subpopulations existing within a single tumour — observing specific alterations as early events (e.g., *EGFR and CDKN2A/B/p14ARF*) and later events (e.g., *PDGFRA and PTEN*) during GBM progression [16].

GBM progression may be driven by the cooperation of multiple heterogenous tumour-cell sub-populations, with different mutational and phenotypical properties. Patterns of co-invasion have been observed — with more invasive cells acting as the leader, and sub-populations of poorly invasive cells as the followers. This 'division' of labour may facilitate not only tumour invasion but also proliferation [5]. Additionally, co-operation of multiple heterogenous tumour-cell populations drives treatment resistance. A specific monotherapy may only eliminate a fraction of the tumour cells, while others remain intact, and eventually will induce relapse. The surviving population may not be a single resistant cancer clone but rather a heterogeneous population of malignant cells with 'favourable' genetic aberrations that allow them to survive the initial treatment.

Currently, no molecular sub-type of GBM is predictive of treatment response, and choosing a single sub-type can be challenging in some GBMs due to intra-tumoral heterogeneity, as well as 'sub-type-switching' during later stages of tumour progression [6]. In order to understand GBM progression and treatment response, mathematical models should consider the impact of GBM heterogeneity, and key genetic and phenotypic properties that influence aggressive invasion patterns and treatment resistance. If we can recognise specific patterns of intra-heterogeneity and inter-heterogeneity, we may in the future be able to further stratify patients and better select an appropriate therapeutic strategy [16].

2.3.   *Histopathogenesis of GBM*

2.3.1.   *WHO 2021 classification of gliomas and other CNS tumours*

GBMs arise from neuro-progenitor cells [1], which have the ability to proliferate and differentiate into different glial cell types. In the developing CNS, it is important to note that neuro-progenitor cells exhibit a high migratory behaviour [5]. This may in part explain why malignant glioma cells commonly feature a blockade of differentiation (i.e., 'stemness').

In recent years, molecular biomarkers have gained significant clinical relevance in providing both ancillary and defining diagnostic information. The *2021 WHO Classification of CNS tumours (CNS5)*, which superseded the 2016 classification, has moved towards the consideration of molecular changes important for the accurate classification of CNS neoplasms (biomarkers) and away from histological features (pathological markers) [Table 1] [5]. For some tumour families, *CNS5* has grouped tumours according to the genetic changes that enable a complete diagnosis (e.g., *IDH and H3 status*); by looser oncogenic associations, such as *MAPK* pathway alterations; by histological and histogenetic similarities despite variations in molecular signature (e.g., *Other Gliomas, Glioneuronal Tumours, and Neuronal Tumours*); or, for many, by using molecular features to define new types and sub-types (e.g., *Medulloblastoma*). (For more details on key diagnostic genes, molecules, pathways, and/or combinations in gliomas, glioneuronal tumours, and neuronal tumours, see Table 2 of WHO CNS classification 2021 (WHO CNS5)) [17]. This hybrid taxonomy is likely only an intermediate stage to an even more precise future classification [17].

The role of molecular diagnostics has now been more fully incorporated into CNS tumour classification to aid clinical decision-making. For example, glioblastomas were previously diagnosed based on the histologic findings (Table 1) and included both IDH-mutated (10%) and IDH wild-type (90%) tumours, which had highly variable biology and prognoses. The new classification of these tumours takes into account molecular findings which are related to prognosis. Following WHO CNS5, glioblastomas comprise only IDH wild-type tumours. All IDH-mutant diffuse astrocytic tumours are now considered a single type (astrocytoma and IDH-mutant) and are graded as 2, 3, or 4, i.e., IDH-mutant astrocytomas with poorly prognostic molecular alterations (e.g., CDKN2A/B homozygous deletion) will have a WHO CNS grade of 4, even in the absence of microvascular proliferation or necrosis. Classifying tumours on a molecular-based prognostic pattern is beneficial for clinical trial design (as a more homogenous population can be studied); it should similarly assist with mathematical modelling design.

2.3.2. *IDH mutation status*

IDH mutations are common in low-grade gliomas (LGG), with a prevalence of ~80% [18]. IDH mutation status is also an important prognostic feature [18], with IDH-mutant tumours conferring a more favourable outcome than IDH-wild-type counterparts (median OS 65 vs. 20 months) [19]. IDH status is also used to sub-divide GBMs into IDH-wild-type GBM and IDH-mutant GBM, corresponding to primary GBM (which arise *de novo*) and secondary GBM (which arise from Grade II tumours that have mutated), respectively. They are associated with different molecular signatures and clinical presentations (Table 2). IDH mutations occur more frequently in secondary GBMs (generally associated with better prognosis and occur in younger individuals); whereas IDH-wild-type (primary) GBMs define *de novo* high-grade gliomas (HGGs). IDH-mutant (secondary) GBMs are associated with significantly greater median OS than

Table 2. Features of IDH-wild type and IDH-mutant glioblastomas.

Tumour type	Primary GBM (90%)	Secondary GBM (10%)
Clinical presentation	No prior evidence of precursor Poorer prognosis Age >45	Evidence of precursor lower-grade glioma Better prognosis Age <45
Molecular features	*IDH-wild type* • EGFR amplification • TERT promoter mutations • PTEN deletion • MGMT promoter methylation (30–50%) • BRAFV600E mutation • LOH 10q • LOH 10p	*IDH-1 or −2 mutation (>70%)* • TP53 mutation • ATRX mutation • PDGFRA amplification • LOH 10q • LOH 19q

Notes: Primary GBM develop rapidly without prior clinical evidence of a lower-grade precursor. Secondary GBMs typically develop from an existing lower-grade glioma. Abbreviations: IDH = isocitrate dehydrogenase; EGFR = epidermal growth factor receptor; TERT = telomerase reverse transcriptase; PTEN = phosphatase and tensin homolog; MGMT = O^6-methylguanine-DNA methyltransferase; BRAF = murine sarcoma viral oncogene homolog B; ATRX = alpha thalassemia X-linked intellectual disability syndrome gene; PDGFRA = platelet-derived growth factor receptor A; LOH = loss of heterozygosity.

IDH-wild-type GBMs (primary) (31 vs. 15 months) [19]. Unfortunately, most clinical trials investigating novel agents for GBM pre-date the revised WHO classification of GBMs and so likely contained both IDH-wild-type and IDH-mutant GBM, which is a significant confounder to clear interpretation of results. Future clinical studies will assess outcomes based on IDH status, with clinicians particularly keen to treat patients with IDH-wild-type tumours due to the poor prognosis this entails. However, the risk is that there will be fewer clinical trials designed for rarer IDH-1 mutant astrocytomas (especially grade 4); Jiang *et al.* [18] and Aoki *et al.* [54] both have used the clinical relevance of IDH mutation status to develop mathematical models (see Sections 5.8 and 5.9). This ability to model rare tumour types is another potential advantage of mathematical modelling in allowing researchers to predict outcomes and develop clinical trial options for this population of patients also.

Several concepts have attempted to explain why IDH status influences GBM outcome. Interestingly, IDH mutation does not always correlate with OS [19]. Gain-of-function mutations which offer survival advantage may be clonally selected for by cancer cell subpopulations. Such pro-oncogenic mutations in IDH can promote DNA methylation and block cellular differentiation. This results in the development of a *CpG island methylator phenotype* (featuring increased mutagenesis), as well as promotion of cancer cell 'stemness' [20]. IDH mutations can also supply the excessive growth demands of GBM by promoting metabolic adaptation (anaerobic glycolysis), via increased expression of *hypoxia-induced-factor-1a* (HIF-1a).

2.3.3. *1p/19q co-deletion status*

In addition to IDH status, 1p/19q status also plays a key role in glioma classification and enables the identification of the sub-type of LGG which may progress to a secondary GBM. 1p/19q co-deletion is also associated with better response to radiotherapy and TMZ, as well as longer progression-free survival (PFS) and OS [21]. Despite its clinical relevance, little is understood about the mechanism underlying the benefit of 1p/19q co-deletion. Yao *et al.* hypothesised that the better prognosis and higher sensitivity to treatment of 1p/19q co-deleted gliomas may be related to less acidity in the tumour microenvironment, following their observation of 1p/19q co-deleted gliomas to be less acidic than their counterparts [21].

2.3.4. *MGMT methylation status*

O6-methylguanine-DNA methyltransferase (MGMT) is a methylating enzyme often over-expressed in GBM. MGMT promoter methylation, and subsequent MGMT under-expression, renders a tumour cell more sensitive to the effects of DNA-alkylating agents, such as TMZ. Consequently, MGMT methylation is considered a favourable prognosis marker associated with longer survival outcomes [22].

In summary, it is becoming apparent that the most accurate mathematical models of GBM growth will need to incorporate the molecular biomarker profile of individual patients' tumours to provide the most accurate prognostic model of growth.

2.4. *The hallmarks of cancer and GBM*

Understanding the connections between clinically observable glioma behaviour and underlying molecular and cellular processes remains a major challenge. To rise to this challenge, we must better understand the mechanisms that contribute to glioma invasion. It is well established that tumour progression is aided by the sequential acquisition of the different *Hallmarks of Cancer* — first described by *Hanahan and Weinberg* [23,24]. This section focusses on the cancer hallmarks relevant to the maintenance and progression of GBM and the associated favourable genetic and epigenetic alterations which enable this aggressive cancer to thrive. Though the list of hallmarks summarised in the following is not exhaustive, mathematicians would be encouraged to incorporate as many of these relevant underlying processes as possible into their models of tumour growth, being also aware that this would lead to more complex models. Nevertheless, due to the limitations of human understanding of the complex interactions between the different hallmarks of cancers, it is necessary to investigate these interactions with the help of mathematical/computational models.

2.4.1. *Sustained proliferative signalling*

Arguably, the most important cancer cell trait is the ability to sustain chronic proliferation. To do this, cancer cells utilise existing mechanisms which maintain growth homeostasis in normal tissue. Such pathways involve the binding of stimulatory growth factors to cell-surface receptors which are comprised of an extra-cellular domain and intra-cellular tyrosine kinase domain. The latter domain triggers intra-cellular signalling pathways which regulate specific biological responses, such as cell division, proliferation, and motility [24]. The proliferative and invasive nature of GBM is the foundation of the *Proliferation-Invasion (PI) Model* (Section 5.1) and other mathematical models that have branched from the original PI model.

When genes involved in pro-growth signalling pathways acquire pro-cancerous genetic alterations (becoming oncogenes), pro-proliferative cellular responses can occur. Cancer cells become 'addicted' to such oncogenes for their survival. Growth factor signalling can become dysregulated following increased expression of the aforementioned cell-surface receptor proteins (*e.g., secondary to*

EGFR gene amplification), making the cancer cell hyper-responsive to growth factors. Genetic mutations that modify such receptors can also enable them to trigger downstream signalling independent of the presence of growth factors *(e.g., EGFR mutation)* [24]. Additionally, natural inhibitors/regulators of pro-growth signalling pathways may become inactivated *(e.g., PTEN)*.

EGFR: *Epidermal growth factor receptor* (EGFR) regulates the growth and proliferation of multiple cell types. The most common EGFR mutation is EGFRvIII, with substantial evidence suggesting its key role in gliomagenesis. However, attempts to target EGFR in GBM have yet to show therapeutic benefit. The lack of efficacy of EGFR inhibitors in GBM clinical trials *(e.g., Erlotinib)* [25], suggests that more complex/a combination of molecular signatures *(e.g., co-existing PTEN mutation)* associated with individual tumours may need to be identified for clinically effective targeting of growth factors in GBM. A recent mathematical model developed by Stein *et al.* focussed on the effect of the dosing of another anti-EFGR TKI, Lapatinib, on a EGFR-mutant GBM cell line. This model provides a potential method for comparing treatment schedules for optimal dosing in GBM, in a bid to improve the poor clinical translation of EGFR inhibitors seen thus far [26].

PTEN: The tumour suppressor gene PTEN *(phosphatase and tensin homolog)* opposes the mitogenic signalling mediated by *phosphatidylinositol 3-OH kinases (PI3K)* and has important roles in regulating cell proliferation, invasion, apoptosis, and DNA damage repair [27]. PTEN loss occurs in 5–40% of glioma cases and is linked to malignant progression. Additionally, reduced sensitivity to both radiotherapy and chemotherapy has been observed in GBM with PTEN loss [27]. The impact of PTEN mutation on OS remains uncertain; however, some studies have shown a correlation with poor prognosis in glioma [28].

2.4.2.   *Evading growth suppressors*

In addition to 'putting on the accelerator' by sustaining autonomous growth signalling (described earlier), cancer cells thrive if they additionally 'tamper with the breaks'. This involves tumour suppressors proteins which negatively regulate cellular growth and proliferation.

p53: Mutation of the gene encoding tumour suppressor p53, *TP53*, is the most frequent genetic aberration in human cancer. In response to multiple cellular stress signals, activated p53 governs the decisions of cells to proliferate or to enter pro-senescence or pro-apoptotic programmes. Other well-established functions of p53 include the following: DNA-repair, differentiation, metabolism, and angiogenesis. How p53 'decides' which cellular response to induce is thought to be dependent on tissue type, cell type, or the nature of the stress signal [29]. This may include intracellular signals (*e.g., DNA-damage and hypoxia*), extracellular signals (*e.g., nutrient availability, cell adhesion molecules, and cytokines*), as well as other oncogenic signalling pathways (*e.g., Ras and PI3K*) influenced by the co-existence of carcinogenic mutations.

GBMs with *TP53* mutations are associated with resistance to both DNA-damaging chemotherapeutics and radiotherapy [30]. This resistance may be explained by the correlation of inactivated p53 with cells more tolerant of DNA damage and a higher threshold for the induction of apoptosis, as well as cells of a more aggressive and 'stem-like' phenotype. The influence of p53 on GBM resistance is considered in Stamatakos *et al.*'s mathematical model (see Section 5.7). Attempts to exploit the p53 pathway have yet to show significant success in GBM treatment, but approaches are currently in development.

TGF-β: The *transforming growth factor-beta* (TGF-β) superfamily of high homologous, multi-functional cytokines includes TGF-β1, -β2, and -β3. Through downstream signalling (involving SMADs), TGF-β can influence a myriad of cellular responses including proliferation, differentiation, invasion, angiogenesis, and immunosuppression [31]. TGF-β can act as either a tumour suppressor or a tumour promotor dependent upon genetic and epigenetic changes within the cancer cell. Pro-oncogenic TGFβ drives GBM carcinogenesis by inducing proliferation and an invasive phenotype. Elevated TGFβ1 and TGFβ2 expression is typically observed in malignant gliomas and correlates with poor prognosis. Additionally, loss of TGFβ's tumour suppressor function has been observed in HGG [4].

GBM cell invasion requires the degradation of the adjacent ECM. TGFβ increases the levels of several matrix metalloproteinases (MMPs) which digest components of the ECM while decreasing the levels of tissue inhibitors of MMPs. This results in ECM degradation and thus, invasion. TGFβ also can induce the *Epithelial-to-Mesenchymal Transition* (EMT), a process which enables the acquisition of favourable cancer cell traits [24]. In order to successfully invade and metastasise, cancer cells alter in their shape as well as in their degree of adhesion to each other, adjacent cells, and the ECM [24]. In response to molecular cues (*e.g.*, $TGF\beta$), glioma cells acquire a mesenchymal (elongated, wedge-like) phenotype to promote ECM penetration and migration [5]. TGFβ can also mediate microtubule development, a key component of GBM invasion, through downstream signalling [32]. TGFβ1 can induce angiogenesis both directly and indirectly via enhanced expression of the pro-angiogenic protein vascular endothelial growth factor (VEGF). Blocking the TGFβ pathway may help combat GBM invasion. However, evasion of the anti-proliferative effects of TGF-β by cancer cells of these effects is now appreciated to be far more elaborate than simple shutdown of its signalling circuitry. This may explain why the use of TGF-β inhibitors for GBM is yet to be successful in the clinical setting [33, 34]. GBM secrete TGFβ to induce immunosuppression within the tumour microenvironment, as TGF-β has the ability to down-regulate M1 TAM (tumour-associated macrophages) and cytotoxic T-lymphocyte activity [35]. Khajanchi *et al.*'s mathematical model, which focusses on the interplay of glioma cells and the immune system, includes the immunosuppressive function of TGFβ (see Section 5.10).

2.4.3. *Angiogenesis*

Like any normal tissue, cancer cells require adequate nutrition and oxygenation, as well as a means of disposing of cellular waste products and carbon dioxide. The process of angiogenesis addresses these needs by utilising pre-existing neovascularisation mechanisms that are required during embryogenesis. However, the proliferating vessels that result from angiogenesis are in fact 'faulty', with significantly larger diameters and thicker basement membranes than those in normal brain tissue. The most frequently discussed angiogenesis inducer and inhibitor are *vascular endothelial growth factor-A* (VEGF-A) and TSP-1, respectively [24]. VEGF can be upregulated both by hypoxia and by oncogenic signalling. Additionally, inactivated VEGFs can be sequestered in the ECM and are subject to release and activation by ECM-degrading proteases. TSP-1 also binds transmembrane receptors displayed by endothelial cells and thereby evokes suppressive signals that can counteract pro-angiogenic stimuli [24].

During uncontrolled glioma proliferation, hypoxic regions develop at locations farthest from the original vascular supply of the tumour. Within hypoxic regions, glioma cells favour certain behaviours, such as invasion and neoangiogenesis (features used in the histopathological diagnosis of WHO IV GBM, see Table 1). These features are often spatially and temporally related, with sites of neovascularisation indicative of hypoxic and necrotic regions. Mathematical models that consider hypoxia and angiogenesis include the *PINHA model* and those built on the 'Go or Grow' hypothesis (see Sections 5.1–5.5).

2.4.4. *Tumour-promoting inflammation*

Monocytes circulate in the bloodstream and are recruited into tumours in response to several tumour-derived chemoattractants. Once inside the tumour, monocytes differentiate into tumour-associated macrophages (TAMs) and then accumulate in hypoxic/necrotic areas. Histological analyses have shown TAMs to be the predominant infiltrating immune cells in gliomas, accounting for ~30–50% of the tumour mass. Such inflammatory cells contribute to cancer progression by supplying bioactive molecules to the tumour microenvironment, including growth factors, survival factors that limit cell death, pro-angiogenic factors, and enzymes that invasion and metastasis through degradation of the ECM [5]. Additionally, TAMs can secrete chemicals (e.g., reactive oxygen species) that are actively mutagenic for nearby cancer cells, accelerating their genetic evolution towards states of heightened malignancy [24]. Khajanchi *et al.*'s model takes into consideration the role of the interaction between glioma cells and TAMs (see Section 5.10).

2.4.5. *Evading immune destruction*

A key role of the immune system is to detect and eradicate developing cancers. Cancer cells can escape immune destruction through the immunosuppressive interaction between cancer cell-surface molecules and receptors expressed on the T-cell surface, such as cytotoxic T lymphocyte-associated antigen-4 (CTLA-4) and programmed cell death protein-1 (PD-1) [36]. These ligands are overexpressed in many cancer cells and are termed 'immune checkpoints' as they 'put the brakes' on the T-cell anti-tumoural response. CTLA-4 stops the activation of naive T-cells, whereas PD-1 prevents activated T-cells from recognising and responding to cancer-specific cell surface molecules [36]. In recent years, immune checkpoint inhibitors (ICIs) have shown success in breast, skin and lung cancers [36], but are yet to show significant clinical benefit in GBM. This may be in part due GBM heterogeneity. To improve the efficacy of ICIs in GBM treatment, biomarkers that can screen for 'suitable' patients need to be developed. The main markers used in directing ICI use include PD-L1 expression, mutation burden, levels of tumour-infiltrating lymphocytes, and microsatellite instability status.

2.4.6. *Genomic instability*

Tumour cells have the ability to increase their rates of mutation. Cancer cells benefit from this mechanism as it increases the likelihood of acquiring a genetic or epigenetic change which confers a specific sub-clone of cancer cells a selective advantage, enabling their outgrowth and eventual dominance in a local tissue environment. Later in the course of tumour progression, when hyperproliferation combined with increased genetic instability spawn distinct clonal subpopulations, clonal heterogeneity arises [24]. The loss of function of p53 [24] and mutation of the ATRX gene [37] are examples of mutations that contribute to genomic instability and thus favour GBM progression. In light of this hallmark, one specific model takes into account the relationship between mutational burden and the malignant transformation (MT) rate of GBM (see Section 5.10).

2.4.7. *The tumour microenvironment*

Both the tumour stroma and microenvironment contain a myriad of distinct cell types and extra-cellular components. Each have the ability to influence adjacent glioma cells by partaking in different neuronal interactions which promote invasion [38]. Invasion of glioma cells involves four distinct steps: (1) detachment from the primary tumour, a process triggered by downregulation of cell–cell adhesion molecules and microenvironmental changes, (2) integrin-mediated adhesion to the ECM, (3) protease-mediated ECM degradation, and (4) migration through the extension of a prominent leading cytoplasmic protrusion, followed by a burst of forward movement of the cell body. MNO may allow a better understanding of invasion and the key mediators involved in glioma invasion and to better predict which targeted agents may be of potential therapeutic use.

The ECM: The ECM in the brain mainly consists of the polysaccharide hyaluronan and proteoglycan-based matrix, mostly hyaluronic acid-binding secreted chondroitin sulfate proteoglycans of the lectican family. The brain's ECM also lacks many ECM elements found in other organs, including collagens, fibronectin, type I laminin, and supporting stromal tissue. The unique composition of the brain's ECM may explain why many other tumours do not metastasise to the brain and why primary brain tumours (such as GBM) *do not metastasise* outside the brain, perhaps due to lack of a 'suitable' microenvironment to host the disseminated tumour cells [39]. To enable *local invasion* of the brain parenchyma, GBM cells produce and secrete MMPs. MMPs induce proteolysis of different ECM components and create routes along which glioma cells can migrate. The composition of the substances within the brain parenchyma may influence specific paths/patterns of GBM invasion and is taken into consideration by Suveges *et al.* [52] mathematical model (see Section 5.6).

Integrins: Integrins are transmembrane receptors on the glioma cell cytoskeleton which detect and interact with different ligands in the ECM (*e.g., fibronectin, collagen, and laminin*) to promote a promigratory response. Active integrins also promote changes in the glioma cell cytoskeleton by interacting with actin filaments and the Talin adaptor protein, which in turn activates Focal Adhesion Kinase (FAK). The role of integrins and communication between the tumour invasion front and ECM is considered by Angihortri *et al.*'s model (see Section 5.11).

Tumour Microtubules: GBM cells can modify their cytoskeleton to create finger-like, highly dynamic membrane protrusions that communicate with the tumour microenvironment to mediate intercellular communication and in modulating cell adhesion. These protrusions are known as *tumour microtubules*. Microtubules are a sub-type of filopodia and have key roles in tumour cell responses to the gradients of insoluble (haptotaxis) and soluble (chemotaxis) components of the tumour microenvironment [40]. The role of microtubules in GBM invasion is considered by some novel mathematical models (Sections 5.6 and 5.12).

3. Macroscopic Growth Patterns and Morphology of GBM

3.1. *Macroscopic tumour features*

The most significant characteristic of GBMs is their diffuse invasion of the normal brain parenchyma. GBMs typically have poorly defined borders as a result and will present as single, irregularly shaped lesions [41]. GBMs are also highly heterogenous on the macroscopic level, featuring necrotic regions ('soft' and yellow in colour), abnormally 'firm' and white regions, and other regions exhibiting marked cystic degeneration and haemorrhage [41], which makes realistic modelling difficult. 95% of GBMs arise from the supratentorial cerebral hemispheres, with only a small percentage occurring in cerebellum, brainstem, and spinal cord [41].

3.2. *Pseudopalisades*

Uncontrolled glioma proliferation leads to blood vessel occlusion and/or collapse. This induces peri-vascular tumour cell hypoxia and necrosis, which typically form lines with peri-focally increased cell density, termed *pseudopalisades*. Pseudopalisades are common features of GBM. When present around necrotic foci, pseudopalisades are indicative of severe hypoxia and are linked to waves of glioma cells actively migrating away from such oxygen-deficient regions. Experimental studies suggest that greater degrees of tumour hypoxia results in increased migration and invasion, and strongly correlate with tumour malignancy — a key factor for mathematical modelling methods of GBM to consider [5].

3.3. *The infiltration front*

A 'sharp invasion front' has been described to lead GBM tumour propagation – the part of the tumour in contact with healthy brain parenchyma. The predilection of glioma cells to invade into adjacent 'healthy' brain tissue by following specific growth patterns seems to be guided along pre-existing tracks of least resistance, defined by the architecture and molecular composition of the brain parenchyma and associated ECM. Common paths include along white matter tracts, basal lamina of cerebral vessels, or in between the glia limitans[1] and pia mater [39]. Blood vessels guide invading glioma cells via laminin- and collagen-IV-mediated integrin engagement, whereas white matter tracks guide glioma cells through cell–cell contacts and mechanisms regulating cell–ECM adhesion forces [5].

Serial MRI imaging helps demonstrate patterns of tumour growth and can assist mathematical modellers to mimic and analyse potential contributing factors to the predilection for specific glioma migration patterns. For example, Swanson's model revealed augmented diffusion rates of malignant cells in white matter, compared to those in grey matter [42]. Jbabdi's group then further generalised the concept that glioma cells migrate faster in white matter by taking into account the anisotropy as well as heterotopy of the brain tissue, dealing with the fact that glioma cell migration is facilitated in the direction of white matter fibres [43]. As white matter tracks are best visualised radiologically by following the isotropic water molecules along them with diffusion tensor imaging (DTI) (a variant of diffusion-weighted imaging (DWI) which utilises a tissue water diffusion rate for image production [44]), the Jbabdi group's work was augmented by the DTI technique.

4. How Can Mathematical Modelling Address Clinical Challenges in GBM?

Despite years' worth of research into GBM, there are still multiple clinical challenges that collectively contribute to the poor overall prognosis for GBM patients. It is also well established that very

---

[1]The glia limitans is a 'barrier' structure designed to limit CNS infiltration by blood leukocytes and immune molecules. It is a thin tight-junction barrier composed of astrocytic foot processes. It is the outermost layer covering the brain parenchyma and spinal cord and lies directly beneath the pia mater (the innermost layer of the meninges) [45].

few or no GBMs are truly eradicated/'cured' with initial resection and systemic therapies (e.g., chemoradiotherapy, targeted agents, immunotherapies). In light of these facts, tumour stabilisation and radiographic response, as well as meaningful prolongation of *quality* life (deemed so by the patient, subjectively), are the current goals in designing treatment of progressive GBM.

The field of MNO is gaining more credence as clinical scientists collaborate with mathematicians to improve predictions of tumour growth and response to standard treatment protocol, as well as novel GBM therapies. New therapies are continually in development, such as nanoparticle drug delivery, tumour-treating fields, immunotherapies, and focused ultrasound to open the blood–brain barrier or activate photosensitisers to promote tumour cell death. In theory, any of these novel anti-cancer agents can have its effects modelled mathematically, whether outcomes are measured by tissue biopsy histopathological analysis, radiographic, and clinical response (PFS or OS). Some of these aspects are address in more detail in a different chapter of this volume, focussed on immunotherapies for cancer. Examples of clinical challenges that may be overcome by the application of MNO, to improve the precision treatment for newly diagnosed and progressive GBM, are discussed in this section of the chapter.

4.1. *Extent of safe surgical resection*

Neurosurgeons have to question not only 'should we resect or not?' (i.e., is the patient fit enough or likely to benefit from surgery) but also 'how much should be resected?' To achieve their aim of gross total resection (GTR), the surgeon must surpass many challenges. First, due to the highly infiltrative nature of GBM, tumour areas visible on contrast-enhanced MRI are assumed to be infiltrated by tumour cells at time of diagnosis but it is not always possible to distinguish normal brain from tumour intra-operatively. This uncertainty has been helped by the use of intra-operative dyes that localise to tumour cells, such as 5-ALA to allow fluorescent-guided resection [46]. Second, any benefit obtained from a more extensive resection is nullified if the post-operative neurological deficit is greater than the pre-operative deficit. Alterations in post-operative neurological status is associated with poorer OS [47]. Third, determining the extent of GBM invasion pre-operatively is best achieved with MRI; however, there is a debate over whether such techniques underestimate the aggressivity of GBMs, with some 'invisible' areas of diffuse infiltration not being detected. Fourth, the neoplasia visible on MRI can invade eloquent or vital brain areas (from the moment of diagnosis), making GTR impossible: surgery needs to be safe rather than simply removing all abnormal tissue [47]. Current imaging techniques also do not reflect the on-going microscopic behaviour of the glioma cells at the invasion front, simply offering a 'snap-shot' of information about the tumour location. It is therefore hoped that mathematical models that utilise optimal real-time imaging techniques will enable clinicians to better distinguish the characteristics and parameters of an individual's tumour and subsequently guide delicate surgical equipoise. These real-time techniques are still in development and out with the scope of this chapter, such as intra-op ultrasound scanning and MRI, spectroscopy, OCT, and histopathological sampling.

4.2. *Development of predictive molecular biomarkers*

The presence of different epigenetic and genetic alterations between and within (inter-tumoural and intra-tumoral heterogeneity) individual tumours can contribute to the differential responses to GBM treatments. Within a single GBM tumour, some sub-populations of genetically and functionally distinct glioma cells will be more sensitive to TMZ or radiotherapy; however, some may have existing (or adapt) mechanisms that enable them to survive such treatments (i.e., 'fitter' sub-populations with favourable characteristics). Other challenges that reduce GBM treatment efficacy include, the presence of the BBB (precluding the delivery of many drugs into the brain), an immunosuppressive microenvironment, and the adaptation/utilisation of signalling networks that can result in treatment resistance [6].

Chemotherapy and/or radiotherapy may offer a subtle increase in survival. However, such survival is associated with significant treatment-related toxicities (*e.g., systemic toxicities, radiotherapy-induced neurocognitive injury, and radiation necrosis*) which impact quality of life [6]. MNO may be able to help clinicians determine which patients the benefit of a specific treatment (such as radiotherapy) would outweigh the potential toxicities and to determine the shortest duration of treatment necessary to induce a maximal response, with minimal negative impact on quality of life.

Approximately two-thirds of recurrent GBMs appear within 2cm of the initial tumour margin [48]. There is currently no established theory behind this. However, intra-tumoural heterogeneity has been experimentally shown to exist between primary and recurrent GBMs — the survival and proliferation of previously undetected sub-clones originating from the primary tumour perhaps explaining the appearance of a molecularly distinct recurrence within close proximity to the initial margin. Determining molecular characteristics of the recurrent GBM cell population, and incorporating these into mathematical models, will perhaps determine which primary tumours contain sub-clones that are likely to survive and proliferate. Thus, MNO may identify the tumours which require more extensive resection and/or more aggressive post-operative treatment regimens, which may be targeted to any identified patient-specific biomarkers.

4.3. *Non-invasive approaches*

Assessment of tumour heterogeneities on a molecular level requires an invasive biopsy. Clinicians desire a non-invasive and less traumatic method to estimate the risk of cancer progression. Patient-specific mathematical modelling (based on multi-scale parameter estimation from available data) could be used to evaluate tumour response to chemotherapy and radiotherapy in individual patients and to estimate patients' OS among groups with different cancer heterogeneities. Modelling is also crucial to investigate the proliferation/migration pattern of individual GBM tumours and to predict the time-evolution of such patterns.

4.4. *Integration of patient-specific data*

Only by utilising advanced molecular and imaging-based diagnostics will we achieve a comprehensive prediction of tumour behaviour, which cannot be achieved by simple imaging or histological analysis alone. Continual, integrated analysis of these complementary and complex data streams should be made possible by MNO [49]. This will require a concerted effort to invent and deploy new analytical approaches and visualisation technologies in order to generate a single flow of information that travels with a patient from diagnosis and throughout their treatment journey [49].

5.   Mathematical and Computational Models of GBM

By utilising measurements from serial imaging techniques, and putting them into simulation, mathematical and computational models of GBM allow for the identification of individualised tumour proliferation and invasion rates about an individual's tumour. Therefore, MNO has the potential to have a profound impact on how we practice personalised medicine [40]. Patient-specific models can be used to overcome imaging limitations, improve prognostic predictions, stratify patients, and assess treatment response *in silico* [2]. In the following, we discuss some of the models developed over the last decades to reproduce various aspects of GBM evolution. We have simplified the description of the mathematical models discussed in the following section for the benefit of clinicians without a background in higher mathematics. These models are summarised in Table 3.

5.1.   *Proliferation-invasion (PI) model*

The classical concept of proliferating cancer cells to have the capacity to both invade and metastasise can be simplified for gliomas, due to their lack of metastases. Based on this basic concept, the proliferation-invasion (PI) model was developed [50]. The PI model is a partial differential equation which describes the rate of change of tumour cell density in time as being equal to the net migration rate (D, mm^2/year), plus the net proliferation rate (ρ, year^{-1}) of the tumour cells. These parameters are obtained on a patient-specific basis using routine clinical imaging prior to treatment. The PI model can be used to determine the velocity of growth, as well as an 'invisibility index' (ratio of D/ρ), representing the glioma cell population which is not quantifiable or visible upon radiographic imaging. Because the group later discovered that malignant glioma cells can migrate up to 100-fold faster in white matter than in grey, the PI model now incorporates the differential motility of glioma cells through grey and white matter into the model to provide predictions that are specific to the patient's tumour architecture [2].

Table 3. Mathematical modelling of glioblastoma multiforme — A summary of models in development.

Model	Considerations of tumour biology	Future prospects
PI model	Proliferation-invasion	Prediction of tumour growth on an individual basis
PIRT model	Proliferation-invasion for radiotherapy effectiveness	Personalisation of radiotherapy regimens according to predicted tumour response *in silico*. Future scope to influence the personalisation of treatment regimens (e.g., *adjuvant treatment for tumours deemed 'more aggressive'*)
PINHA model	Proliferation-invasion-hypoxia-necrosis-angiogenesis	Prediction of tumour growth as well as spatial distribution of intra-tumoral hypoxia on an individual basis. Future scope to influence the personalisation of treatment regimens (e.g., *adjuvant treatment for tumours deemed 'more aggressive'*)
3D modelling of brain microfibres	Tumour microenvironment, ECM composition and degradation	Predict the course of tumour progression based on the composition of an individual tumour's surrounding parenchyma and associated ECM. Used in combination with imaging techniques such as DTI and MR-Spectroscopy. Future scope to influence the personalisation of treatment regimens (e.g., *adjuvant treatment for tumours deemed 'more aggressive'*)
ISOG model	P53 mutation status (tumour suppressor dysfunction)	Prediction of individual tumour response to radiotherapy using p53 mutation status. Future scope to determine which patients will be responsive to radiotherapy
Whole slide images to infer IDH mutation status	IDH mutation status (involved in metabolic reprogramming, hypermethylator phenotype, dedifferentiation)	Prediction of IDH mutation status ($+/-$ prognosis) through utilisation of a more cost-effective, timely technique. Future scope to influence the personalisation of treatment regimens (e.g., *adjuvant treatment for tumours deemed 'more aggressive'*)

(*Continued*)

Table 3. (*Continued*)

Model	Considerations of tumour biology	Future prospects
Malignant transformation rate	IDH mutation status (involved in metabolic reprogramming, hypermethylator phenotype, dedifferentiation), 1p19q co-deletion, tumour microenvironment, genomic instability	Prediction of the rate of malignant transformation (+/− prognosis) of LGGs using IDH and 1p19q co-deletion status. Future scope to influence the personalisation of treatment regimens (e.g., *adjuvant treatment for tumours deemed 'more aggressive'*)
Spatio-temporal model	Immune evasion (M1 TAMs and TGF-β)	Prediction of GBM migration pattern through analysis of the interactions with the immune system. Future scope to influence the personalisation of treatment regimens (e.g., *adjuvant treatment for tumours deemed 'more aggressive'*). Also, future scope to influence the use of immunotherapeutics
Tumour microtubules and tumour invasion front	Invasion, tumour microenvironment, ECM composition and degradation, epithelial-mesenchymal transition	Prediction of GBM migration pattern through analysis of the tumour invasion front and ECM interactions. Future scope to influence the personalisation of treatment regimens (e.g., *adjuvant treatment for tumours deemed 'more aggressive'*)

Notes: Abbreviations: PI = proliferation-invasion model; PIRT = proliferation-invasion for radiotherapy effectiveness (RT) model; PINHA = proliferation-invasion-hypoxia-necrosis-angiogenesis; ECM = extra-cellular matrix; DTI = diffusion tensor imaging; ISOG = *in silico* oncology group model; IDH = isocitrate dehydrogenase; LGGs = low grade gliomas; TAMs = tumour-associated macrophages; TGF-β = transforming growth factor beta; GBM = glioblastoma multiforme.

5.2. *PIRT model*

Rockne *et al.* incorporated the classic linear-quadratic model (LQ model) for radiation (RT) effectiveness into the PI model. This resulted in the extended PI model, PIRT. The group found minimal difference (2.4 mm) between simulated and actual tumour volumes post-RT, illustrating the PI model to accurately predict post-RT tumour size [50]. The PIRT model is considered one of the most clinically relevant models, validating the prognostic capacity of a new patient-specific response metric called 'Days Gained Score' (see Section 6.2.1). PIRT was the first MNO model to estimate radiobiological parameters for individual patients *in vivo*, providing the basis for personalised predictions of response to radiotherapy treatment [50].

5.3. *PINHA model*

Further analysis of the PI model revealed a strong correlation between hypoxic conditions and the ρ/D ratio (invisibility index). As previously mentioned, we know that a rapidly dividing tumour that outgrows its blood supply can develop regions of hypoxia. This results in the development of necrotic areas within the tumour, as well as activation of the pro-survival mechanism, angiogenesis. This leads to the development of the inclusive PIHNA (*Proliferation-Invasion-Hypoxia-Necrosis-Angiogenesis*) model. The PINHA model investigated the dynamics between glioma cells and their microenvironment, illustrating that genetic mutations are not a necessity for malignant progression of GBM — the latter can be a result of the interaction of the tumour cells alone (of a given net invasion rate and proliferation rate) with their environment. The PIHNA model can also be used to predict a patient's spatial distribution of intra-tumoral hypoxia [50].

5.4. *'Go or Grow' hypothesis*

There is significant evidence to suggest that the two distinct states of proliferation and invasion are mutually exclusive in GBM cells. This 'either-or' behaviour of glioma cells is referred to as the *migration-proliferation dichotomy (the 'Go-or-Grow' hypothesis)*. Tumour cells are thought to 'switch' to an invasive phenotype (migrates rapidly, proliferates slowly) from a proliferative phenotype (proliferates rapidly, migrates slowly) when their microenvironment does not suffice in either nutrients or oxygen (metabolic stress), and thus, they migrate to find such sources to survive [2].

The validity of this hypothesis is greatly debated within the field of MNO, with some experts implying that it is too simple, and considers too few parameters. However, the 'Go-or Grow' hypothesis inspired the development of models based on the link between hypoxia and invasiveness [50]. One such group applied the hypothesis into a model which analysed the speed and shape of travelling wave solutions of GBM growth, in which tumour cell motility and proliferation were considered as separate processes. It was found that the shape of the travelling wave varied depending on the type of attractor that the equilibrium point is. If the non-negative equilibrium point was a stable spiral, the wave profile featured a prominent 'bump'. If it was a stable node, the resulting wave profile was monotonic [51]. Because the density of the proliferating and migrating cells in the tumour core is determined by this non-negative equilibrium point, the group could then find tumours where there were more proliferating cells in the centre or more migrating cells in the centre. The presence of a stable spiral corresponded to a higher density of cells near the moving boundary (as opposed to a further behind the wave front). The presence of a stable node was associated with the cell density near the moving boundary to be the same as the cell density in the tumour core [51].

5.5. *Infiltrative morphology*

Specific morphological features, such as pseudopalisades, are associated with glioma invasiveness and aggressiveness [5]. For example, hypoxic and necrotic regions (rich in pseudopalisades) correlate with *invasive* glioma cell behaviour, whereas cells in normoxic regions are more *proliferative*. This has been confirmed by mathematical simulations of travelling waves of glioma cells migrating away from central hypoxia regions closely resembling the actual observed histological patterns of pseudopalisades. A link has also been established between the time scale of formation, lifetime, and persistence of pseudopalisades, with their distance from occluded functional blood vessels. Simulations have also shown palisading waves to occur at faster rates, and in the specific direction of, regions with plentiful oxygen supply, rather than pure random motion. This indicates that vascular occlusion may accelerate glioma invasion and that tumour vasculature normalisation is a strategy to reduce migration [5].

5.6. *3D modelling of brain microfibres*

Most published mathematical models of GBM focus on single-scale 2D dynamics and cannot capture the complex multi-scale tumour invasion patterns in the 3D brain. As previously described, GBM invasion relies on cell adhesion to the ECM, degradation of the ECM, and altered cell contractility/motility. Additionally, differences in the invasive phenotype of GBM differ between grey and white matter — owing to their differences in architecture, molecular composition, and densities.

Suveges *et al.* investigated the relationship between distribution and orientation of microfibres that comprise the tumour and surrounding brain tissue, and the 3D invasion patterns of tumours. The study found that microfibre rearrangements influence changes in the tumour boundary over time. The cancer cells' movement is not only influenced by the scans (through the anisotropic diffusion term) but also biased by crucial non-local adhesions such as cell–cell and cell–fibre ECM adhesion, the latter of which is naturally interconnected to tissue structural changes [52].

In their model, the fibrous ECM phase described all major fibrous proteins (such as collagen and fibronectin) whose microscale distribution induces the spatial orientation of the ECM fibres. The non-fibrous ECM phase describes every other ECM component, such as non-fibrous proteins, enzymes, polysaccharides, and extracellular calcium ions [52]. Diffusion Tensor Imaging (DTI) and T1-weighted scans (which measure the diffusion of water molecules) were used to produce a tumour diffusion tensor *Dt(x)*, a fully anisotropic diffusion term. *Anisotropic diffusion* is a method to improve the precision of tumour edge detection — it can remove noise from radiographic images to 'smooth' the image intensity, without 'blurring' the tumour edges. T1-weighted images provided white-grey matter densities, allowing the calculation of different diffusion rates according to tumour location. DTI provided information about the underlying brain structure, as well as higher diffusion rates along specific directions based on how water molecules behave within the brain. Current DTI scans lack the resolution required to construct a unique fibre distribution within a microdomain. *Suveges'* group set fibre distributions to be either random or orientated based on whether they were positioned in grey or white matter, respectively. However, to genuinely capture (and not assume) the fibre distributions within underlying brain structures, better resolution DTI scans are required, or, in the future, this technique could be combined with other emerging technologies, such as MR-elastography [52].

5.7. *In silico oncology group (ISOG) model*

Stamatakos *et al.* developed a 4D model of imageable tumour response to radiotherapy *in vivo* based on the LQ model, called the *In silico Oncology Group (ISOG)* model. The ISOG model is a stochastic model that enables the simulation of radiation response in GBM patients [53]. It is clinically relevant as it takes into account molecular characteristics of each patient, for example, p53 mutation status. A number of studies associate p53 mutations with increased radio-resistance and poorer outcome for GBM patients. Furthermore, radiotherapy provides a selective advantage to GBM cells expressing mutant p53. The observed radio-resistance of cells expressing mutant p53 is attributed to its ability to confer a deficit in G1 checkpoint, and a resultant increase in cell-cycle distribution within the radio-resistant S-phase, in response to irradiation [53].

5.8. *Whole slide images to infer IDH mutation status*

As previously mentioned, IDH mutational status can help predict patient outcome. Consideration of IDH mutation status is therefore key in clinical treatment planning. However, confirmation of IDH mutation status is both time consuming and expensive. Additionally, current sequencing techniques can only identify a small proportion of IDH mutations. In light of these factors, Jiang *et al.* developed end-to-end deep learning models using whole slide images (WSIs) of adults diagnosed with diffusely infiltrating WHO grade 2 gliomas to predict prognosis and IDH mutation status [18]. By obtaining IDH mutation status directly from histopathological slides (WSI-inferred IDH mutation status), these models represent a readily available tool that could significantly reduce time and cost. The group's novel WSI models, combined with demographic and clinical features, where shown to be strong predictors of prognosis and IDH mutations, with an area under the curve (AUC) of up to 0.784 and

0.739 (ROC curve analysis), respectively [18]. The group summarised that histological information only partly explains variance in prognosis, and the addition of demographic, clinical, and genetic/molecular information to such methods will further improve prediction of prognosis [18].

5.9. *Malignant transformation rate*

Aoki *et al.* developed a model that took both IDH mutation and 1p19q codeletion status into consideration. This study was the first to clarify the relationship between treatment success and malignant transformation (MT) rate in IDH-mutant LGGs. The group modelled tumour progression using serial tumour volume data (obtained from imaging) and treatment history of IDH-mutant LGGs with or without additional 1p/19q codeletion [54]. The analysis showed tumour mutational burden to correlate positively with MT. Chemotherapy and radiotherapy were shown to significantly suppress tumour growth but to increase the MT to 1.8–2.8 times greater than that before treatment [54]. The model then illustrated prompt adjuvant chemotherapy to successfully prolong MT-free survival in *small* volume IDH-mutant LGGs (<50 cm^3). In *larger* volume IDH-mutant LGGs, optimal treatment differed according to genetic alterations. Adjuvant therapies delayed MT in the IDH-mutant/1p19 non-codel but accelerated the MT in IDH-mutant/1p19q code tumoursl [54]. By uncovering that IDH-mutant/1p19q codel LGGs could represent a patient group requiring more extensive treatment (*e.g., adjuvant therapies*), this model represents a potential method of MNO-guided patient stratification, through which we can improve OS in patients with IDH mutations.

Notably, an additional *PI3K* mutation in IDH-mutant/1p19q codel tumours was not associated with MT (with all *PI3K* mutations present prior to MT) but increased the net post-operative proliferation rate and decreased MT-free survival, in comparison to *PI3K*-wild-type/IDH-mutant/1p19qcodel tumours [54]. This suggests that although not involved in tumorigenesis, *PI3K* mutations acquired during tumour expansion do influence tumour progression and may represent another predictive molecular marker that can be utilised by MNO.

5.10. *Spatio-temporal model*

GBM migratory patterns can be influenced through the interaction of glioma cells with immune cells and other immune system components. Tumour-associated macrophage (TAM) populations are highly heterogenous within in the GBM tumour microenvironment with disseminated M1 and M2 sub-populations. Macrophages can also easily move through pseudopodia, allowing their migration [35]. The interaction between GBM and the immune system is highly complex. Nevertheless, immunotherapy is currently a main focus of glioma therapy research, with the hope of developing methods to strengthen the immune system in order to combat malignant gliomas. Developing models of the glioma-immune system response can help us to better understand the complexities of these interactions and to develop better treatment strategies that can potentially improve patient prognosis and quality of life [35].

Khajanchi *et al.* developed a mathematical model which depicts the spatiotemporal dynamics of glioma cells, TAMs, cytotoxic-T-lymphocytes, TGF-β (immunosuppressive), and IFN-γ (immunostimulatory) through a system of five coupled reaction–diffusion equations. While the M1 TAM activity is down-regulated by TGF-β, it is activated by IFN-γ and can go on to suppress the activity of glioma cell populations. The researchers explained that, because GBM exhibits spatio-temporal heterogeneity, dispersive glioma-immune interactions will also exhibit these spatial variations. Therefore, the model utilised reaction–diffusion modelling to show how the glioma cell population and immune components spread over the domain and how this migration evolves in response with various parameters. Simulation of the model did indeed show the glioma cell population, TAMs, as well as T-lymphocytes to readily disperse with time [35].

5.11. *Tumour microtubules (TM) and tumour invasion front*

Angihortri *et al.* [39] developed a mathematical model that analysed tumour microtubules (TMs), metalloproteases (MMPs), and integrins to predict the behaviour of the tumour invasion front [40]. The researchers illustrated that microtubules are not randomly scattered but are concentrated around the tumour front, presumably to influence the direction of migration. Integrins have also been shown to co-localise with TMs and concentrate within the GBM invasion front [40]. The same is true for the localisation of MMPs (e.g., *MMP2 and MT1-MMP*). This observation correlates with the known association between significantly elevated MMP levels (a mechanism which favours ECM degradation) and GBM invasiveness.

6. Future Directions and Scope of Mathematical Modelling of GBM

6.1. *Overcoming limitations of imaging and histopathology*

Currently, clinical assessment of gliomas relies on non-invasive MRI and computed tomography (CT). CT provides morphological information of gliomas and is used as an early screening tool (e.g., *for patients with intractable headaches*), but early-stage tumours are often missed. MRI is significantly more sensitive and has become the gold standard imaging modality in neuro-oncology. However, neither technique accurately quantifies the full extent of invasion, recurrence, or progression during post-treatment surveillance, making the detection of 'invisible tumour' a key aim of MNO. For example, the PI model has shown concentrations of diffusely invading glioma cells to extend well beyond the threshold of MRI detection [2]. In addition, the aforementioned standard imaging techniques do not provide any molecular or functional information about the underlying tumour biology. By integrating mathematics, molecular markers, and different novel imaging techniques, we can simultaneously determine true tumour anatomy, underlying biological processes, molecular composition, and most likely pattern of growth on a patient-specific basis. The development of a tool which reflects dynamic progression of tumour features in real time, in 3D, and with optimal resolution would be a significant step forward in clinical neuro-oncology.

It is important to consider that there is significant variation between the imaging parameters used to try and delineate areas of tumour recurrence after resection. T2-weighted *Fluid-Attenuated Inversion Recovery* (FLAIR) signal can illustrate GBM progression which is not picked up as 'enhancing' tissue by T1-weighted MRI with contrast. This phenomenon is termed *non-enhancing tumour progression* [55]. *The Macdonald Criteria (1990)* was historically used to determine post-resection tumour response, using contrast enhancement as a surrogate marker of progression. The *Macdonald Criteria* used tumour measurements, obtained from post-resection MRI with gadolinium contrast, to stratify treatment response into 4 categories: complete response (CR), partial response (PR), stable disease (SD), and progressive disease (PD). *The Macdonald Criteria* measured *contrast-enhancing tumour progression* but did not take any non-enhancing disease into account. To address this limitation, the *Response Assessment in Neuro-Oncology* (RANO) working group proposed updated response criteria for HGGs in 2010 [55]. The RANO criteria definition of progression is not only a 25% increase in contrast-enhancing area over baseline or best response but also includes any significant enlargement of non-enhancing T2/FLAIR signal on MRI that was attributed to tumour growth. The new response criteria have subsequently made clinicians aware that removal of all 'enhancing' tissue does not constitute a surgical cure and are why T2/FLAIR MRI is now routinely used to reliably detect and measure tumour recurrence [55]. Additionally, previous researchers, such as Young *et al.*, have highlighted that conventional MRI signs used to distinguish pseudoprogression from early progression fail to offer a high negative predictive value for pseudoprogression. Subependymal enhancement was found to be the only sign to predictive for early progression ($p = 0.001$) with 38.1% sensitivity, 93.3% specificity, and 41.8% negative predictive value. The other 10 signs investigated had no predictive value for early progression ($p = 0.06 - 1.0$) [56].

We hope that incorporating a multitude of our best imaging techniques for GBM with patient-specific models will help us to overcome imaging-associated limitations and better predict and monitor tumour behaviour.

MR-spectroscopy (MRS) uses proton signals to determine relative concentrations of target metabolites. It has shown to be capable of detecting IDH mutations, as well as assessing response to various therapies. MRS has also given rise to the study of metabolomic signatures in tumours (metabolomics) and the use of imaging technology to extrapolate molecular tumour data (radiomics). However, the resolution of MRS is much lower than standard MRI. Functional imaging techniques like positron emission tomography (PET) scans are useful in providing deeper insights into the biology of gliomas, as well as detect changes within a neoplasm. This information is complemented by MRI, as PET scans lack anatomic context and have relatively low spatial resolution [5]. MRS and/or PET imaging is often used by clinicians trying to try and distinguish whether areas of new contrast enhancement seen on standard of care serial MRI imaging demonstrates true disease progression or pseudoprogression (the latter is usually due to the inflammation caused by radiotherapy or alterations in tumour-BBB characteristics from immunotherapy, which can cause identical FLAIR and contrast imaging changes to true tumour regrowth) [57].

Diagnosis and classification of glioma is based on histopathology, i.e., the microscopic examination of tissue sections by an experienced neuropathologist. Histopathology can also provide further information at the single-cell level that is extremely important to analyse intra-tumoural heterogeneity. However, biopsy specimens only provide a 'snap-shot' of dynamic biological processes occurring within only a portion of the tumour. Therefore, because the data obtained are limited in both space and time, biopsy specimens will undoubtedly miss subtle alterations arising in this highly heterogeneous cancer [5]. Thus, though histopathology is vital to MNO, it is now an adjunct to the more clinically relevant molecular signature of tumours discussed in Section 2.3 of this chapter.

6.2. *Applications of mathematical modelling in GBM*

Listed in the following are five aspects of care of GBM patients in which MNO has been utilised with the aim of better informing clinical decision-making and guiding the patient towards maximum possible benefit. These are summarised in Table 4. The field of MNO is still developing, and an integrated approach to these differing models will hopefully result in MNO being a standard tool used in the neuro-oncologist's armamentarium for treatment of GBM.

6.2.1. *Survival outcomes — Days gained score*

An effective demonstration of clinical utility of MNO is the use of the untreated virtual control (UVC). Because untreated gliomas have a

Table 4. A summary of the potential benefits of mathematical neuro-oncology on the clinical approach to glioblastoma multiforme treatment.

Advantage offered by MNO	Clinical challenges addressed	Further details
Prediction of growth pattern and identification of which patients will be responsive to treatment	• Lack of tools to predict which patients may require and benefit from additional therapy.	*'Days Gained' score accounts for the relative growth kinetics of individual tumours. It is prognostic of OS and time to tumour recurrence. It can enable the determination of patients who will have a survival benefit from treatment.*
Prediction of pseudoprogression	• The current standard of care after detecting post-treatment tumour progression is to imminently alter therapeutic regimens. However, current imaging techniques cannot distinguish pseudoprogression from true progression.	*The potential of pseudoprogression masquerading as true progression complicates clinical decision making in GBM. Therefore, there is a great need to accurately distinguish between the two. Patients with pseudo progression have been found to have significantly higher Days Gained scores.*
Identification of patient groups responsive to targeted therapies	• Treatment resistance and intra-tumoral and inter-tumoral heterogeneity. • Future development of personalised medicine.	*The 'PINHA' model has the potential to identify which GBM patients will benefit from adjuvant Bevacizumab therapy.*
Identification of patient groups responsive to different adjuvant radiotherapy regimens	• Should peritumoral oedema be included in the measurement of gross tumour volume? • Future development of biologically guided personalised radiotherapy treatment plans.	*MNO models could help elucidate which patients, according to their molecular, imaging and clinical characteristics, would benefit the most from different adjuvant radiotherapy approaches.*

Table 4. (*Continued*)

Advantage offered by MNO	Clinical challenges addressed	Further details
Determination of the optimal degree of resection for individual patients	• Current imaging techniques alone do not take into account molecular and functional information about the tumour biology. • Additionally, there is often suboptimal resolution to accurately determine the degree of tumour invasion and thus, the appropriate extent of resection required.	*MNO models tuned with patient-specific parameters could help determine the optimal amount of tissue to resect in order to maximise survival.* *The development of a model which accurately simulates GTR and STR by reflecting dynamic progression of tumour features over time, in three dimensions, and with optimal resolution would be a significant step forward in clinical neuro-oncology.*

Notes: MNO = mathematical neuro-oncology; OS = overall survival; PINHA = proliferation-invasion-hypoxia-necrosis-angiogenesis model; GBM = glioblastoma multiforme; GTR = gross total resection; STR = subtotal resection.

predictable pattern of growth, the UVC approach is simple to apply. By using a UVC, a model can describe the inherent, untreated disease behaviour in a specific patient and use this as a baseline for future comparisons. Deviations from the predicted UVC behaviour can be used as a metric of response to therapy. The *Days Gained* score is a tool which measures treatment-induced reduction in tumour growth. The score is calculated at the first post-radiotherapy MRI and, as well as considering the UVC, accounts for the relative growth kinetics of the individual tumour [50]. This tool is predictive of time to recurrence and may therefore aid the determination of which patients will benefit from radiotherapy [2].

6.2.2. *Extent of resection*

Surgical equipoise over GBM management is not only at the point of deciding on whether tumour imaging is demonstrating true progression or pseudoprogression. There is still debate as to the survival benefit of sub-total resection (STR) versus gross total resection (GTR); the amount of high-level evidence available remains limited but suggests that GTR offers a better chance of survival [47, 58]. MNO tuned with patient-specific parameters provides a valuable insight into this clinical debate and could help determine the optimal amount of tissue to resect in order to maximise survival. Swanson *et al.* (2008) simulated surgical resection using the PI model. This model incorporated the contrast-enhanced T1-weighted MRI tumour volume and radial velocity of tumour growth. The model was able to predict the survival curve for biopsy, STR, and GTR groups. The group stated that although GTR was shown to provide a survival benefit over biopsies or STR, this may be partially due to the preferential selection of patients with smaller tumours for GTR [2]. It is hoped that if we can incorporate patient-specific tumour measurements into a model that is predictive of the extent of resection, we will be to achieve the best survival outcome for individual patients with different tumour size and location.

6.2.3. *Adjuvant radiotherapy regime*

There is no single approach that is effective for all GBM patients due to its heterogeneity. MNO models could help elucidate which patients, according to their molecular, imaging, and clinical characteristics, would benefit from radiotherapy and which specific regimen would be most effective. *In silico* models which take into account the patient-specific description of tumour growth and response may also be used to generate biologically guided treatment plans which optimise radiation therapy (i.e., *the maximisation of normal tissue sparing and minimisation of tumour burden at appropriate time points*) [2].

There is currently no consensus on the target delineation for GBM patients who require adjuvant radiotherapy, over whether it is necessary to treat all locations of potential microinvasion, and whether the target volume of GBM should include peritumoral oedema. The reasoning behind including peritumoral oedema is that the oedema may be an infiltrative area. The reasoning behind excluding peritumoral oedema is that there is no significant difference in recurrence patterns with or without oedema. Another important consideration is that increasing the target volume also increases the volume of normal brain tissue exposed to irradiation. At present, the radiotherapy protocols of the *Radiation Therapy Oncology Group* (RTOG) and the *European Organisation for Research and Treatment of Cancer* (EORTC) have different irradiation protocols which are used in GBM (Table 5). RTOG includes peri-tumoral oedema in the measurement of gross tumour volume (GTV), whereas EORTC excludes it. A clinical trial has not yet been carried out to make a direct comparison between the two strategies proposed and recommended by RTOG and EORTC, respectively. MNO could be used to enable the comparison of these radiation strategies and determine whether the GTV should be inclusive of peritumoral oedema. By using MNO and machine learning to characterise the kinetics and molecular features of the tumour, we may be able to better differentiate peritumoral oedema from tumour infiltration and either decrease or increase (respectively) the measurement of the GTV as required. This could be used to guide clinicians to offer the best individualised radiotherapy regimen based on a set of pre-determined clinical criteria [50].

6.2.4. *Personalised treatment with anti-angiogenic therapy*

Treatment with Bevacizumab (an anti-angiogenic agent) has been approved for the treatment of recurrent/progressive GBM in the USA, as it provides improved disease control compared to historical controls as measured by best imaging response and progression-free survival at 6 months. However, there is no evidence for improvement in OS [60] and it is thought that the improved imaging response is due to reduced tumour vascularisation rather than actual tumour response. There is also insufficient evidence to show benefit of first-line Bevacizumab in combination with TMZ in progressive GBM [60]. Interestingly, the PIHNA model tried to explain the inefficacy of the addition of Bevacizumab to standard TMZ in previous studies. Patients who were not eligible for GTR were found to possibly benefit from the addition of Bevacizumab to their treatment regime. Thus, the PINHA model has the potential to identify which GBM patients will benefit from Bevacizumab [50].

6.2.5. *Predicting pseudoprogression*

Pseudoprogression is a clinical phenomenon defined by increased contrast enhancement within 100 days of chemo- or radiotherapy

Table 5. GBM radiotherapy protocols of Radiation Therapy Oncology Group (RTOG) or European Organisation for Research and Treatment of Cancer (EORTC) [59].

Radiation strategy	RTOG	EORTC
Protocol	Stage 1: 46Gy in 23 fractions Stage 2: 14Gy in 7 fractions	60Gy in 30 fractions
Gross tumour volume (GTV)	GTV1 = T1-weighted MRI enhancement area + resection cavity + abnormal signal area in T2-weighted and FLAIR MRI phase GTV2 = T1-weighted MRI enhancement area + resection cavity	GTV = T1-weighted MRI enhancement area + resection cavity (*does not include peri-tumoral oedema*)
Clinical target volume (CTV)	CTV1 = 2 cm expansion from GTV1 (*or 2.5 cm if no oedema present around tumour*) CTV2 = 2 cm expansion from GTV2	CTV = 2 cm expansion from GTV
Planning target volume (PTV)	PTV1 = 0.3–0.5 cm expansion from CTV1 PTV2 = 0.3–0.5 cm expansion from CTV2	PTV = 0.3–0.5 cm expansion from CTV

Notes: The first stage of the RTOG protocol comprises 46 Gy in 23 fractions. Gross tumour volume 1 (GTV1) includes the postoperative T1-weighted MRI enhancement area, resection cavity, and abnormal signal area in the T2-weighted and fluid-attenuated inversion recovery (FLAIR) MRI phases. Clinical target volume 1 (CTV1) is defined as a 2 cm expansion from GTV1. If there is no oedema around the tumour, 2.5 cm from GTV1 is added. Planning target volume 1 (PTV1) is expanded 0.3–0.5 cm from CTV1 and varies in different centres. The second stage is irradiation with 14 Gy in seven fractions. GTV2 includes the enhancing area of T1-weighted MRI and the resection cavity. CTV2 is expanded 2 cm from GTV2. PTV2 is the same range as in the first stage. The EORTC protocol is comprised of one target volume of 60 Gy in 30 fractions. GTV includes the T1-weighted MRI enhancement area and resection cavity but does not intentionally include the peritumoral oedema area. CTV is obtained by GTV extended 2 cm. PTV is treated with 0.3–0.5 cm expansion (depending on centre). (Abbreviations: RTOG = Radiation Therapy Oncology Group; EORTC = European Organisation for Research and Treatment of Cancer; Gy = Grays; MRI = magnetic resonance imaging; FLAIR = fluid-attenuated inversion recovery).

that spontaneously resolves with no subsequent change in treatment. The increased contrast enhancement occurs secondary to the ability of these cytotoxic therapies to increase vascular permeability [61]. Approximately 50% of patients will experience contrast enhancement on MRI within 1 month of radiotherapy, a feature which characteristic of GBM recurrence. However, 50% of these cases will actually have pseudoprogression, as opposed to true recurrence [61]. Because the current standard of care after detecting recurrence is to imminently alter therapeutic regimens, the uncertainty posed by the potential presence of pseudoprogression influences and complicates clinical decision-making. Currently, clinicians are unsure whether to reoperate on these enhancing areas (if safe), offer second line/experimental chemotherapy, or simply rescan after two months. The former two options have risks and side effects (affecting quality of life in people with limited life expectancy) and the latter option may mean that the tumour increases exponentially in size during the two months and the option of safe surgery is lost or further neurological deficit has occurred. Therefore, there is an urgent need to find a method to accurately distinguish between the two. Although there is currently no method to predict which patients will and will not exhibit pseudoprogression (due to a lack of understanding of the causal biological mechanisms), the *Days Gained* score has been shown to potentially discriminate pseudoprogression in individual patients. Patients with pseudoprogression were found to have significantly higher *Days Gained* scores, connecting model-based metrics of response to patient-specific clinical outcomes [2]. It is the hope of the authors that future mathematical models are combined with large datasets of post chemo-radiotherapy MRI scans from patients who *either* go on to have a tissue diagnosis confirming true recurrence at sites of enhancement *or* the enhancement resolves without treatment confirming pseudoprogression. Matching such models to outcomes will then help develop MNO into a tool which distinguishes pseudoprogression from actual progression and allows clinicians to decide on best treatment.

7. Concluding Remarks

This chapter has illustrated that the aggressiveness of GBM is due to its high invasive capacity and significant intra- and inter-tumoral heterogeneity. Developing mathematical models which attempt to 'map' macroscopic growth patterns of GBM and predict treatment response must therefore take into account various multi-scale aspects: (1) key genetic and epigenetic aberrations (e.g., p53 status) and biological factors (e.g., hypoxia and nutrient availability), (2) mechanical interactions between the tumour and its microenvironment, as well as (3) molecular and kinetic properties of the tumour invasion front. Exploration of the use of MNO in GBM will hopefully help the development of a computational tool that captures the interplay of both microscopic and macroscopic factors that drive GBM evolution.

Many MNO models which combine both clinical and imaging data have shown significant predicative abilities, but such models remain to be perfected. For example, incorporating modern and non-invasive techniques (e.g., the detection of circulating tumour DNA (ctDNA) and MR-spectroscopy) may further improve the accuracy of *in silico* modelling of GBM. Additionally, each individual model has its own pros and cons. There has not yet been a direct comparison to confirm the superiority of one over another; however, it may be that some are more applicable to certain clinical situations. We suggest the future lies with the development of hybrid models. This is because GBM invasion is influenced by such a multitude of biological factors — of which only a select few (or none) are considered in individual models. We recommend that mathematicians work together to create a model that considers as many, if not all known, aspects of GBM tumour biology on the microscopic/molecular level, in order to more accurately predict macroscopic behaviour and subsequently, improve clinical decisions and outcomes (see Fig. 1). Several molecular factors, such as the four molecular sub-types of GBM discussed previously in this chapter, and MGMT methylation status are now used to refine GBM survival prediction. The predictive value of MNO models should therefore be compared to (and perhaps combined with) these existing prognostic tools.

Because the mathematical models described in this chapter utilise patient-specific parameters, they address the key feature of GBM that makes it so difficult to treat and predict clinical outcome: its heterogeneity. It is hoped that the use of MNO approaches will enable the integration of any relevant patient-specific data at critical points in the patient journey, providing an unprecedented level of comprehensive decision-making to guide the selection of the most

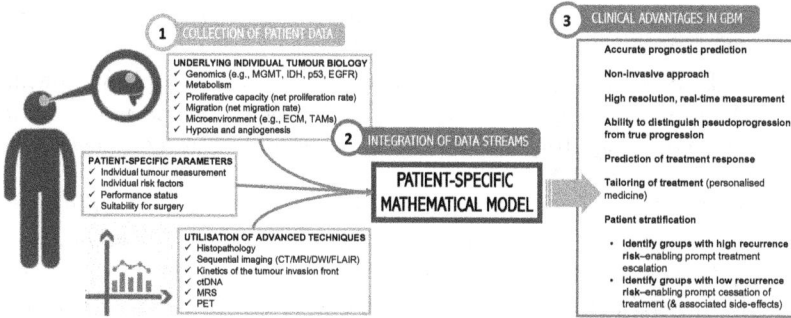

Fig. 1. The clinical advantages of mathematical modelling using patient-specific parameters.

Notes: The use of mathematical modelling should enable the integration of separate data streams at critical points in the patient journey. This includes data obtained from high resolution imaging techniques, molecular analysis of the underlying tumour biology (e.g., angiogenesis, proliferation, invasion, microenvironment, hypoxia, and metabolism), and patient-specific parameters (e.g., tumour measurement at diagnosis, location, and mutations) with the latter addressing the key issue of heterogeneity in GBM treatment. Using these data streams in combination, to create a patient-specific mathematical model that is highly representative of the individual's tumour on both the macroscopic and microscopic levels, will enable the development of an unprecedented level of comprehensive decision-making to guide the selection of the most appropriate treatment and support the management of GBM. This will also enable constant refinement and improvements in clinical decision-making [49]. (Abbreviations: MGMT = O^6-methylguanine-DNA; IDH = isocitrate dehydrogenase; EGFR = epidermal growth factor receptor; ECM = extracellular matrix; TAMs = tumour-associated macrophages; ctDNA = circulating tumour DNA; MRS = MR-spectrometry; PET = positron emission tomography).

appropriate treatment for patients with GBM. The knowledge gained through the management of each patient should be analysed iteratively over time with teams of clinicians and mathematicians working together, enabling constant refinement and improvements in clinical decision-making. This chapter can therefore conclude that MNO represents an exciting prospect for GBM patients in the modern era of precision medicine and personalised neuro-oncology.

References

[1] A. C. Tan, D. M. Ashley, G. Y. López, M. Malinzak, H. S. Friedman, and M. Khasraw, Management of glioblastoma: State of the art

and future directions, *CA: A Cancer Journal for Clinicians.* **70**(4), 299–312 (2020).

[2] A. L. Baldock, R. C. Rockne, A. D. Boone, M. L. Neal, A. Hawkins-Daarud, D. M. Corwin, *et al.,* From patient-specific mathematical neuro-oncology to precision medicine, *Frontiers in Oncology.* **3**, 1–9 (2013).

[3] A. Brodbelt, D. Greenberg, T. Winters, M. Williams, S. Vernon, and V. P. Collins, Glioblastoma in England: 2007-2011, *European Journal of Cancer.* **51**(4), 533–42 (2015).

[4] J. L. Birch, B. J. Coull, L. C. Spender, C. Watt, A. Willison, N. Syed, *et al.,* Multifaceted transforming growth factor-beta (TGFβ) signalling in glioblastoma, *Cellular Signalling* (Elsevier Inc.). **72**, 109638 (2020).

[5] J. C. L. Alfonso, K. Talkenberger, M. Seifert, B. Klink, A. Hawkins-Daarud, K. R. Swanson, *et al.,* The biology and mathematical modelling of glioma invasion: A review, *Journal of the Royal Society Interface* (Royal Society Publishing). **14**, 1–15 (2017).

[6] P. Y. Wen, M. Weller, E. Q. Lee, B. M. Alexander, J. S. Barnholtz-Sloan, F. P. Barthel, *et al.,* Glioblastoma in adults: A Society for Neuro-Oncology (SNO) and European Society of Neuro-Oncology (EANO) consensus review on current management and future directions, *Neuro-Oncology.* **22**(8), 1073–1113 (2020).

[7] R. Stupp, W. P. Mason, M. J. van den Bent, M. Weller, B. Fisher, M. J. B. Taphoorn, *et al.,* Radiotherapy plus concomitant and adjuvant temozolomide for glioblastoma, *New England Journal of Medicine.* **352**(10), 987–996 (2005).

[8] I. M. Germano, M. Ziu, P. Wen, D. R. Ormond, and J. J. Olson, Congress of neurological surgeons systematic review and evidence-based guidelines update on the role of cytotoxic chemotherapy and other cytotoxic therapies in the management of progressive glioblastoma in adults, *Journal of Neuro-Oncology.* **158**(2), 225–253 (2022).

[9] O. Rominiyi, A. Vanderlinden, S. J. Clenton, C. Bridgewater, Y. Al-Tamimi, and S. J. Collis, Tumour treating fields therapy for glioblastoma: current advances and future directions, *British Journal of Cancer.* **124**(4), 697–709 (2021).

[10] T. J. Brown, M. C. Brennan, M. Li, E. W. Church, N. J. Brandmeir, K. L. Rakszawski, *et al.,* Association of the extent of resection with survival in glioblastoma, *JAMA Oncology.* **2**(11), 1460 (2016).

[11] F. Ringel, H. Pape, M. Sabel, D. Krex, H. C. Bock, M. Misch, *et al.,* Clinical benefit from resection of recurrent glioblastomas: results of a multicenter study including 503 patients with recurrent glioblastomas undergoing surgical resection, *Neuro-Oncology.* **18**(1), 96–104 (2016).

[12] B. Suchorska, M. Weller, G. Tabatabai, C. Senft, P. Hau, M. C. Sabel, *et al.*, Complete resection of contrast-enhancing tumor volume is associated with improved survival in recurrent glioblastoma—results from the DIRECTOR trial, *Neuro-Oncology.* **18**(4), 549–556 (2016).

[13] F. W. Kreth, N. Thon, M. Simon, M. Westphal, G. Schackert, G. Nikkhah, *et al.*, Gross total but not incomplete resection of glioblastoma prolongs survival in the era of radiochemotherapy, *Annals of Oncology.* **24**(12), 3117–3123 (2013).

[14] R. Daneman and A. Prat, The blood–brain barrier, *Cold Spring Harbor Perspectives in Biology.* **7**(1), 1–18 (2015).

[15] N. Bergmann, C. Delbridge, J. Gempt, A. Feuchtinger, A. Walch, L. Schirmer, *et al.*, The intratumoral heterogeneity reflects the intertumoral subtypes of glioblastoma multiforme: A regional immunohistochemistry analysis, *Frontiers in Oncology.* **10**, 1–10 (2020).

[16] A. Sottoriva, I. Spiteri, S. G. M. Piccirillo, A. Touloumis, V. P. Collins, J. C. Marioni, *et al.*, Intratumor heterogeneity in human glioblastoma reflects cancer evolutionary dynamics, *Proceedings of the National Academy of Sciences.* **110**(10), 4009–4014 (2013).

[17] D. N. Louis, A. Perry, P. Wesseling, D. J. Brat, I. A. Cree, D. Figarella-Branger, *et al.*, The 2021 WHO classification of tumors of the central nervous system: A summary, *Neuro-Oncology.* **23**(8), 1231–1251 (2021).

[18] S. Jiang, G. J. Zanazzi, and S. Hassanpour, Predicting prognosis and IDH mutation status for patients with lower-grade gliomas using whole slide images, *Scientific Reports.* **11**(1), 16849 (2021).

[19] B. Kaminska, B. Czapski, R. Guzik, S. Król, and B. Gielniewski, Consequences of IDH1/2 mutations in gliomas and an assessment of inhibitors targeting mutated IDH proteins, *Molecules.* **24**(5), 968 (2019).

[20] S. Agnihotri and G. Zadeh, Metabolic reprogramming in glioblastoma: The influence of cancer metabolism on epigenetics and unanswered questions, *Neuro-Oncology.* **18**(2), 160–172 (2016).

[21] J. Yao, A. Hagiwara, C. Raymond, S. Shabani, W. B. Pope, N. Salamon, *et al.*, Human IDH mutant 1p/19q co-deleted gliomas have low tumor acidity as evidenced by molecular MRI and PET: A retrospective study, *Scientific Reports.* **10**(1), 11922 (2020).

[22] H. G. Vuong, T. Q. Nguyen, T. N. M. Ngo, H. C. Nguyen, K. M. Fung, and I. F. Dunn, The interaction between TERT promoter mutation and MGMT promoter methylation on overall survival of glioma patients: A meta-analysis, *BMC Cancer.* **20**(1), 897 (2020).

[23] D. Hanahan and R. A. Weinberg, The hallmarks of cancer, *Cell.* **100**(1), 57–70 (2000).

[24] D. Hanahan and R. A. Weinberg, Hallmarks of cancer: The next generation, *Cell.* **144**(5), 646–674 (2011).

[25] K. J. Hatanpaa, S. Burma, D. Zhao, and A. A. Habib, Epidermal growth factor receptor in glioma: Signal transduction, neuropathology, imaging, and radioresistance, *Neoplasia.* **12**(9), 675–684 (2010).

[26] S. Stein, R. Zhao, H. Haeno, I. Vivanco, and F. Michor, Mathematical modeling identifies optimum lapatinib dosing schedules for the treatment of glioblastoma patients, *PLOS Computational Biology.* **14**(1), e1005924 (2018).

[27] J. A. Benitez, J. Ma, M. D'Antonio, A. Boyer, M. F. Camargo, C. Zanca, *et al.*, PTEN regulates glioblastoma oncogenesis through chromatin-associated complexes of DAXX and histone H3.3, *Nature Communications.* **8**(1), 15223 (2017).

[28] H. Yang, F. Han, R. Hu, J. Liu, J. Sui, X. Xiang, *et al.*, PTEN gene mutations correlate to poor prognosis in glioma patients: A meta-analysis, *OncoTargets and Therapy.* **9**, 3485–3492 (2016).

[29] M. P. Khoury and J. C. Bourdon, P53 isoforms: An intracellular microprocessor? *Genes and Cancer.* **2**, 453–465 (2011).

[30] Y. J. Lee, H. W. Seo, J. H. Baek, S. H. Lim, S. G. Hwang, and E. H. Kim, Gene expression profiling of glioblastoma cell lines depending on TP53 status after tumor-treating fields (TTFields) treatment, *Scientific Reports.* **10**(1), 1–11 (2020).

[31] J. Han, C. A. Alvarez-Breckenridge, Q. E. Wang, and J. Yu, TGF-β signaling and its targeting for glioma treatment, *American Journal of Cancer Research.* **5**(3), 945–955 (2015).

[32] J. V. Joseph, C. R. Magaut, S. Storevik, L. H. Geraldo, T. Mathivet, M. A. Latif, *et al.* TGF-β promotes microtube formation in glioblastoma through thrombospondin 1, *Neuro-Oncology.* **24**(4), 541–553 (2022).

[33] A. A. Brandes, A. F. Carpentier, S. Kesari, J. M. Sepulveda-Sanchez, H. R. Wheeler, O. Chinot, *et al.* A phase II randomized study of galunisertib monotherapy or galunisertib plus lomustine compared with lomustine monotherapy in patients with recurrent glioblastoma, *Neuro-Oncology.* **18**(8), 1146–1156 (2016).

[34] A. Wick, A. Desjardins, C. Suarez, P. Forsyth, I. Gueorguieva, T. Burkholder, *et al.*, Phase 1b/2a study of galunisertib, a small molecule inhibitor of transforming growth factor-beta receptor I, in combination with standard temozolomide-based radiochemotherapy in patients with newly diagnosed malignant glioma, *Investigational New Drugs.* **38**(5), 1570–1579 (2020).

[35] S. Khajanchi and J. J. Nieto. Spatiotemporal dynamics of a glioma immune interaction model, *Scientific Reports.* **11**(1), 22385 (2021).

[36] N. Zhang, L. Wei, M. Ye, C. Kang, and H. You, Treatment progress of immune checkpoint blockade therapy for glioblastoma, *Frontiers in Immunology.* **11**, 1–6 (2020).

[37] S. Haase, M. B. Garcia-Fabiani, S. Carney, D. Altshuler, F. J. Núñez, F. M. Méndez, *et al.*, Mutant ATRX: Uncovering a new therapeutic target for glioma, *Expert Opinion on Therapeutic Targets.* **22**(7), 599–613 (2018).

[38] F. S. Varn, K. C. Johnson, T. E. Wade, T. M. Malta, T. S. Sabedot, F. P. Barthel, *et al.*, Longitudinal analysis of diffuse glioma reveals cell state dynamics at recurrence associated with changes in genetics and the microenvironment (2021). bioRxiv. 2021.05.03.442486.

[39] S. Agnihotri, K. E. Burrell, A. Wolf, S. Jalali, C. Hawkins, J. T. Rutka, *et al.*, Glioblastoma, a brief review of history, molecular genetics, animal models and novel therapeutic strategies, *Archivum Immunologiae et Therapiae Experimentalis (Warsz).* **61**(1), 25–41 (2013).

[40] M. Conte, S. Casas-Tintò, and J. Soler, Modeling invasion patterns in the glioblastoma battlefield, *PLOS Computational Biology.* **17**(1), e1008632 (2021).

[41] F. Hanif, K. Muzaffar, K. Perveen, S. M. Malhi and S. U. Simjee, Glioblastoma multiforme: A review of its epidemiology and pathogenesis through clinical presentation and treatment, *Asian Pacific Journal of Cancer Prevention.* **18**(1), 3–9 (2017).

[42] K. R. Swanson, E. C. Alvord, and J. D. Murray, A quantitative model for differential motility of gliomas in grey and white matter, *Cell Proliferation.* **33**(5), 317–329 (2000).

[43] S. Jbabdi, E. Mandonnet, H. Duffau, L. Capelle, K. R. Swanson, M. Pélégrini-Issac, *et al.*, Simulation of anisotropic growth of low-grade gliomas using diffusion tensor imaging, *Magnetic Resonance in Medicine.* **54**(3), 616–624 (2005).

[44] L. R. Ranzenberger, M. J. Das, and T. Snyder, *Diffusion Tensor Imaging* (StatPearls Publishing, Treasure Island, FL, 2023).

[45] F. J. Quintana, Astrocytes to the rescue! Glia limitans astrocytic endfeet control CNS inflammation, *Journal of Clinical Investigation.* **127**(8), 2897–2899 (2017).

[46] W. Stummer, U. Pichlmeier, T. Meinel, O. D. Wiestler, F. Zanella, H. J. Reulen, *et al.*, Fluorescence-guided surgery with 5-aminolevulinic acid for resection of malignant glioma: A randomised controlled multicentre phase III trial, *The Lancet Oncology.* **7**(5), 392–401 (2006).

[47] F. Revilla-Pacheco, P. Rodríguez-Salgado, M. Barrera-Ramírez, M. P. Morales-Ruiz, M. Loyo-Varela, J. Rubalcava-Ortega, *et al.*,

Extent of resection and survival in patients with glioblastoma multiforme, *Medicine.* **100**(25), e26432 (2021).

[48] B. Campos, L. R. Olsen, T. Urup, and H. S. Poulsen, A comprehensive profile of recurrent glioblastoma, *Oncogene.* **35**(45), 5819–5825 (2016).

[49] K. Aldape, K. M. Brindle, L. Chesler, R. Chopra, A. Gajjar, M. R. Gilbert, *et al.*, Challenges to curing primary brain tumours, *Nature Reviews Clinical Oncology.* **16**(8), 509–520 (2019).

[50] M. Protopapa, A. Zygogianni, G. S. Stamatakos, C. Antypas, C. Armpilia, N. K. Uzunoglu, *et al.*, Clinical implications of in silico mathematical modeling for glioblastoma: A critical review, *Journal of Neuro-Oncology* (Springer, New York LLC). **136**(1), 1–11 (2018).

[51] T. L. Stepien, E. M. Rutter, and Y. Kuang, Traveling waves of a go-or-grow model of glioma growth, *SIAM Journal on Applied Mathematics.* **78**(3), 1778–1801 (2018).

[52] S. Suveges, K. Hossain-Ibrahim, J. D. Steele, R. Eftimie, and D. Trucu, Mathematical modelling of glioblastomas invasion within the brain: A 3d multi-scale moving-boundary approach, *Mathematics.* **9**(18), 1–16 (2021).

[53] D. D. Dionysiou, G. S. Stamatakos, N. K. Uzunoglu, K. S. Nikita, and A. Marioli, A four-dimensional simulation model of tumour response to radiotherapy in vivo: Parametric validation considering radiosensitivity, genetic profile and fractionation, *Journal of Theoretical Biology.* **230**(1), 1–20 (2004).

[54] K. Aoki, H. Suzuki, T. Yamamoto, K. N. Yamamoto, S. Maeda, Y. Okuno, *et al.*, Mathematical modeling and mutational analysis reveal optimal therapy to prevent malignant transformation in grade II IDH-mutant gliomas, *Cancer Research.* **81**(18), 4861–4873 (2021).

[55] P. Y. Wen, S. M. Chang, M. J. van den Bent, M. A. Vogelbaum, D. R. Macdonald, and E. Q. Lee, Response assessment in neuro-oncology clinical trials, *Journal of Clinical Oncology.* **35**(21), 2439–2449 (2017).

[56] R. J. Young, A. Gupta, A. D. Shah, J. J. Graber, Z. Zhang, W. Shi, *et al.*, Potential utility of conventional MRI signs in diagnosing pseudoprogression in glioblastoma, *Neurology.* **76**(22), 1918–1924 (2011).

[57] I. Law, N. L. Albert, J. Arbizu, R. Boellaard, A. Drzezga, N. Galldiks, *et al.*, Joint EANM/EANO/RANO practice guidelines/SNMMI procedure standards for imaging of gliomas using PET with radiolabelled amino acids and [18F]FDG: Version 1.0, *European Journal of Nuclear Medicine and Molecular Imaging.* **46**(3), 540–557 (2019).

[58] T. J. Brown, M. C. Brennan, M. Li, E. W. Church, N. J. Brandmeir, K. L. Rakszawski, *et al.*, Association of the extent of resection with survival in glioblastoma, *JAMA Oncology.* **2**(11), 1460 (2016).

[59] L. Zheng, Z. R. Zhou, Q. Yu, M. Shi, Y. Yang, X. Zhou, *et al.*, The definition and delineation of the target area of radiotherapy based on the recurrence pattern of glioblastoma after temozolomide chemoradiotherapy, *Frontiers in Oncology.* **10**, 1–8 (2021).

[60] E. Winograd, I. Germano, P. Wen, J. J. Olson, and D. R. Ormond, Congress of neurological surgeons systematic review and evidence-based guidelines update on the role of targeted therapies and immunotherapies in the management of progressive glioblastoma, *Journal of Neuro-Oncology.* **158**(2), 265–321 (2021).

[61] B. M. Ellingson, C. Chung, W. B. Pope, J. L. Boxerman, and T. J. Kaufmann, Pseudoprogression, radionecrosis, inflammation or true tumor progression? Challenges associated with glioblastoma response assessment in an evolving therapeutic landscape, *Journal of Neuro-Oncology* (Springer, New York LLC). **134**, 495–504 (2017).

[62] K. Swanson, R. Rostomily, and E. Alvord, A mathematical modelling tool for predicting survival of individual patients following resection of glioblastoma: a proof of principle, *British Journal of Cancer.* **98**, 113–119 (2008).

Chapter 3

Multi-Scale Aspects of Immune Responses to Solid Cancers: Mathematical and Computational Modelling Perspectives

Raluca Eftimie[*]

*Laboratoire de mathématiques de Besançon,
Université de Franche-Comté,
Besançon, France
raluca.eftimie@univ-fcomte.fr*

Immunotherapy has now become a standard therapeutic approach against cancers (in addition and complementary to surgery, chemotherapy, radiotherapy, and targeted therapies). However, due to the complex interactions between immune cells and cancer cells, until now very few such immunotherapy approaches have led to significant results. Mathematical models of immune responses to cancer have been developed over the years to shed light on some of these complex immune–cancer interactions that usually take place across multiple spatial and temporal scales. The focus of this chapter is to briefly review some of these mathematical

---

[*]The author is also an Honorary Professor at School of Science and Engineering, University of Dundee, Dundee, UK. Email address: r.a.eftimie@dundee.ac.uk.

modelling approaches while emphasising the multi-scale aspect of the models. We do not aim to offer a comprehensive discussion of all mathematical models in the literature but rather to emphasise the different classes of continuum multi-scale models developed over the past decades (and in particular over the last few years) in the context of cancer–immune interactions. The review is build step by step: (i) first we discuss some biological aspects related to cell-level immune responses to cancers and then mention current immuno-therapeutic approaches targeting various molecules, (ii) next we present general mathematical equations for deterministic continuum models for cancer–immune interactions (where the multi-scale aspect is presented explicitly or implicitly), and for each of these different classes of mathematical models, we discuss in detail one particular model published in the past five years, and (iii) finally, we conclude by discussing some open problems related to available multi-scale data and model parametrisation.

1. Introduction

The role of immune system in cancers has been recognised since the 19th century, as recorded by various anecdotal stories that reported the shrinkage of various solid malignant tumours following patient infection with different pathogens [1] (e.g., bacteria and bacterial products that became known as Coley's toxins [2]). However, the exact mechanisms though which the immune system (stimulated or not by external pathogens) recognises and destroys the cancerous cells has started to be identified only in the 20th century. Nevertheless, despite the intensive research carried out on this topic over the past century, successful anti-cancer immunotherapies (i.e., treatments that help the immune system fight cancers) are still relatively few and are mainly directed to some specific cancers (e.g., melanoma, lymphoma, and bladder cancer) [1]. Other cancers, including glioblastoma and pancreatic cancers, do not seem to respond to immunotherapies and are still very hard to treat.

The complex, heterogeneous, and time-evolving cancer microenvironment is the main reason for which immunotherapies do not work for all patients and all types of cancers [3,4]. The cancer microenvironment is composed of a variety of cancer and immune cells embedded in an extracellular matrix (ECM), which interact in complex ways that could lead to either cancer inhibition/elimination or cancer proliferation and spread [4]. These cancer–immune interactions occur

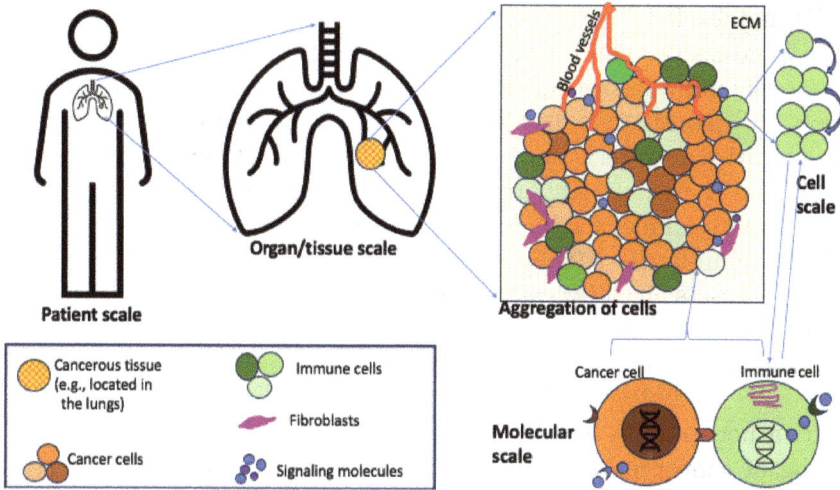

Fig. 1. Description of multi-scale aspects during cancer–immune interactions (shown a caricature depiction of a lung cancer): from molecular scale (e.g., DNA mutations inside cell nucleus and receptors on cell surface) to cell scale (e.g., cell proliferation or death), tissue scale (e.g., the interactions between the different cell types and extracellular matrix (ECM) that could lead to cell invasion into surrounding tissue), and even patient scale (e.g., different systems affected by the spread of cancerous cells).

across multiple scales: microscale (molecular/genetic scale; e.g., signalling pathways cells and cell receptors), mesoscale (cellular scale; e.g., cell proliferation and death), and macroscale (tissue/organ scale; e.g., cell invasion into new tissue and biomechanical forces); see also Fig. 1. Thus, understanding the cancer–immune dynamics (to improve current immunotherapies) requires understanding the dynamics at every single scale, as well as understanding how the dynamics at one scale influences the dynamics at a different scale (i.e., understanding the connections between the different scales).

In an attempt to shed light on the multi-scale interactions between cancer cells and the anti-cancer/pro-cancer immune responses, numerous mathematical models have been derived over the past years; see the reviews in [5–11] and the references therein. We note that all these reviews of mathematical models for immune–cancer interactions that have been published over the past years each focus on specific aspects: from the temporal dynamics (described by ordinary differential equations (ODEs)) of tumour and immune cells [5] to

ODE models for cancer immunotherapies (including pharmacokinetic and pharmacodynamic models) [8], models that focus on immune responses for various diseases (including cancer, but not restricted to it) [6], continuum models that focus on single cells, multi-cells and multi-scale interactions between cells [9], multi-scale agent-based and hybrid models [11], models focussed on temporal vs. spatio-temporal dynamics for the interactions between cancer cells and specific immune cells [10], or even a summary of different databases with datasets at different scales (molecular, cellular, and tissular levels) [7].

The goal of this brief review is not to recapitulate the published reviews (most of which focussing anyway on single-scale modelling) but rather to focus on the multi-scale (across space and time) modelling of cancer–immune interactions that took place over the past 20–30 years (when the various multi-scale aspects of tumour–immune interactions started to be revealed experimentally), which gave rise to new open problems related to model parametrisation across scales. To achieve this, we structured the review as follows. In Section 2, we review briefly some multi-scale aspects in cancer immunology and immunotherapies for cancer, in Section 3, we review briefly the current mathematical modelling approaches aimed at addressing various multi-scale biological questions, while in Section 4, we discuss some current open problems related to modelling available data and models parametrisation. We conclude in Section 5 with a brief summary and future perspectives on the evolution of this field.

2. Brief Review of Multi-Scale Aspects in Cancer Immunology

Throughout the rest of this chapter we interchangeably use the words cancer and tumour, with the specification that by "tumours" we refer exclusively to solid malignant tumours. In the following, we briefly review the pro-tumour and anti-tumour roles of various immune cell populations found in the tumour microenvironment, with the aim to emphasise the multi-scale processes involved in these tumour–immune interactions.

2.1. The immune composition of the tumour microenvironment

The tumour microenvironment (TME) is the environment that forms and surrounds the solid tumour; it includes not only tumour cells but also immune cells, stromal cells (including fibroblasts), blood vessels, and extracellular matrix (ECM) [12, 13]. The components of the TME interact continuously via cytokines, chemokines, growth factors, and matrix remodelling enzymes to support tumour progression and escape of anti-tumour therapies. Since tumour progression can, in principle, be controlled by immune cells that infiltrate the tumour [14], in the following we summarise the main innate and adaptive immune cells that can be found in the TME. We note that different types of solid tumours are formed of different types of immune cells, in different percentages [15]. Thus understanding the interactions between immune cells and tumour cells in one TME might not always be informative for a different TME; instead, we need to understand the basic principles of these multi-scale interactions that are valid for all TMEs. To this end, in the following we focus on a few immune cell populations that have been found in high numbers in different solid tumour tissues: T cells (both cytotoxic $CD8^+$ T cells and helper $CD4^+$ T cells), B cells, Natural Killer (NK) cells, and macrophages. The following discussion provides (i) a few general information about each of these cell types and (ii) some numbers quantifying these cell distributions inside various solid tumours (to emphasise the heterogeneity of these cell infiltrates into different TME).

Note that we emphasise the different percentages of these immune cells inside various tumours since over the years such immune cells (and cell percentages) have been used as prognostic biomarkers for tumour evolution. In particular, a digital pathology-based assay called *Immunoscore* was developed over the last two decades [16, 17] to improve the prognostic performance of cancer classification by considering also the immune infiltrates inside tumours. The *Immunoscore* uses the densities of different T cell subsets (CD3 & CD8; or CD3 & CD45RO; or CD8 & CD45RO) inside the tumour and at the invasive margin, not only to classify colorectal cancers but also as a prognostic and predictive value for colon cancer patients.

(Note here that CD3 is an antigen present on the surface of all T lymphocytes, CD8 is an antigen present on the surface of cytotoxic T cells, and CD45RO is an antigen expressed by memory $CD4^+$ T cells.) This *Immunoscore* has received international validation for the classification of colon cancer [18]. While the *Immunoscore* concept could apply to all solid cancers, eventually by including other immune cells specific to other cancers [19], it still needs to receive official validation for these other cancers:

- **T cells** are one of the main immune cell population (part of the adaptive immune response) involved in the fight against tumours. The two main classes of T cells are the $CD4^+$ T cells (which secrete cytokines and chemokines that regulate different anti-tumour immune responses, but can also kill tumours directly) and the $CD8^+$ T cells (which have direct potent cytotoxic effects against tumour cells). Their infiltration within a solid tumour has been usually associated with improved survival prognosis [20] (although the presence of a sub-population of $CD4^+$ T cells, the Treg cells that maintain tolerance within the immune system, is associated with poor prognosis). Despite this, the unpredictability of tumour evolution is also caused by the fact that TMEs are infiltrated not only by the tumour-specific T cells but also by large numbers of bystander non-tumour specific T cells that cannot recognise cancer cells in a T cell receptor (TCR)-dependent manner [21]. The heterogeneity of the phenotypes of T cell populations infiltrating TMEs has an impact on immunotherapies for cancers, as is discussed in Section 2.2.

  Examples of percentages of infiltrates: Various tumour types are characterised by different percentages of T cell infiltrates. For example, T cells can represent approximately 16% of the mass of Diffuse Large B-Cell Lymphoma (DBLCL)(with 6.1% $CD8^+$ T cells and 5.4% $CD4^+$ T cells) [22] or more than 54% of the mass of Head and Neck Squamous Cell Carcinoma (HNSCC) (with 52.72% formed of $CD8^+$ T cells and 2.35% $CD4^+$ T cells) [23]. In Non-Small Cell Lung Cancers (NSCLC), the T cells represent 47% of all immune infiltrates into the tumour (of which 26% are $CD4^+$ T cells and 22% represent $CD8^+$ T cells) [24].

- **B cells** are responsible for the humoral immunity component of the adaptive immune response. These cells recognise circulating tumour antigens and respond by secreting antibodies and cytokines. They also present antigens to T cells (the CD4$^+$ T cells). Various studies have shown that B cells are the main partners of T cells in anti-tumour immunity [25], and B cell and T cell aggregations inside the TME are positively associated with better tumour prognosis. However, there are also studies that suggest that B cell infiltration is associated with a worse prognosis [25] (due in part to the presence of regulatory B cells, Breg).

Examples of percentages of infiltrates: The B cells are the second most-common type of immune cell infiltrated into NSCLC (representing 16% of all infiltrates) [24]. These cells can also account for approximately 17.26% of all lymphocytes infiltrating melanomas, 23.05% of lymphocytes infiltrating breast tumours, and 31.76% of lymphocytes infiltrating brain tumours [15].

- **Natural Killer (NK) cells:** These cells belong to the same family of lymphocytes as T and B cells, but they are actually part of the innate immune system. The NK cells have critical roles in the early detection and killing of cancer cells, without any activation against cancer antigens (in contrast to the T cells discussed earlier). Their presence in the peripheral blood has been positively associated with better prognosis in various tumours: from melanomas to breast cancers, colorectal cancers, etc. [26].

  Examples of percentages of infiltrates: NK cells seem to be found in high percentages in brain tumours (where they formed 14.23–50.45% of all infiltrating lymphocytes); they are found in lower percentages in tumours such as melanomas (0.3–7.35%, with and average of 3.14%) or breast cancers (0–10.44%, with an average of 5.84%) [15].

- **Macrophages** are one of the main cell populations in the TME, with a significant role in modulating the environment to prevent or promote tumour growth. These innate immune cells form a very heterogeneous and plastic cell population, with the two extreme phenotypes being represented by (i) the anti-tumour and pro-inflammatory M1 cells and (ii) the pro-tumour and anti-inflammatory M2 cells. During tumour progression, the tumour-associated macrophages (TAMs) are switching their phenotype from an M1-dominated phenotype during early tumour stages to an M2-dominated phenotype during late tumour stages, in response to changes in the tumour microenvironment (i.e., changes in the concentration of various cytokines and growth factors, inflammation, and hypoxia) [27]. However, one can have also the reversed switch: appropriate cytokines (e.g., interleukin-12 (IL-12), interferon gamma (IFN-γ), and tumour necrosis factor (TNF)) could induce a change from an M2 phenotype towards an M1 phenotype [27]. Finally, we emphasise that the heterogeneity of the macrophage population is given not only by these M1 and M2 cells but also by cells with a whole range of mixed M1/M2 phenotypes, which can have an impact on the aggressiveness of cancer [28].

Examples of percentages of infiltrates: These cells can represent up to 30–50% of the tumour mass for glioblastoma [29] or between 20–40% of hepatocellular carcinoma [30]. Nevertheless, other studies showed that monocytes represent only 3.5% of leukocytes infiltrating brain tumours [15], 85% of leukocytes infiltrating breast tumours [15], and 11.06% of leukocytes infiltrating melanomas [15]. In NSCLC, macrophages represent only 4.5% of all immune cell infiltrates [24].

Despite the high anti-tumour potential of any of the immune cells mentioned earlier, clinical results have shown that in all clinical situations, tumours have evaded this immune control. Therefore, to understand and eliminate these tumour evasion mechanisms, one needs to understand the cell-level interactions between these immune cells and tumour cells, which are controlled by various molecular-level aspects [31] (see also Fig. 1): from loss of tumour antigen expression and reduced antigen recognition by immune cells to expression of checkpoint inhibitors on immune cell membranes (e.g., PD-1 and CTLA4) and over-production of tumour-promoting cytokines and growth factors (e.g., IL-10, VEGF, and TGF-β). These molecular aspects are currently targeted by different immuno-therapeutic approaches, which are discussed in the following sub-section.

2.2. *Immunotherapies for cancer: Multi-scale aspects*

The immune cells mentioned earlier (which can identify various tumour antigens) are the targets for new potential immunotherapies, some more advanced than others [32]. However, the multi-scale aspect of tumour–immune interactions (via cytokines and growth factors secreted by various cells or via receptors on cell surfaces;

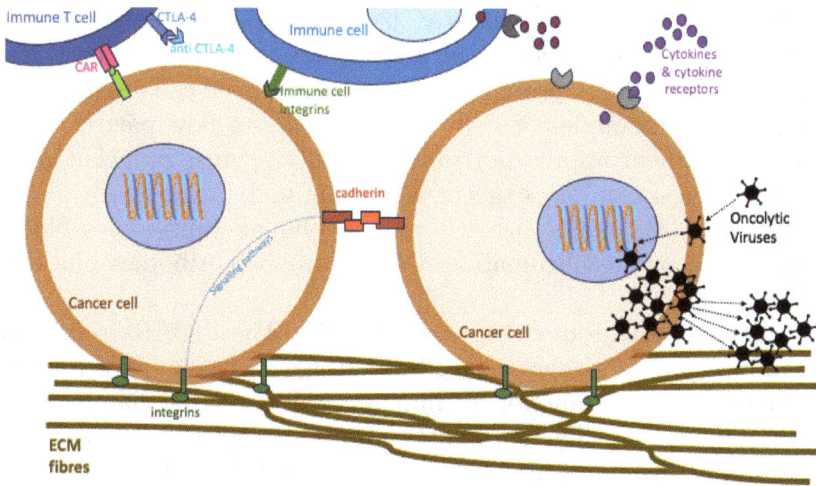

Fig. 2. Description of some of the molecular-level aspects involved in cell dynamics. (i) Cell–cell and cell–ECM interactions via cell surface adhesion molecules (such as cadherins or integrins). Cells can interact with each other also via cytokines (secreted by the cells themselves or by other cells in the environment). (ii) The main anti-cancer immunotherapies involve cytokines, immune checkpoint inhibitors (e.g., anti CTLA-4), cell receptors (CARs), or oncolytic viruses (OVs).

see Fig. 2), which is currently not fully understood, is one of the main factors impacting the success of cancer immunotherapies.

In the following, we summarise some of the current immunotherapies for human cancers by focussing on the molecular aspects targeted by these therapies (see also Fig. 2). However, we note that some of these molecular-level therapies are part of other cell-based therapies (e.g., the chimeric antigen receptor therapy discussed in the following is part of the adoptive transfer-based therapy that involves the *ex vivo* expansion of immune cells that recognise tumour antigens, followed by their reinjection into patients) [31]:

- **Immune checkpoint inhibitors:** The checkpoint proteins on immune cells act as switches for the immune responses to ensure that normal cells are not attacked. However, these proteins can be used by the cancer cells to ensure that they are not attacked. The immune checkpoint inhibitors are drugs (based on monoclonal antibodies) that work by blocking checkpoint proteins, thus allowing immune cells to identify and target the cancer cells [3].

The main checkpoints targeted in anti-cancer therapies are the cytotoxic T lymphocyte-associated protein 4 (CTLA-4) and programmed cell death protein 1 (PD1)/programmed cell death ligand 1 (PDL1). Examples of such drugs, which are now part of standard treatment approaches to many cancers, such as melanomas, breast cancers, or lung cancers, are ipilimumab (an antibody blocking CTLA-4), pembrolizumab and nivolumab (antibodies blocking PD1), or atezolizumab and durvalumab (antibodies blocking PDL1) [33].

- **Chimeric antigen receptors (CAR):** These CARs represent a new class of drugs that allow antigen binding to cells and can redirect the function of immune cells towards that particular antigen [34]. These receptors target naive cell surface antigens that do not require peptide processing or recognition of HLA expression (which are common mechanisms for immune escape). Various tumours (with various antigens) have been the subject of this immunotherapy approach: from colorectal cancers to glioblastomas, ovarian cancers, breast cancers, B cell malignancies, etc. [34]. Until now, mainly the T cells have been targeted with CAR (CAR-T cells). However, more recently, other immune cells have started to be targeted with CAR: NK cells (CAR-NK cells) [35] and macrophages (CAR-macrophage) [36]. These new approaches have their own positive and negative aspects. For example, the CAR-NK therapy seems to cause fewer side effects compared to CAR T-cell therapy, which can lead to neurotoxicity or to the cytokine release syndrome [35], but as a downside, this CAR-NK therapy lacks *in vivo* persistence [31]. Also the CAR-macrophage therapy has different limitations caused, for example, by (i) lack of expansion properties of macrophages and (ii) the plasticity of tumour-associated macrophages that adapt their phenotype in response to the environmental stimuli (as discussed earlier).

- **Cytokine modulation:** Cytokines are proteins secreted by cells, which act as signals to coordinate cell growth, cell functions, and overall cell–cell communication (over short and medium spatial ranges). Over the past four decades, there has been significant interest in using cytokines to enhance the anti-tumour immune responses [37]. The two cytokines that have been FDA-approved so far are the interleukin-2 (IL-2) (against melanoma and renal cell carcinoma) and interferon-α (IFN-α) (against melanoma, follicular lymphoma, and Kaposi's sarcoma) [3]. More recent studies have suggested the use of pro-inflammatory cytokines such as interleukin-12 (IL-12) to reprogram the tumour-associated macrophages (TAMs) with a pro-tumour M2-like phenotype towards an anti-tumour M1-like phenotype [38]. There are various factors that limit the efficacy of cytokines as immunotherapy agents: from the lack of specificity of cytokine action (e.g., IL-2 can promote the cytotoxic activity of NK cells and CD8$^+$ T cells and also promote the maintenance of CD4$^+$ Treg subpopulation [39] and the induction of immunological checkpoints CTLA-4 and PD1/PDL1 [37, 39]) to the cytokine toxicity at high doses required for effective intra-tumoural concentrations [37].

- **Oncolytic viruses (OVs):** These are natural viruses or engineered viruses that selectively replicate inside cancer cells and destroy them, while leaving non-cancerous cells intact [3]. OVs can also act as cancer vaccines that induce immunogenic cell death, followed by the release of tumour-associated antigens and the activation of anti-tumour specific immune responses [40]. The best known example of such an OV-based anti-tumour drug is the Talimogene laherparepvec (T-VEC). This widely used drug, based on a modified herpes simplex virus, is FDA-approved for the treatment of melanoma. A few other oncolytic viruses are approved in different countries for the treatment of bladder cancer (the adenovirus-based Nadofaragene firadenovec drug) or for the treatment of glioblastoma (the herpex simplex virus-based Teserpaturev drug) [40]. OVs offer huge promises for future anticancer therapies since (i) they can be engineered to kill tumour cells directly and (ii) modulate the anti-tumour immune responses. However, there are still many challenges in developing efficient oncolytic viruses: these range from ensuring a balance between anti-viral immunity (that usually eliminates the OV on a short time scale) and anti-tumour immunity mediated by OVs (that requires a longer time to develop), to restrictions on the use of mouse models for OVs designed to be active in humans (as mouse cells could be resistant to viruses), to challenges with the use of human endemic viruses to which patients might have pre-existent immunity that prevents viral replication or even regulatory (i.e., drug approval) challenges [40].

We note that some of these immunotherapies are combined with classical therapies, such as chemotherapy or radiotherapy, with the goal of enhancing tumour immunogenicity [3]. Moreover, some of these therapies can be used in combinations (concurrently or sequentially): e.g., by combining different checkpoint inhibitors, combining checkpoint inhibitors with oncolytic viruses, and combining checkpoint inhibitors with chemotherapy or radiotherapy [31]. Such combination therapies are most efficient when the mechanisms through which different therapies eliminate tumour cells are different so that multiple pathways are targeted at the same time.

In the following, we review briefly some classes of mathematical models that take into consideration these different multi-scale interactions between immune cells and tumour cells inside the TME to propose hypotheses related to the mechanisms behind the temporal and spatio-temporal dynamics observed experimentally/clinically and hypotheses that could explain tumour escape or control by immune cells (in the presence/absence of different therapies). Due to the large amount of literature on this topic, the focus of this review is on mathematical models that describe the interactions between tumour cells and some of the immune cells mentioned earlier.

3. Brief Review of Multi-Scale Mathematical Models

Before reviewing various multi-scale models developed over the past decades, we need to mention what is understood by *multi-scale models* since there are different approaches in the field. All these different modelling approaches try connect the dynamics of the components of the tumour microenvironment across different scales (molecular scale–cell scale; cell scale–tissue scale; or molecular–cell–tissue scales; see also Fig. 1) while considering either implicitly or explicitly the different spatial and temporal scales:

- **Implicit multi-scale models** are usually described by deterministic equations (ordinary differential equations (ODEs) or partial differential equations) for the changes in the densities of cells (i.e., cancer cells and immune cells) and changes in the concentrations of molecules (e.g, cytokines and receptors on cell surface) secreted by the cells. For these models, the only suggestion that the authors investigate multi-scale dynamics inside the TME is the different orders of magnitudes for the parameters modelling the kinetics of cells (at cell scale) and parameters modelling the kinetics of molecules (at molecular scale). For example, at cell scale, the 144 days that represent the mean doubling time of melanoma cells [41] translates into a cell proliferation rate of $\ln(2.0)/(144\,\text{day}) = 0.0048/\text{day}$. In contrast, at molecular scale, the average receptor-ligand dissociation rate is $2.92 \times 10^{-5}/\text{s}$ at $0°C$ and 0.014 at $25°C$ [42] which translates into a rate $2.5228/\text{day}$ at $0°C$ or $1209.6/\text{day}$ at $25°C$. Hence, models that consider cell proliferation and cell–cell interactions through receptor–ligand binding also consider a difference of at least two orders of time magnitudes between the values of parameters describing cell kinetics and those describing receptor kinetics. Similarly, the movement of receptors on cell surface (molecular-level dynamics) occurs over spatial domains at least one order of magnitude smaller than the movement of cells inside tissue (cell-level and tissue-level dynamics).

- **Explicit multi-scale models** incorporate specific molecular-level variables into (i) equations for the cell-level variables (that assures a two-way feedback between scales) or even into (ii) cell-level variables themselves. These molecular-level variables can be continuous (e.g., macrophages are characterised by a phenotype sub-variable that varies continuously between the M1 and M2 extremes) or discrete (e.g., one can focus only on macrophages with M1 phenotype and macrophages with M2 phenotype). Note that when the cell-level variables depend on molecular-level variables, we refer to these models as kinetic models or structured-population models (where the cell-level variable is structured by a molecular state described by the molecular-level variable). When the molecular-level variables are discrete, the models usually reduce to implicit ODE models, where the different model compartments are characterised by different discrete-variable states (see also Remark 2). The molecular-level variables are usually described by explicit space/time scales much smaller than the space/time scales of cell-level variables.

In the following, we summarise the main classes of mathematical models that investigate multi-scale dynamics inside the tumour microenvironment. We focus only on the continuum models (for temporal/spatio-temporal changes in the densities of cells and molecules) and ignore the discrete models (that focus on the dynamics of individual cells) or hybrid models (that connect the dynamics of individual cells with the dynamics of densities of molecules distributed over the spatial domains or the density of the extracellular matrix in the environment, all of which influence individual cell dynamics). Note that there are other studies in the literature that cover multi-scale discrete and hybrid models of cancer [9, 43]. In the following, we present the general equations for these different classes of continuum models. For each class of models, we start by referencing various studies that developed such models but discuss in more detail one specific example published in the last 5 years that incorporates (implicitly or explicitly) some of the immunotherapies mentioned in the previous section.

Ordinary differential equation (ODE) models: The multiscale models described by ODEs are usually of implicit type and focus on the time evolution of different variables at molecular scale or cellular scale. In this case, the different spatial scales are ignored, while the different time scales are considered implicitly through the different magnitudes of the parameters. The general equations for these models (corresponding to a system containing n cellular/molecular species) are as follows:

$$\frac{d\mathbf{u}}{dt} = \mathbf{f}(\mathbf{u}, t), \quad \text{with} \quad \mathbf{u} = (u_1, \ldots u_i, \ldots, u_n), \quad n > 0, \quad (1)$$

where $u_i(t)$ describes the density of the ith species considered in the biological system, at time t. Moreover, $\mathbf{f} = (f_1, \ldots, f_i, \ldots, f_n)$ is a (nonlinear) function describing the interactions between the various species considered in the system, which lead to growth/decay of the various species. There is a huge mathematical literature of ODE models for different interactions between cells and molecules in the context of cancer evolution [5, 6, 44–49]. In the following, we discuss in more detail an implicit model derived by Yu and Jang [48] that focussed on the cell-level dynamics of CD4$^+$ T cells and tumour cells and the molecular-level dynamics of CTLA-4 proteins expressed on the surface of CD4$^+$ T cells.

Example. Since in Section 2.2 we discussed immunotherapies focussed on immune checkpoint inhibitors, now we present in more detail a 4-equations ODE model for the dynamics of a generic tumour cell population and a population of CD4$^+$ T cells, as mediated by the concentration of a major cytokine, the IFNγ, and the density of CTLA-4 proteins expressed on the surface of CD4$^+$ T cells that inhibits the function of these T cells. Using the mathematical notation in equation (1), we can represent these variables as $u_1(t)$ (tumour cells), $u_2(t)$ (CD4$^+$ T cells), $u_3(t)$ (IFNγ cytokine), and $u_4(t)$ (CTLA-4 protein). The nonlinear functions that describe the interactions between these variables are as follows:

$$f_1(u_1, u_2, u_3, u_4) = ru_1\left(1 - \frac{u_1}{K}\right) - \frac{\delta u_1 u_3}{m + u_1}, \tag{2a}$$

$$f_2(u_1, u_2, u_3, u_4) = \frac{\beta u_1 u_3}{(u_1 + \eta)(1 + \nu u_4)} - au_2 + I_2(t), \tag{2b}$$

$$f_3(u_1, u_2, u_3, u_4) = \frac{\alpha u_1 u_2}{1 + bu_4} - \mu u_3 + I_3(t), \tag{2c}$$

$$f_4(u_1, u_2, u_3, u_4) = cu_2 - du_4. \tag{2d}$$

The above functions describe the following: (I) the logistic growth of tumour cells (at rate r up to carrying capacity K), the direct tumour killing by IFNγ (at rate δ, but in a saturated manner with half-saturation constant m); (II) the activation of immune cells by tumour cells and IFNγ and their subsequent proliferation (at a rate β), the inhibition of immune cells activation/proliferation by CTL4-A protein (with inhibition coefficient ν), the apoptosis of immune cells (at a rate a); (III) the secretion of IFNγ by immune cells in the presence of tumour cells (at a rate α), the inhibition of IFNγ production by CTLA-4 expression (with inhibition coefficient b), the degradation of IFNγ (at a rate μ); (IV) the expression of CTLA-4 by the immune cells (at a rate c) and the degradation of these proteins at a rate d. The I_2 term describes a time-dependent influx of activated T cells into the system, while the $I_3(t)$ term describes a time-dependent influx of IFNγ into the system, as a result of different immunotherapy approaches.

The authors then parametrise the model using some values taken from the literature and perform a global sensitivity analysis (using Partial Rank Correlation Coefficients (PRCC) with Latin Hypercube Sampling (LHS)) to investigate the impact of parameters on model outcomes. They also perform various numerical simulations to show model dynamics as the I_2 and I_3 immunotherapies are varied. While the authors state that they validated their model using some experimental data for the cytotoxic effect of CD4$^+$ T cells on murine melanoma [50], the validation method is unclear. The authors seem to have randomly adjusted model parameters based on some experimental knowledge, without actually fitting their model to the data to identify the parameters.

Partial differential equation (PDE) models: The multi-scale models for tumour–immune interactions described by PDEs usually include implicit time/space multi-scale dynamics [51]. The general equations for these models (corresponding to a system containing n cellular/molecular species) are as follows:

$$\frac{\partial \mathbf{u}(t, \mathbf{x})}{\partial t} = \nabla \cdot (D(\mathbf{u})\nabla \mathbf{u} - A(\mathbf{u})\mathbf{u}) + \mathbf{f}(\mathbf{u}), \quad \text{with}$$

$$\mathbf{u} = (u_1, \ldots, u_i, \ldots, u_n), \quad n > 0. \tag{3}$$

Again, we denote by $u_i(t, \mathbf{x})$, $i = 1, \ldots, n$, the density of the ith species considered in the biological system, at time t and space point $\mathbf{x} = (x, y)$ in a 2D space domain (or $\mathbf{x} = x$ in 1D). Moreover, $D(\mathbf{u})$ is a diffusion coefficient (for chemicals/molecules) or a random-walk coefficient (for cells). It can be constant or depend on the density of some/all species considered in the system. The term $A(\mathbf{u})$ describes the velocity of the transport (directed movement) of species $\mathbf{u}$ through space. Again, it can be a constant, or it can depend locally/non-locally on the densities of these species $\mathbf{u}$. Finally, the function $\mathbf{f} = (f_1, \ldots, f_i, \ldots, f_n)$ describes the growth/decay of theses species as a result of different interactions between these species. In the following, we focus on a particular PDE model [51] describing the implicit multi-scale interactions between glioma cells, macrophages, cytotoxic T cells, and two cytokines (TGFβ and IFNγ) secreted by the cells.

Example. In Khajanchi and Nieto [51] the authors introduced a 5-equations PDE model for the spatio-temporal dynamics of glioma cells, M1 macrophages and CD8$^+$ T cells, in response to two cytokines: TGFβ and IFNγ. (Again, this model captures implicitly the cell-scale/molecular-scale interactions in the TME.) Using the notation in equation (3), the model by Khajanchi and

Nieto [51] focussed on the following five variables: $u_1(t; x, y)$ (glioma cells), $u_2(t; x, y)$ (macrophages), $u_3(t; x, y)$ (cytotoxic CD8$^+$ T cells), $u_4(t; x, y)$ (TGFβ cytokine), and $u_5(t; x, y)$ (IFNγ cytokine). It was assumed that cells exhibit random movement and cytokines can diffuse [51], and thus the vector with the diffusion coefficients is $D(\mathbf{u}) = (D_G, D_M, D_C, D_T, D_I)$. Moreover, it was assumed that cells/cytokines do not display any directed movement, and thus $A(\mathbf{u}) = 0$ in equation (3). Finally, the reaction term $\mathbf{f} = (f_1, f_2, f_3, f_4, f_5)$ in equation (3) is given by the following components [51]:

$$f_1(u_1, u_2, u_3, u_4, u_5) = r_1 u_1 \left(1 - \frac{u_1}{u_{G\,\text{max}}} \right) - \frac{(\alpha_1 u_2 + \alpha_2 u_3)u_1}{(e_1 + u_4)(u_1 + k_1)},$$
$$\tag{4a}$$

$$f_2(u_1, u_2, u_3, u_4, u_5) = r_2 u_2 \left(1 - \frac{u_2}{u_{M\,\text{max}}} \right) + a_1 \left(\frac{u_5}{k_4 + u_5} \right)$$
$$\times \left(\frac{1}{u_4 + e_2} \right) - \alpha_3 \frac{u_1 u_2}{k_2 + u_1}, \tag{4b}$$

$$f_3(u_1, u_2, u_3, u_4, u_5) = \frac{a_2 u_1}{k_5 + u_4} - \mu_1 u_3 - \alpha_4 \frac{u_1}{k_3 + u_1} u_3, \tag{4c}$$

$$f_4(u_1, u_2, u_3, u_4, u_5) = s_1 + b_1 u_1 - \mu_2 u_4, \tag{4d}$$

$$f_5(u_1, u_2, u_3, u_4, u_5) = b_2 u_3 - \mu_3 u_5. \tag{4e}$$

The earlier reaction terms incorporate the following assumptions: (I) tumour cells grow logistically (at rate r_1, up to a carrying capacity $u_{G\,\text{max}}$) and are eliminated (in a saturated manner with the half-saturation constant k_1) by macrophages (at rate α_1) and T cells (at rate α_2), and this tumour elimination is impeded by the action of TGFβ (with coefficient e_1); (II) macrophages grow logistically (at rate r_2, up to carrying capacity $u_{M\,\text{max}}$), are activated by IFNg (at rate a_1) and down-regulated by TGFβ (with coefficient e_2), and are inactivated (at rate α_3) by the presence of tumour cells; (III) the cytotoxic T cells are recruited into glioma (with antigenicity rate a_2) and this recruitment is inhibited by TGFβ (with coefficient k_5), cells die at a rate μ_1 and are inactivated (at a rate k_4) by the presence of glioma cells; (IV) TGFβ is produced at constant source rate s_1 by cells in the environment and also at a rate b_1 by the glioma cells and

decay at a rate μ_2; (V) IFNγ is produced at a rate b_2 by the T cells
and decays at a rate μ_3.

This model has been parametrised with values taken from the
published literature, and a global sensitivity analysis (using again the
PRCC-LHS approach) has been performed for the temporal dynamics of the model (i.e., the spatial component was ignored for this
sensitivity analysis). Numerical simulations were then performed to
investigate the spatio-temporal dynamics of the model in 1D and
2D spatial domains. The simulations showed spherical densities of
tumour cells, macrophages and T cells that spread faster/slower
through the domain, depending on the parameter values.

Mixed ODE-PDE models: Many mathematical models for
cancer–immune interactions do combine PDEs and ODEs to describe
the dynamics of the tumour microenvironment, as not all variables
vary with respect to both time and space [52–58]. For example, the
tissue-level dynamics of the extracellular matrix (ECM) is usually
assumed to vary only with respect to time due to local degradation and remodelling by molecules secreted by various cells [59,60].
Similarly, some molecules on cell surfaces (e.g., integrin receptors)
are usually assumed to vary only with respect to time [60]. Again,
many of these mixed ODE/PDE models consider implicit multi-scale
interactions [54–56], but some are actually explicit multi-scale models [52, 53, 57, 58] (since they take into consideration ECM dynamics at tissue level, cell dynamics at cell level, and the dynamics
of molecules secreted by cells at cell/sub-cell level modelled with
the help of microdomains inside the tissue). However, these explicit
multi-scale models are usually extremely complex. For this reason,
in the following example, we briefly mention one such model without
actually showing the model equations, which would take too much
space to describe them here (and thus would defy the purpose of this
brief review).

Example. A multi-scale moving boundary framework initially introduced in Trucu *et al.* [61] in the context of tumour invasion was later
extended [57,58] to incorporate also the dynamics of M2 macrophages
infiltrating the solid tumour. The explicit multi-scale model [57]
that focusses on tissue-scale and cell-scale dynamics models the
changes in the densities of tumour cells, macrophages, and the two
components of the extracellular matrix (the fibrous and non-fibrous

component). The tissue-level dynamics describes the random and directed movement of cancer cells and macrophages inside the tissue (where the directed cell movement is the result of a non-local spatial flux caused by cell–cell and cell–matrix adhesive interactions), as well as on cell proliferation and death inside the tissue. The macroscale (tissue-level) dynamics of the two ECM components (fibrous and non-fibrous) is described by ODEs showing the degradation and secretion/remodelling of ECM. The fibrous component of the ECM has also a representation at the microscale (cell scale) [57], where its spatial distribution inside a cell-scale microdomain inside the tumour tissue is rearranged due to cancer and macrophages cell fluxes. This microscale rearrangement then translates into changes in the density and orientation of ECM fibres at macroscale (i.e., tissue scale). Also, at the microscale, there is the diffusion and production (by cancer cells and macrophages) of matrix-degrading enzymes (e.g., matrix metalloproteinases) that degrade de ECM on other cell-scale microdomains on the invasive tumour boundary. This microscale ECM degradation of each of these microdomains determines the direction and magnitude of the movement of tumour boundary into the surrounding tissue (at tissue scale). Numerical simulations of this multi-scale moving-boundary model [57] have shown a variety of tumour growth and invasive 2D patterns with M2 macrophages usually positioned at the invasive boundary. In contrast to the PDE model by Khajanchi and Nieto [51] discussed earlier, which had an implicit multi-scale structure (for the dynamics of cells and cytokines secreted by cells) and showed spherical spread of cells, in this explicit multi-scale moving-boundary model, the boundary of the tumour is very irregular, as observed in real tumours. This suggested that the explicit microscale dynamics at the invasive tumour boundary might be critical for the invasive patterns of tumour cells into the surrounding tissue. However, due to the complexity of this multi-scale model and the lack of multi-scale data to parametrise it, the parameters were randomly chosen and the model offered only qualitative results (although the simulation results had a biological realism).

Kinetic models: Another class of mathematical models that include explicitly multi-scale aspects of the dynamics inside the tumour microenvironment is represented by the kinetic models [62–68]. In these models, the cell variables usually depend not only on time and space but also on an internal variable (denoted here by "a") describing sub-cellular (i.e., molecular) dynamics. This variable could be the density of integrin receptors on cell surface [67, 68], the phenotype of macrophages [65, 66] or more generally the anti-tumour activation status of immune cells [62, 63] or the mutation level of tumour cells [63, 65]. In general, these kinetic models are suitable to describe the time evolution of various heterogeneous cell populations inside the tumour microenvironment: from heterogeneous tumour cells with different molecular signatures that have different sensitivity levels to treatments [69] to macrophages phenotypic heterogeneity [70] or the phenotypic heterogeneity of infiltrating T cells that are not all tumour-specific (i.e., do not recognise tumour-associated antigens) [21].

These kinetic models are described by the following general integro-partial differential equations:

$$\frac{\partial \mathbf{u}(t; a; \mathbf{x})}{\partial t} + \nabla_{\mathbf{x}}\left(\mathbf{u}T(\mathbf{u})\right) + \nabla_a\left(\mathbf{u}C^e[\mathbf{u}]\right)$$

$$= C^i[\mathbf{u}](t; a; \mathbf{x}) + \mathbf{u}(t; a; \mathbf{x})PD[\mathbf{u}] + IO[\mathbf{u}](t; a; \mathbf{x}), \qquad (5)$$

where $\mathbf{u}(t; a; \mathbf{x}) = (u_1(t; a; \mathbf{x}), \ldots, u_i(t; a; \mathbf{x}), \ldots, u_n(t; a; \mathbf{x}))$ describes the distribution of $n > 0$ cellular/molecular species u_i, $i = 1, \ldots, n$, at time t and space $\mathbf{x} = (x, y)$ (here in 2D) and characterised by an internal variable a. The term $T(\mathbf{u})$ gives the velocity of the movement through the spatial domain and the term $C^e[\mathbf{u}]$ gives the progression velocity through the internal variable space a in response to external factors, while the term $C^r[\mathbf{u}]$ describes the progression through the internal variable space due to random probabilities (i.e., internal to the system). Interactions between different species (u_i and u_j) that lead to changes in the microscopic state (i.e., internal variable $a \in A \subseteq [0, \infty)$) of either species are called conservative interactions, while interactions between different species that lead to changes in the population size of the involved species are called non-conservative interactions. Note that in equation (5) the term $\nabla_a(\mathbf{u}C^e[\mathbf{u}]) = (\nabla_a(u_1 C_1^e[\mathbf{u}]), \ldots, \nabla_a(u_i C_i^e[\mathbf{u}]), \ldots, \nabla_a(u_n C_n^e[\mathbf{u}]))$ describes conservative interactions between species u_i with internal state "a"

and other species u_j with internal states "b": $u_i(t; a; \mathbf{x}) C_i^e[\mathbf{u}] = u_i(t; a; \mathbf{x}) \sum_{j=1}^n \int_A \phi_{ij}^e(a, b) u_j(t; b; \mathbf{x}) db$ (where ϕ_{ij}^e is a conservative action function). The second conservative term is given by $C_i^r[\mathbf{u}] = \sum_{j=1}^n \int_A \int_A \phi_{ij}^r(b, c; a) u_i(t; b; \mathbf{x}) u_j(t; c; \mathbf{x}) db \, dc$ (with ϕ_{ij}^r a conservative action function) and describes the evolution of species u_i towards the internal state a following interactions between the same species u_i with initial internal state b with species u_j that has internal state c. The term $PD[\mathbf{u}] = (PD_1[\mathbf{u}], \ldots, PD_i[\mathbf{u}], PD_n[\mathbf{u}])$ describes Proliferation/Decay dynamics as a result of interactions between species u_i (with internal state "b" that could be also "a") and species u_j (with internal state "c"): $PD_i[\mathbf{u}](t; a; \mathbf{x}) = \sum_{j=1}^n \int_A \int_A \psi_{ij}(b, c; a) u_i(t; b; \mathbf{x}) u_j(t; c; \mathbf{x}) db \, dc$, with $\psi_{ij}(b, c; a)$ a non-conservative action function. Finally, the term $IO[\mathbf{u}] = (IO_1[\mathbf{u}], \ldots, IO_i[\mathbf{u}], \ldots, IO_n[\mathbf{x}])$ describes the Influx/Outflux of different species (hence, no bilinear interactions between different species, as seen in the $PD[\mathbf{u}]$ terms discussed earlier).

Remark 1. Note that equations (5) can be reduced to integro-differential equations if we ignore the movement through space ($T(\mathbf{u}) = 0$) and the externally induced progression through the activity space ($C[\mathbf{u}] = 0$).

Remark 2. When we assume that the internal activity state "a" is a discrete variable (i.e., it takes one single constant value or a finite set of constant values), then the above integro-differential or integro-partial differential equations reduce to ODEs or PDEs (since $u_i(t; a; \mathbf{x}) := u_i^a(t; \mathbf{x})$, $\forall i = 1, \ldots, n$).

Example. In the following, we discuss in more detail a simple kinetic model introduced in Eftimie and Gibelli [65] to describe the interactions between a heterogeneous tumour cell population characterised by a continuum of mutation states $a \in [0, 1]$ (with $a = 0$ describing weakly aggressive tumour cells and $a = 1$ describing highly aggressive cells) and a heterogeneous macrophage cell population characterised by a continuum of phenotype states $a \in [-1, 1]$ (with $a = 1$ describing cells with an M1-like anti-tumour phenotype and $a = -1$ describing cells with an M2-like pro-tumour phenotype). The model [65] that describes the temporal evolution of the probability distribution functions $u_1(t, a)$ (for macrophages) and $u_2(t, a)$ (for tumour cells) assumes that $T(\mathbf{u}) = 0$, $C^e[\mathbf{u}] = 0$, and

$$C_1^r[u_1, u_2] = \lambda_1 \int_{-1}^{1} \int 0^1 \phi_{12}^r(b, c; a) u_1(t; b) u_2(t; c) db \, dc, \quad (6a)$$

$$C_2^r[u_1, u_2] = \lambda_2 \int_{-1}^{0} \int_{0}^{1} \phi_{21}^r(b, c; a) u_1(t; b) u_2(t; c) db \, dc, \quad (6b)$$

In addition, the non-conservative terms in the general kinetic equation (5) are given as follows:

$$PD_1[u_1, u_2] = -\lambda_1 u_1(t; a) \int_0^1 u_2(t; b) db$$

$$+ \alpha u_1(t; a) \left(1 - \frac{\int_{-1}^1 u_1(t, b) db}{K_1} \right) \int_0^1 u_2(t; b) db, \quad (7a)$$

$$PD_2[u_1, u_2] = -\lambda_2 u_2(t; a) \int_{-1}^0 u_1(t; b) db$$

$$+ \beta^f u_2(t; a) \int_{-1}^0 u_1(t; b) db \left(1 - \frac{\int_0^1 u_2(t, b) db}{K_2} \right)$$

$$- \gamma u_2(t; a) \int_0^1 u_1(t; b) db, \quad (7b)$$

and

$$IO_1[u_1, u_2] = -\mu^d u_1(t; a),$$

$$IO_2[u_1, u_2] = \beta^n u_2(t; a) \left(1 - \frac{\int_0^1 u_2(t, b) db}{K_2} \right). \quad (8)$$

The above terms contain the following biological assumptions: (I) polarisation/repolarisation of macrophages occurs at rate λ_1; macrophages proliferate logistically (up to a carrying capacity K_1) at a rate α and die at a rate μ^d; (II) tumour cells progress through the internal state space (i.e., mutate) at a rate λ_2, proliferate logistically (up to carrying capacity K_2) at a rate β due to interactions between tumour cells and some external nutrient (at rate β^n) as well as inter-actions between tumours and M2-like macrophages with state $a < 0$

(at rate β^f) and are destroyed at a rate γ by M1-like macrophages (i.e., cells with state $a > 0$).

This kinetic model has been partially parametrised: the immune-related parameter values have been estimated using murine experimental data, while most of the cancer-related parameters have been chosen randomly, to test the range of simulation outcomes for various types of tumours (from melanoma to non-small cell lung cancer) with different population growth rates and different anti-tumour immune responses. Numerical simulations with this multi-scale model have shown that enhanced tumour heterogeneity (i.e., spread through the internal variable space describing enhanced mutations) is associated with macrophage heterogeneity (i.e., spread through the internal variable space describing the phenotype). This theoretical result is in line with various experimental studies that emphasise phenotypic heterogeneity in tumour cells [71] and tumour-associated macrophages [72], due to common factors such as metabolism.

4.   Open Problems

There are various open problems related to modelling immune responses in the context of cancer: from the development and simulations of 3D multi-scale mathematical models (to match the current interest in biomedical research of shifting from 2D to 3D cell culture experiments [73]), to single-scale and multi-scale data availability for parameter estimation, to performing uncertainty analysis on the results of these multi-scale models, or to modelling and investigating the delicate balance between inflammatory immune responses and biomechanical responses. In the following, we discuss in more detail two such open problems related to data: (i) data availability and model parametrisation and (ii) attempts to develop digital twins that ensure a real-time connections between numerical simulations and data:

(i) **Data availability and model parametrisation:** The great majority of explicit multi-scale models for tumour–immune interactions that exist in the literature are not properly parametrised and validated using appropriate data and thus can only be used to explore the qualitative behaviour of the biological systems

investigated. In fact, the majority of parameters used by such
models are taken from the published experimental literature or
from the mathematical literature, without any discussion as to
whether the various experiments that generated the data are
actually compatible with each other. For example, it is not
uncommon to find mathematical studies where some parameters
have values obtained from murine experiments and other values
obtained from human experiments (even if not all cell kinetics are similar in mice and humans; see, for example, the half-
life of different macrophage subsets in mice and humans [74]).
One of the reasons for this issue is that most of the biologi-
cal/clinical experiments generate single-scale data (see Gondal
and Chaudhary [7] for a summary of different databases with
molecular/cellular/tissue scale data) and combining data from
different experiments to parametrise multi-scale mathematical
models is not a trivial problem. The obvious solution would be
to generate more multi-scale data (across multiple spatial and
temporal scales) and to make these data available to all interested researchers. In fact, current experimental approaches (e.g.,
multi-region cell/tissue sampling, single-cell sequencing) aim to
provide information on spatial and temporal heterogeneity of
immune and cancer cells inside the tumour microenvironment
(TME) [69]. Other approaches focus on the use of innovative 3D
microfluidic systems to create organ-on-a-chip (OOC) biological models that allow high-resolution and real-time imaging to
gather new data on the interactions between immune cells and
cancer cells [75]. However, these systems are still in their early
days and don't provide yet multi-scale data of the form required
by the mathematical models discussed earlier (such experimental
systems usually provide either cell-level data or molecular-level
data). In any case, all these multi-scale mathematical models
should be accompanied by sensitivity and uncertainty analysis
studies to quantify the variability in the model outcomes given
the variability in the parameter values.

(ii) **Towards digital twins — connecting simulations and
data in real time:** The availability of single-scale and multi-
scale data is an important step towards the development of
digital twins for cancer research — a hot research topic these
days [76, 77]. We are not there yet — at least not for cancer

immunotherapy research — since such digital twins approaches need to use real-time data to parametrise the mathematical models, which in turn could offer fast real-time feedback on clinical treatment approaches. As mentioned earlier, a first step in this direction has been made with the development of OOC which provide real-time data [75]. These OOC reproduce simple sub-systems of the TME (e.g., interactions between tumour cells and immune cells, in the presence/absence of various anti-cancer drugs) and for now the real-time data obtained with these OOC is mostly single-scale data. Nevertheless, such multi-scale data will eventually be produced, and the AI approaches that are currently revolutionising the field of biomedicine will likely be integrated with multi-scale modelling approaches to estimate model parameters for these high-dimensional complex systems [78].

5.   Conclusion

Investigating the multi-scale aspects of tumour–immune interactions in the context of continuously changing tumour microenvironment is a challenge that cannot be solved only through experimental approaches. Mathematical modelling combined with computer simulations have been successfully used over the years to investigate qualitatively and even quantitatively different single-scale biological systems to propose hypotheses about possible biological mechanisms behind the observed behaviours. These approaches are now being used to investigate multi-scale biological systems. However, a lack of multi-scale spatio-temporal data (mainly due to the complexity of the continuously changing tumour microenvironment and to our lack of understanding how different biological sub-systems are connected across different spatial and temporal scales) is slowing down progress in this field, which currently focusses only on qualitative simulation results.

The direction of the research in this field is quite clear: combining *in vitro*/*ex vivo*/*in vivo* experiments that generate quantitative data, with *in silico* models and simulations for real-time predictions on the evolution of the disease and the success of the treatment for each individual patient. As discussed in the Introduction section, different solid tumours are composed of different immune cells in different percentages, which influence differently the evolution of the disease and the success of the treatment, and thus mathematical models and their computer simulations need to reflect the composition of the TME for each individual patient. However, this requires multi-scale data for the parametrisation of the multi-scale mathematical models, and such patient-specific data are not yet available.

Acknowledgements

RE acknowledges support from a French Agence Nationale de Recherche (ANR) grant (No. ANR-21-CE45-0025-01) and a University of Franche-Comté *"Chrysalide: soutien aux nouveaux arrivants"* (2022) grant.

References

[1] S. Oiseth and M. Aziz, Cancer immunotherapy: A brief review of the history, possibilities, and challenges ahead, *Journal of Cancer Metastasis and Treatment.* **3**, 250–261 (2017).

[2] E. McCarthy, The toxins of William B. Coley and the treatment of bone and soft-tissue sarcomas, *Iowa Orthopedic Journal.* **26**, 154–158 (2006).

[3] Y. Murciano-Goroff, A. B. Warner, and J. Wolchock, The future of cancer immunotherapy: Microenvironment-targeting combinations, *Cell Research.* **30**, 507–519 (2020).

[4] H. Rad, J. Monkman, M. Warkiani, R. Ladwa, K. O'Byrne, N. Rezaei, *et al.*, Understanding the tumour microenvironment for effective immunotherapy, *Medicinal Research Reviews.* **41**(3), 1474–1498 (2021).

[5] R. Eftimie, J. Bramson, and D. Earn, Interactions between the immune system and cancer: A brief review of non-spatial mathematical models, *Bulletin of Mathematical Biology.* **73**, 2–32 (2011).

[6] R. Eftimie, J. Gillard, and D. Cantrell, Mathematical models for immunology: Current state of the art and future research directions, *Bulletin of Mathematical Biology.* **78**, 2091–2134 (2016).

[7] M. Gondal and S. Chaudhary, Navigating multi-scale cancer systems biology towards model-driven clinical oncology and its applications in personalised therapeutics, *Frontiers in Oncology.* **11**, 712505 (2021).

[8] A. Sancho-Araiz, V. Mangas-Sanjuan, and I. Trocóniz, The role of mathematical models in immuno-oncology: Challenges and future perspectives, *Pharmaceutics.* **13**, 1016 (2021).

[9] S. Makaryan, C. Cess, and S. Finley, Modelling immune cell behaviour across scales in cancer, *WIREs Systems Biology and Medicine.* **12**(4), e1484 (2020).

[10] G. Malbacher, K. Reihmer, and H. Frieboes, Mathematical modelling of tumour-immune cell interactions, *Journal of Theoretical Biology.* **469**, 47–60 (2019).

[11] K. Norton, C. Gong, S. Jamalian, and A. Popel, Multiscale agent-based and hybrid modelling of the tumour immune microenvironment, *Processes (Basel).* **7**(1), 37 (2019).

[12] N. Anderson and M. Simon, The tumour microenvironment, *Current Biology.* **30**(16), R921–R925 (2020).

[13] R. Baghban, L. Roshangar, R. Jahanban-Esfahlan, K. Seidi, A. Ebrahimi-Kalan, M. Jaymand, *et al.*, Tumour microenvironment complexity and therapeutic implications at a glance, *Cell Communication and Signaling.* **18**, 59 (2020).

[14] H. Gonzales, C. Hagerling, and Z. Werb, Roles of the immune system in cancer: From tumour initiation to metastatic progression, *Genes & Development.* **32**(19–20), 1267–1284 (2018).

[15] E. Holl, V. Frazier, K. Landa, G. Beasley, E. Hwang, and S. Nair, Examining peripheral and tumour cellular immunome in patients with cancer, *Frontiers in Immunology.* **10**, 1767 (2019).

[16] J. Galon, B. Mlecnik, G. Bindea, H. Angell, A. Berger, C. Lagorce, *et al.*, Towards the introduction of the "Immunoscore" in the classification of malignant tumours, *The Journal of Pathology.* **232**(2), 199–209 (2014).

[17] J. Galon and A. Lanzi, Immunoscore and its introduction in clinical practice, *The Quarterly Journal of Nuclear Medicine and Molecular Imaging.* **64**(2), 152–161 (2020).

[18] F. Pagés, B. Mlecnik, F. Marliot, G. Bindea, F.-S. Ou, C. Bifulco, *et al.*, International validation of the consensus immunoscore for the classification of colon cancer: A prognostic and accuracy study, *The Lancet.* **391**(10135), 2128–2139 (2018).

[19] H. Angell, D. Bruni, J. Barrett, R. Herbst, and J. Galon, The immunoscore: Colon cancer and beyond, *Clinical Cancer Research.* **26**, 332–339 (2020).

[20] E. Spurrell and M. Lockley, Adaptive immunity in cancer immunology and therapeutics, *Ecancermedicalscience.* **8**, 441 (2014).

[21] S. Meier, A. Satpathy, and D. Wells, Bystander T cells in cancer immunology and therapy, *Nature Cancer.* **3**, 143–155 (2022).

[22] M. Autio, S.-K. Leivonen, O. Brück, S. Mustjoki, J. Jørgensen, M.-L. Karjalainen-Lindsberg, *et al.*, Immune cell constitution in the tumour microenvironment predicts the outcome in diffuse large B-cell lymphoma, *Haematologica*. **106**(3), 718–729 (2021).

[23] A. Caruntu, L. Moraru, M. Surcel, A. Munteanu, C. Tanase, C. Constantin, *et al.*, Assessment of immune cell populations in tumour tissue and peripheral blood samples from head and neck squamous cell carcinoma patients, *Analytical Cellular Pathology*. (Amsterdam). **2021**, 2328218 (2021).

[24] B. Stankovic, H. Bjørhovde, R. Skarshaug, H. Aamodt, A. Frafjord, E. Müller, *et al.*, Immune cell composition in human non-small cell lung cancer, *Frontiers in Immunology*. **9**, 3101 (2018).

[25] E. Zhang, C. Ding, S. Li, X. Zhou, B. Aikemu, X. Fan, *et al.*, Roles and mechanisms of tumour-infiltrating B cells in human cancer: A new force in immunotherapy, *Biomarker Research*. **11**, 28 (2023).

[26] I. Chan and A. Ewald, The changing role of natural killer cells in cancer metastasis, *Journal of Clinical Investigation*. **132**(8), e143762 (2022).

[27] A. Boutilier and S. Elsawa, Macrophage polarisation states in the tumour microenvironment, *International Journal of Molecular Sciences*. **22**, 6995 (2021).

[28] K. Pe, R. Saetung, V. Yodsurang, C. Chaotham, K. Suppipat, P. Chanvorachote, *et al.*, Triple-negative breast cancer influences a mixed M1/M2 macrophage phenotype associated with tumor aggressiveness, *PLoS One*. **17**(8), e0273044 (2022).

[29] G. Wang, K. Zhong, Z. Wang, Z. Zhang, X. Tang, A. Tong, *et al.*, Tumour-associated microglia and macrophages in glioblastoma, *Frontiers in Immunology*. **13**, 964898 (2022).

[30] H. Zheng, X. Peng, S. Yang, X. Li, M. Huang, S. Wei, *et al.*, Targeting tumour-associated macrophages in hepatocellular carcinoma: Biology, strategy, and immunotherapy, *Cell Death Discovery*. **9**, 65 (2023).

[31] S. Vu, P. Vetrivel, J. Kim, and M.-S. Lee, Cancer resistance to immunotherapy: Molecular mechanisms and tackling strategies, *International Journal of Molecular Sciences*. **23**(18), 10906 (2022).

[32] T. Gajewski, H. Schreiber, and Y.-X. Fu, Innate and adaptive immune cells in the tumour microenvironment, *Nature Immunology*. **14**(10), 1014–1022 (2013).

[33] C. Robert, A decade of immune-checkpoint inhibitors in cancer therapy, *Nature Communications*. **11**, 3801 (2020).

[34] M. Sadelain, R. Brentjens, and I. Riviere, The basic principles of chimeric antigen receptor (car) design, *Cancer Discovery.* **3**(4), 388–398 (2013).

[35] L. Zhang, Y. Meng, X. Feng, and Z. Han, CAR-NK cells for cancer immunotherapy: From bench to bedside, *Biomarker Research.* **10**, 12 (2022).

[36] S. Wang, Y. Yang, P. Ma, Y. Zha, A. Lei, and N. Li, CAR-macrophage: An extensive immune enhancer to fight cancer, *eBioMedicine.* **76**, 103873 (2022).

[37] K. Conlon, M. Milijkovic, and T. Waldmann, Cytokines in the treatment of cancer, *Journal of Interferon & Cytokine Research.* **39**(1), 6–21 (2019).

[38] F. van Dalen, M. van Stevendaal, F. Fennemann, M. Verdoes, and O. Ilina, Molecular repolarisation of tumour-associated macrophages, *Molecules.* **24**(1), 9 (2019).

[39] T. Jiang, C. Zhou, and S. Ren, Role of il-2 in cancer immunotherapy, *Oncoimmunology.* **5**(6), e1163462 (2016).

[40] S. Shalhout, D. Miller, K. Emerick, and H. Kaufman, Therapy with oncolytic viruses: Progress and challenges, *Nature Reviews Clinical Oncology.* **20**, 160–177 (2023).

[41] J. A. Carlson, Tumour doubling time of cutaneous melanoma and its metastasis, *The American Journal of Dermatopathology.* **25**(4), 291–299 (2003).

[42] S. Chesla, P. Selvaraj, and C. Zhu, Measuring two-dimensional receptor-ligand binding kinetics by micropipette, *Biophysical Journal.* **75**(3), 1553–1572 (1998).

[43] H. Warner, N. Sivakumar, S. Peirce, and M. Lazzara, Multiscale computational models of cancer, *Current Opinion in Biomedical Engineering.* **11**, 137–144 (2019).

[44] R. Eftimie, J. Bramson, and D. Earn, Modelling anti-tumour Th1 and Th2 immunity in the rejection of melanoma, *Journal of Theoretical Biology.* **265**, 467–480 (2010).

[45] R. Eftimie and C. Barelle, Mathematical investigation of innate immune responses to lung cancer: The role of macrophages with mixed phenotypes, *Journal of Theoretical Biology.* **524**, 110739 (2021).

[46] F. Hoffman, D. Gavaghan, J. Osborne, I. Barrett, T. You, H. Ghadially, *et al.*, A mathematical model of antibody-dependent cellular cytotoxicity (adcc), *Journal of Theoretical Biology.* **436**, 39–50 (2018).

[47] N. Mirzaei, S. Su, D. Sofia, M. Hegarty, M. Abdel-Rahman, A. Asadpoure, *et al.*, A mathematical model of breast tumour progression based on immune infiltration, *Journal of Personalized Medicine.* **11**, 1031 (2021).

[48] J.-L. Yu and S.-J. Jang, A mathematical model of tumour-immune interactions with an immune checkpoint inhibitor, *Applied Mathematics and Computation.* **362**, 124523 (2019).

[49] J.-L. Yu, R.-J. Jang, and K.-Y. Liu, Exploring the interactions of oncolytic viral therapy and immunotherapy of anti-CTLA-4 for malignant melanoma mice model, *Cells.* **12**(3), 507 (2023).

[50] S. Quezada, T. Sympson, K. Peggs, T. Merghoub, J. Vider, X. Fan, *et al.*, Tumour-reactive CD4$^+$ T cells develop cytotoxic activity and eradicate large established melanoma after transfer into lymphopenic hosts, *Journal of Experimental Medicine.* **207**(3), 637–650 (2010).

[51] S. Khajanchi and J. Nieto, Spatiotemporal dynamics of a glioma immune interaction model, *Scientific Reports.* **11**, 22385 (2021).

[52] T. Alzahrani, R. Eftimie, and D. Trucu, Multiscale modelling of cancer response to oncolytic viral therapy, *Mathematical Biosciences.* **310**, 76–95 (2019).

[53] T. Alzahrani, R. Eftimie, and D. Trucu, Multiscale moving boundary modelling of cancer interactions with a fusogenic oncolytic virus: The impact of syncytia dynamics, *Mathematical Biosciences.* **323**, 108296 (2020).

[54] V. Bitsouni, M. Chaplain, and R. Eftimie, Mathematical modelling of cancer invasion: The multiple roles of TGF-β pathway on tumour proliferation and cell adhesion, *Mathematical Models and Methods in Applied Sciences.* **27**(10), 1929–1962 (2017).

[55] G. Malbacher, L. Curtis, J. Lowengrub, and H. Frieboes, Mathematical modeling of tumour-associated macrophage interactions with the cancer microenvironment, *Journal for ImmunoTherapy of Cancer.* **6**, 10 (2018).

[56] A. Matzavinos, M. Chaplain, and V. Kuznetsov, Mathemtical modelling of the spatio-temporal response of cytotoxic T-lymphocytes to a solid tumour, *Mathematical Medicine and Biology.* **21**, 1–34 (2004).

[57] S. Suveges, R. Eftimie, and D. Trucu, Directionality of macrophage movement in tumour invasion: A multi-scale moving boundary approach, *Bulletin of Mathematical Biology.* **82**, 1–50 (2020).

[58] S. Suveges, R. Eftimie, and D. Trucu, Re-polarisation of macrophages within collective tumour cell migration: A multiscale moving boundary approach, *Frontiers in Applied Mathematics and Statistics.* **7**, 799650 (2022).

[59] L. Bartha and R. Eftimie, Mathematical investigation into the role of macrophage heterogeneity on the temporal and spatio-temporal dynamics of non-small cell lung cancers, *Journal of Theoretical Biology.* **549**, 111207 (2022).

[60] V. Bitsouni, D. Trucu, M. Chaplain, and R. Eftimie, Aggregation and travelling wave dynamics in a two-population model of cancer cell growth and invasion, *Mathematical Medicine and Biology.* **35**, 541–577 (2018).

[61] D. Trucu, P. Lin, M. Chaplain, and Y. Wang, A multiscale moving boundary model arising in cancer invasion, *Multiscale Modeling and Simulation.* **11**(1), 309–335 (2013).

[62] N. Bellomo and M. Delitala, From the mathematical kinetic, and stochastic game theory to modelling mutations, onset, progression and immune competition of cancer cells, *Physics of Life Reviews.* **5**, 183–206 (2008).

[63] E. de Angelis and B. Lods, On the kinetic theory for active particles: A model for tumour-immune system competition, *Mathematical and Computer Modelling.* **47**(1–2), 196–209 (2008).

[64] A. Bellouquid and M. Delitala. From kinetic theory for active particles to modelling immune competition. In *Selected Topics in Cancer Modelling* (Birkhäuser, Boston, MA, 2008), pp. 1–17.

[65] R. Eftimie and L. Gibelli, A kinetic theory approach for modelling tumour and macrophages heterogeneity and plasticity during cancer progression, *Mathematical Models and Methods in Applied Sciences.* **30**(4), 659–683 (2020).

[66] R. Eftimie, Investigation into the role of macrophages heterogeneity on solid tumour aggregations, *Mathematical Biosciences.* **322**, 108325 (2020).

[67] C. Engwer, M. Knappitsch, and C. Surulescu, A multiscale model for glioma spread including cell-tissue interactions and proliferation, *Mathematical Biosciences and Engineering.* **13**(2), 443–460 (2016).

[68] G. Meral, C. Stinner, and C. Surulescu, On a multiscale model involving cell contractivity and its effects on tumour invasion, *Discrete and Continuous Dynamical Systems - B.* **20**(1), 189–213 (2015).

[69] I. Dagog-Jack and A. Shaw, Tumour heterogeneity and resistance to cancer therapies, *Nature Reviews Clinical Oncology.* **15**, 81–94 (2018).

[70] Z. Xuan, L. Fang, G. Zhang, X. Zhang, J. Jiang, K. Wang, *et al.*, The heterogeneity of tumour-associated macrophages contributes to the recurrence and outcomes of glioblastoma patients, *Journal of Molecular Neuroscience.* **73**, 1–14 (2023).

[71] S. Dashmukh and S. Saini, Phenotypic heterogeneity in tumour progression, and its possible role in the onset of cancer, *Frontiers in Genetics.* **11**, 604528 (2020).

[72] S. Li, J. Yu, A. Huber, I. Kryczek, Z. Wang, L. Jiang, *et al.*, Metabolism drives macrophage heterogeneity in the microenvironment, *Cell Reports.* **39**(1), 110609 (2022).

[73] J. Caleb and T. Yong, Is it time to start transitioning from 2D to 3D cell culture? *Frontiers in Molecular Biosciences.* **7**, 33 (2020).

[74] O. Italiani and D. Boraschi, From monocytes to M1/M2 macrophages: Phenotypical vs. functional differentiation, *Frontiers in Immunology.* **5**, 514 (2014).

[75] F. Mattei, S. Andreone, A. Mencattini, A. Ninno, L. Businaro, E. Martinelli, *et al.*, Oncoimmunology meets organs-on-chip, *Frontiers in Molecular Biosciences.* **8**, 627454 (2021).

[76] R. Eftimie, A. Mavrodin, and S. Bordas, From digital control to digital twins in medicine: A brief review and future perspectives, *Advances in Applied Mechanics.* **56**, 323–368 (2023).

[77] R. Eftimie, Grand challenges in mathematical biology: Integrating multi-scale modelling and data, *Frontiers in Applied Mathematics and Statistics.* **8**, 1010622 (2022).

[78] J. Kutz, Machine learning for parameter estimation, *Proceedings of the National Academy of Sciences of the USA.* **120**(12), e2300990120 (2023).

Chapter 4

From Cancer Evolution to Treatment: Viscoelastic Aspects of Solid Cancers

Ivana Pajic-Lijakovic* and Milan Milivojevic

Faculty of Technology and Metallurgy,
Belgrade University, Belgrade, Serbia
*iva@tmf.bg.ac.rs

Breast cancer is females' most common cancer, with a high mortality rate primarily due to metastasis to secondary sites in the body. The migration of cancer cells from the primary tumor is influenced by physical interactions between cancer cells and surrounding epithelium and the extracellular matrix. Cumulative effects of these interactions arise in the form of physical factors such as solid stress accumulated within a tumor spheroid, tissue surface tension, and the viscoelasticity caused by collective cell migration. The cancer spreading is regulated by solid stress generated in spheroid core region during tumor growth and its interactions with external tissue. Tissue viscoelasticity and surface tension are influenced by strength of cell–cell and cell–extracellular matrix adhesion contacts, intracellular signalling cascades, viscoelasticity of extracellular matrix, and cell contractility in response to microenvironmental conditions. However, the interplay between those factors is still unclear. In order to clarify this issue, it is necessary to consider and compare the rearrangement of various mono-cultured breast cancer and epithelial model systems under *in vitro* conditions like rearrangement of cell spheroids and the fusion of two cell spheroids. In this chapter, focus is on the multi-scale modelling approaches aimed at reproducing and understanding these biological systems.

1. Introduction

Cancer invasion through the extracellular matrix (ECM) and the surrounding tissue is a key step in cancer disease progression [1–4]. The main properties of cancer are (1) sustaining proliferative signalling, (2) evading growth suppressors, (3) activating invasion and metastases, (4) enabling replicative immortality, (5) inducing angiogenesis, and (6) resisting cell death [4]. Cancer spreading is influenced by interplay between (1) biological processes, such as cell signalling and gene expression, and (2) physical interactions between cancer cells and surrounding epithelium and the ECM [1]. Cumulative effects of those physical interactions will be discussed in the context of (1) the solid stress within the spheroid core region, (2) tissue surface tension on the spheroid surface region, and (3) the viscoelasticity of this multicellular system caused by collective cell migration (CCM). It is well known that physical factors such as tumor stroma stiffening and solid stress generated in the core region of tumor spheroid during tumor growth and interactions with external tissue, among other biological factors, influence the cancer spreading [5]. Consequently, the solid stress in the spheroid core and the tension on its surface regulate cell rearrangement within a spheroid via CCM. The accumulated stress within a core region of multi-cellular spheroids corresponds to a few kPa [5]. The cell normal residual stress accumulated in the core region of CT26 cancer cell spheroid (diameter of 240 μm) is about eight times higher than stress at the spheroid surface under externally applied osmotic stress of 5 kPa [6]. Accumulated stress influence cell shape and their migration mode. Thus, cells within a core region are smaller and more rounded in comparison to those within the spheroid surface region [7,8].

The viscoelasticity and tissue surface tension are influenced by (1) the strength of cell–cell and cell–ECM adhesion contacts [7, 9, 10], (2) intracellular signalling cascades [11], (3) the viscoelasticity of

ECM [10, 12], and (4) cell contractility as response to microenvironmental conditions [7]. The viscoelasticity caused by CCM has been treated as behaviour of a viscoelastic liquid and/or viscoelastic solid [12–18].

In order to understand the cancer spreading scenario, it is necessary to consider (1) response of cancer cells to mechanical stress conditions and compare it with the response of epithelial cells, (2) surface tension of active (contractile) and passive (non-contractile) cells (both, cancer and epithelial), and (3) viscoelasticity of collectively migrated cells.

In this chapter, focus is on mono-cultured spheroids of breast cancer and epithelial cells under *in vitro* conditions and critical discussion of the experimental data from the literature. Breast cancer is the worldwide most common cancer in females, with a high mortality rate primarily due to metastasis to secondary sites in the body [19]. When the invasive breast cancer is found only in the breast, the 5-year survival rate of women is expectable in average. Consequently, deeper insight into physical interactions is necessary in order to suppress cancer spreading. We are focussing here on the main characteristics of cell rearrangement caused by (1) rearrangement of mono-cultured breast and epithelial spheroids [7] and (2) fusion of two mono-cultured cell spheroids [20–23] based on rheological and thermodynamic approaches. The cell rearrangement is considered at a time scale of hours which corresponds to CCM. The cell division (which corresponds to a time scale of days) is neglected in this modelling consideration.

2. The Rearrangement of Mono-Cultured Cellular Spheroids: The Main Parameters

The rearrangement of cell spheroids as the result of CCM is influenced by interplay between tissue surface tension and solid stress accumulation within spheroids, while the CCM itself induces additional energy storage or dissipation depending on the long-time viscoelasticity. We are focussing on cell rearrangement, while the total number of cells is approximately constant. Consequently, cell spheroid is treated as a canonical ensemble at a time scale of hours. This assumption is important for further modelling consideration.

Two scenarios of cell rearrangement are possible: (1) guided by the tissue surface tension and (2) guided by the solid stress (Fig. 1).

Higher tissue surface tension induces movement of cells from the spheroid surface region to its core region in order to reduce the surface (Fig. 1(a)). This movement results in (1) decrease in the spheroid volume and surface and (2) increase in the cell packing density accompanied with the additional increase in the solid stress in the spheroid core region. However, if the tissue surface tension is significantly reduced, the cell movement is directed from the spheroid core region to its surface driven by the solid stress (Fig. 1(b)). Cell movement in this case results in (1) increase in the spheroid volume and surface and (2) decrease in the cell packing density accompanied with a decrease in the compressive residual stress in the spheroid

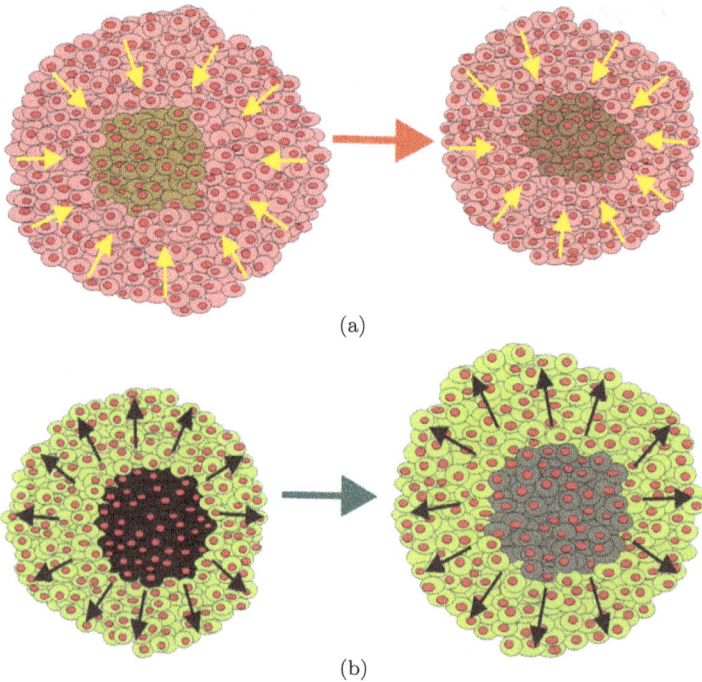

(a)

(b)

Fig. 1. Two scenarios of cell rearrangement, i.e., (a) rearrangement driven by the tissue surface tension and (b) expansion driven by the solid stress.

core region. Besides the rearrangement of spheroids, these scenarios have been recognised during the fusion of two cell spheroids by monitoring the volume and surface of the two-spheroid systems. Before discussing various experimental systems, it is necessary to discuss the cell response under stress and to emphasise the main characteristics of the tissue surface tension for cancer and epithelial cells.

2.1. *Cells response under stress*

While stress reduces movement of some cell types, it has no effect or even enhances movement of the others. The compressive stress of 773 Pa suppresses the movement of human non-tumorigenic breast epithelial cells (MCF-10A) and tumorigenic but not metastatic breast cells (MCF-7) [24]. In contrast, this stress is capable of enhancing the movement of highly aggressive metastatic breast 4T1 cancer cells (4T1) and metastatic mesenchymal breast 231 cancer cells (MDA-MB-231), as well as not metastatic 67NR breast cancer cells (67NR) [24]. Riehl *et al.* [25] considered and compared responses of MDA-MB-231 and metastatic mesenchymal breast 468 cancer cells (MDA-MB-468), as well as the MCF-10A epithelial cells under shear stress of 1.5 Pa. While the shear stress stimulates movement of the MDA-MB-231 cells, this stress has no impact on movement of (MDA-MB-468) and reduces movement of MCF-10A epithelial cells. Therefore, cell response under stress conditions should be discussed in the context of cell mechano-sensitivity.

Cell mechano-sensitivity is influenced by various parameters such as (1) level of E-cadherin [26], (2) stiffness of single-cells [24], and (3) mechanism of cell movement [7, 27]. Mohammed *et al.* [26] indicated that E-cadherin-mediated cell–cell adhesion contacts are the main cause of the MCF-10A epithelial cell movement reduction and the jamming state transition under the compressive stress. Tse *et al.* [24] pointed out that stiffer cells are less mechano-sensitive. It is in accordance with the fact that softer cancer cells are more invasive than stiffer ones [28, 29]. The average Young's modulus decreases from 1.05 kPa for (less invasive) MCF-7 cells to 0.94 kPa for (more invasive) epithelial breast T47D cancer cells (T47D) and to 0.62 kPa for (the most invasive) MDA-MB-231 cells [30]. The single cell stiffness depends on the interplay between cell contractions and the type of cell–cell adhesion contacts. Yousafzai *et al.* [31] found that neighbouring cells within mono-cultured systems significantly alter cell stiffness. The malignant epithelial breast HBL-100 cells (HBL-100) and MCF-7 cells become softer, while the MDA-MB-231 cells become stiffer. Cells which prefer movement with blebs such as MDA-MB-468 cells are more resistant under stress conditions in comparison with the cells which use filopodia during movement through dense adhesive surrounding, such as the MDA-MB-231 cells [27, 29].

Besides solid stress that is generated within the spheroid core region, the surface tension is another key factor which influences cell spreading within the spheroid.

2.2. *Tissue surface tension*

The surface tension, as a specific energy of surface which significantly influences the structural changes of various soft matter systems, represents the characteristic of liquids and amorphous solids [32]. Tissues can behave either as a viscoelastic liquids or viscoelastic solids depending on cell type and microenvironmental conditions [33]. The macroscopic tissue surface tension has been frequently measured during uni-axial compression of cell aggregates between parallel plates by determining the aggregate geometry [34–39]. Two types of macroscopic surface tension can be distinguished, i.e., the static and dynamic surface tensions. The static tissue surface tension is the value of the surface tension in thermodynamic equilibrium state, independent on time, and established after uni-axial compression. The dynamic surface tension depends on the system structural changes during the cellular system relaxation towards the equilibrium state and is time-dependent. The static surface tension has been considered as a product of single-cell state such as cell contractility and the state of cell–cell adhesion contacts [34]. The macroscopic static surface tension of cell aggregate in contact with surrounding liquefied medium γ can be related to the tensions γ_{cc} and γ_{cm} (where γ_{cc} is the cell–cell interfacial tension and γ_{cm} is the cell–medium interfacial tension) and expressed as [38, 39]

$$\gamma = \gamma_{cm} - \frac{1}{2}\gamma_{cc}. \tag{1}$$

In contrast to the static tissue surface tension, the dynamic tissue surface tension is much complex and depends on the rearrangement of the cell aggregate surface region, caused by external or internal loading conditions and can be related to the dilational viscoelasticity [35]. While the static tissue surface tension has been measured for various multicellular cellular systems, the dynamic tissue surface tension has been less elaborated. The dynamic tissue surface tension varies with the volume fraction of migrating cells within the aggregate surface region, the size of migrating cell clusters, and the rate of their changes [35].

Mombach *et al.* [36] considered a change in tissue surface tension during the rounding of 3D chicken embryonic neural retina spheroids. They reported that the tissue surface tension increases from $1.6 \pm 0.6 \, \mathrm{mN/m}$ to $4.0 \pm 1.0 \, \mathrm{mN/m}$ within 9 days. Beysens *et al.* [37] found that the values of the average tissue surface tension for five chicken embryonic tissues varied from 1.6 mN/m (neural retina) to 20 mN/m (limb bud). The tissue surface tension of embryonic carcinoma F9 cell line is $4.74 \pm 0.28 \, \mathrm{mN/m}$ [34]. We would like to emphasise the role of dynamic tissue surface tension in the rearrangement of cell spheroids.

2.2.1. *Tissue surface tension of various cell types*

The tissue surface tension is a product of cumulative effects of cell–cell interactions within the surface region of cell spheroids during CCM. Migrating epithelial cells use adherens junctions (AJs) to mechanically couple each other and also as an important source of signalling that coordinates collective behaviour [40]. One of the main components of AJs are proteins from the cadherin family. While epithelial cells form stronger E-cadherin-based AJs, mesenchymal cells frequently form weak N-cadherin-mediated AJs [40]. The state of cell–cell adhesion contacts is influenced by cell contractility [41] and the state of cell–ECM adhesion contacts (FAs) [10,42]. Cadherin-mediated AJs and integrin-mediated FAs can have either an antagonistic or cooperative relation, which is mediated by their connection to the actin cytoskeleton and results in a balanced force distribution between sites of cell–cell and cell–ECM attachment [42]. The establishing of integrin-mediated FAs stimulates cadherin accumulation which leads to an increase in the cell packing density [9]. Tian *et al.* [10] pointed out that the tension in FAs of the cancer

MDA-MB-231 cells increases on stiffer substrates, while the tension in epithelial MCF-10A cells exhibits no apparent change against the substrate stiffness. This result represents a confirmation of cancer cell adaptability on the microenvironmental conditions.

Devanny *et al.* [7] considered the rearrangement of various breast cell spheroids made by epithelial MCF-10A cells and various mesenchymal cell lines, i.e., MDA-MB-468, along with MDA-MB-231 and MDA-MB-436 cells. While the rearrangement of cancer spheroids occurs primarily via $\beta 1$ integrin-mediated FAs, the rearrangement of MCF-10A cells occurs primarily via cadherin-mediated AJs [7].

Cell contractility influences the state of AJs and FAs, as well as their crosstalk. It was revealed that contractility plays a fundamentally different role in the cell lines in which rearrangement is driven primarily by integrins (MDA-MB-468, along with MDA-MB-231 and MDA-MB-436 cells) compared to those where it is driven by cadherins (MCF-10A) [7]. Epithelial cell contractions enhance the strength of AJs and on that base increase the tissue surface tension. Consequently, migrating clusters of epithelial cells have higher tissue surface tension than resting (non-contractile) epithelial cells. However, contractility of cancer cells, among which integrin mediated adhesion contacts are established, induces an increase in cell–cell repulsions which reduce the tissue surface tension [7]. Warmt *et al.* [43] reported that the contractility of breast cancer cells is more intensive than the contractility of the MCF-10A cells. This important finding points that migrating clusters of cancer cells have lower tissue surface tension in comparison with the resting (non-contractile) cancer cells. Consequently, the distribution of tissue surface tension in the spheroid surface region depends on cell type and the configuration of migrating cells.

3. Fusion of Two Cell Spheroids: The Role of Tissue Surface Tension

The fusion of two cell spheroids represents a simple model system suitable for considering the role of dynamic tissue surface tension in cell rearrangement by monitoring the volume and surface of two-spheroid system vs. time. The tissue surface tension is responsible for a decrease in surface and volume of two-spheroid system by inducing

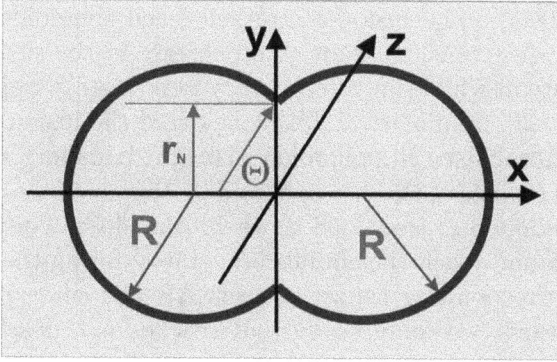

Fig. 2. The geometry of two-spheroid system.

cell movement from the surface towards the core region of this system during the fusion. The surface of two-spheroid system in contact was expressed as [20] $A(\tau) = 4\pi R(\tau)^2(1 + \cos\theta(\tau))$, while the total volume is [22] $V(\tau) = \frac{2\pi}{3}R(\tau)^3(2 + 3\cos\theta(\tau) - \cos^3\theta(\tau))$ (where $R(\tau)$ is the aggregate radius and $\theta(\tau)$ is the fusion angle). The geometry of two-aggregate system is presented in Fig. 2.

In various experimental systems, the volume of two-spheroids in contact $V(\tau)$ can (1) increase for $\frac{V(\tau)}{V_0} > 1$, (2) stay constant for $\frac{V(\tau)}{V_0} = 1$, and (3) decrease for $\frac{V(\tau)}{V_0} < 1$ [20]. The aspect ratio is equal to $AR(\tau) = \frac{d(\tau)}{2r(\tau)}$ (where $d(\tau)$ is the longer axis equal to $d(\tau) = 2R(\tau)(1+\cos\theta)$ and $2r_N(\tau)$ is the shorter axis of multicellular system, while the neck radius is equal to $r_N(\tau) = R(\tau)\sin\theta(\tau)$) [22]. We consider here the rearrangement of two-spheroid system caused by CCM and assumed that the total number of cells is approximately constant, i.e., $N_{cT} \approx$ const. Consequently, the two-spheroid system is treated as a canonical ensemble such that total number of cells N_{cT} is equal to $N_{cT} = N_V(\tau) + N_A(\tau)$ (where $N_V(\tau)$ is the number of cells in the core region and $N_A(\tau)$ is the number of cells in the surface region of two-spheroid system).

3.1. *Two scenarios of the spheroid fusion*

The rearrangement of cancer cell spheroids has been estimated and compared with the rearrangement of epithelial cell spheroids by considering a simple model system, such as the fusion of two cell spheroids [20–23]. The fusion of epithelial cell spheroids, driven by the tissue surface tension, leads to a decrease in the surface of two-spheroid system, while the volume decreases or stays approximately constant [22,23]. Shafiee *et al.* [21] considered the fusion of two confluent skin fibroblast cell spheroids ($440\,\mu$m diameter) and pointed out that the surface of the two-spheroid system decreases 2.18 times, while the volume decreases 2.38 times within 140 h. The surface and volume relax and reach the equilibrium states during the fusion process. The corresponding aspect ratio is AR≈1.1 after 140 h which points out that two-spheroid system reaches out nearly spherical shape.

The volumetric rearrangement of these systems, caused by the work of tissue surface tension, follows two scenarios: (1) total coalescence [21] and (2) arrested coalescence [23,44]. The CCM is intensive at the contact point between two cell spheroids which leads to an increase in the neck radius. In this case, generated two volumetric velocity fronts have opposite directions. The schematic representation of the fusion of two-epithelial spheroids is shown in Fig. 3.

Every cell velocity front is directed from the surface region of one aggregate to the core region of the other. Consequently, local collisions of velocity fronts induce an increase in cell packing density which can lead to the cell jamming state transition [16, 33, 45, 46]. Cell jamming state transitions that occur near the contact point between two spheroids can induce damping effects of the spheroid

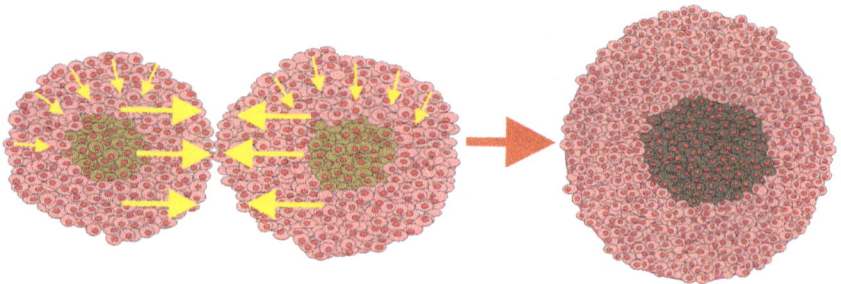

Fig. 3. Fusion of two epithelial spheroids driven by the tissue surface tension. The compaction of two-spheroid system caused by CCM induces an increase in the cell residual stress accumulated in the core region of two-spheroid system.

fusion [44]. This phenomenon is known as the 'arrested coalescence' [23, 44, 47].

Surprisingly, the fusion of cancer cell spheroids follows quite different scenario by increasing the surface and volume after fusion of two-spheroid system. Dechristé *et al.* [22] considered the fusion of two human carcinoma cell spheroids (HCT116 cell line) as a consequence of cell divisions within 70 h. The doubling time of HCT116 cells is 18 h [48]. However, the volume and surface of two-spheroid systems increased even during first 5 h. Within this time period, cell divisions can be neglected, while the surface and volume changes occur primarily via CCM. The surface of two-spheroid systems increases (1) 1.8 times for larger cell spheroids (500 μm diameter) and (2) 2.3 times for smaller spheroids (300 μm diameter) within first 5 h [22]. The increase in the volume of two-spheroid systems is (1) 1.24 times for larger spheroids and (2) 1.12 times for smaller spheroids within 5 h [22]. While the fusion of two confluent skin fibroblast cell spheroids (440 μm diameter) needs 140 h for decreasing the surface about 2.18 times, the fusion of two human carcinoma cell spheroids (HCT116 cell line) (diameter of 500 μm) leads to 1.8 times increase in the surface during only 5 h.

Grosser *et al.* [23] considered and compared the fusion of two breast cell spheroids such as (1) epithelial MCF-10A cell lines and (2) cancerous mesenchymal MDA-MB-436 cells within 60 h. While MCF-10A cells undergo arrested coalescence and the average cell velocity drops to zero, cancer cells kept their velocity approximately constant within this time period and avoided the cell jamming.

These findings point to a different scenario of cell rearrangement for cancer cells in comparison with the epithelial cells as is shown in Fig. 4.

While epithelial cells undergo volumetric rearrangement, driven by the tissue surface tension [21, 23], cancer cells rather perform a surface rearrangement, driven by the solid stress. Interestingly, cancer cells are able to reduce the tissue surface tension and behave as surface active constituents [7]. The main goal of this contribution is to emphasise the possible reason of this interesting phenomenon by accounting for the interplay between the viscoelasticity caused by CCM, surface tension, and the solid stress.

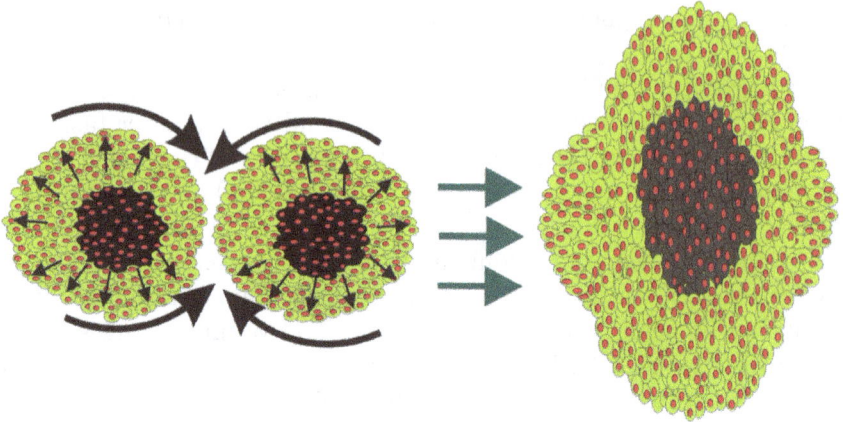

Fig. 4. The fusion of two cancer spheroids.

4. The Fusion of Two-Spheroid Systems and Viscoelasticity

Viscoelasticity and tissue surface tension influence the cell rearrangement during the fusion of two-spheroid systems. The CCM induces
generation of stress (normal and shear). Normal stress is generated
either within a core region of migrating cell clusters or during colli-
sion of clusters caused by uncorrelated motility [18]. Shear stress can
be significant at the biointerface formed between cluster of migrating
cells and surrounding resting cells [49, 50]. The main characteristic
of viscoelasticity caused by CCM is the multi-time nature. Namely,
cell movement and resulted strain and residual stress accumulation
occur at a time scale of hours, while the stress relaxation occurs at
a time scale of minutes [12, 13, 18]. Therefore, accumulation of cell
residual stress has a feedback effect on further cell movement depending on cell type and microenvironmental conditions. Two types of
constitutive behaviour have been discussed in the context of CCM:
viscoelastic liquid and viscoelastic solid. Coordinated movement of
weakly connected cells, in the form of streams, has been treated
as viscoelastic liquids. This type of movement is frequently recognised in spreading of cancer cells [1]. Movement of epithelial cells
during the cell aggregate micropipette aspiration also corresponds
to a viscoelastic liquid [14]. The micropipette aspiration induces

significant energy dissipation during cell rearrangement which has been described by the Maxwell model [14]. The main characteristics of the Maxwell model are that stress can relax under constant strain conditions, while the strain itself cannot relax [51]. Ability of strain to relax corresponds to the viscoelastic solids rather than viscoelastic liquids [51].

However, various *in vitro* model systems of epithelial cells such as (1) free expansion of epithelial monolayers [15], (2) rearrangement of confluent epithelial monolayers [17], and (3) uni-axial compression of cell aggregate between parallel plates behave as viscoelastic solids [13]. This behaviour corresponds to a cell movement in the form of strongly connected cell clusters. Pajic-Lijakovic and Milivojevic proposed [12] the Zener model for describing the constitutive behaviour of these systems based on following characteristics extracted from the experiments:

(a) The cell residual stress change is correlated with the corresponding strain rate for 2D multicellular systems [15, 17].
(b) Stress can relax under constant strain condition during the cell aggregate uni-axial compression between parallel plates [13].
(c) Strain can relax under constant (or zero) stress conditions [13].

The Zener model describes the stress relaxation under constant strain conditions and strain relaxation under constant stress conditions [51]. The fusion of two-spheroid systems behaves similarly as the rounding of epithelial cell spheroids after uni-axial compression [47]. In both cases, those processes are driven by the tissue surface tension. If the volume, surface, as well as, the volumetric and surface strains are capable of relaxing and establishing the equilibrium state, these behaviours point to a viscoelastic solid.

4.1. The constitutive behaviour of two epithelial spheroids in contact during fusion

Shafiee *et al.* [21] considered the fusion of two confluent skin fibroblast cell aggregates and revealed that the volume and surface of two aggregate systems decrease towards the equilibrium states. This finding clearly pointed to a viscoelastic solid behaviour. The Zener model, suitable for describing constitutive behaviour of migrating epithelial cells, is expressed as [12, 50]

$$\widetilde{\sigma}_{ei}(r, t_s, \tau) + \tau_{Ri}\,\dot{\widetilde{\sigma}}_{ei}(r, t_s, \tau) = G_i\widetilde{\varepsilon}_{ei}(r, \tau) + \eta_i\dot{\widetilde{\varepsilon}}_{ei}(r, \tau), \qquad (2)$$

where $i \equiv S, V, S$ is the shear change, V is the volumetric change, t_s is the time scale of minutes, $\widetilde{\sigma}_i$ is the shear or volumetric stress, $\dot{\widetilde{\sigma}}_{ei} = \frac{d\widetilde{\sigma}_{ei}}{dt_s}$, $\widetilde{\varepsilon}_{ei}$ is the epithelial shear or volumetric strain equal to $\widetilde{\varepsilon}_{eS} = \frac{1}{2}(\vec{\nabla}\vec{u}_e + \vec{\nabla}\vec{u}_e^T)$ and $\widetilde{\varepsilon}_{eV} = (\vec{\nabla} \cdot \vec{u}_e)\widetilde{I}$, respectively, $\vec{u}_e$ is the cell displacement field caused by CCM, $\dot{\widetilde{\varepsilon}}_{ei} = \frac{d\widetilde{\varepsilon}_i}{d\tau}$ is the strain rate, G_i is the shear or Young's elastic modulus, and η_i is the shear or bulk viscosity and τ_{Ri} is the corresponding stress relaxation time. Stress relaxation under constant strain condition $\widetilde{\varepsilon}_{e0i}(r, \tau)$ per single short-time relaxation cycle can be expressed starting from the initial condition $\widetilde{\sigma}_{ei}(r, t_s = 0, \tau) = \widetilde{\sigma}_{e0i}$ as

$$\widetilde{\sigma}_{ci}(r, t_s, \tau) = \widetilde{\sigma}_{e0}e^{-\frac{t_s}{\tau_{Ri}}} + \widetilde{\sigma}_{eRi}(r, \tau)^{\text{CCM}}\left(1 - e^{-\frac{t_s}{\tau_{Ri}}}\right), \qquad (3)$$

where $\widetilde{\sigma}_{eRi}(r, \tau)^{\text{CCM}}$ is the cell residual shear or normal stress accumulated during CCM equal to $\widetilde{\sigma}_{eRi}^{\text{CCM}} = G_i\widetilde{\varepsilon}_{e0i}$. The stress relaxation occurs through many short-time stress relaxation cycles under constant strain per cycle, while the strain change occurs at a time scale of hours [18, 50]. This rheological behaviour, described by the Zener model, indicates that dominant viscous behaviour occurs at short-time scale (a time scale of minutes), while elastic behaviour occurs at long-time scale (a time scale of hours).

Total cell residual stress caused by CCM includes the cell shear and normal stress contributions, i.e., $\widetilde{\sigma}_{eR}^{\text{CCM}} = \widetilde{\sigma}_{eRV}^{\text{CCM}} + \widetilde{\sigma}_{eRS}^{\text{CCM}}$.

The movement of epithelial cells from the surface region to the core region of two-spheroid system during fusion is driven by the tissue surface tension force $n_e\vec{F}_{st}^e = n_e\gamma_e\vec{u}_e$ (where γ_e is the surface tension of epithelial cells) [12]. Besides the surface tension force, the surface tension of epithelial cells also influences the viscoelastic force as well. The normal residual stress of the epithelial cells is equal to

$$\widetilde{\sigma}_{eRV}^{\text{CCM}} = \Delta p_e\widetilde{I} + \widetilde{\sigma}_{eV}^{d\,\text{CCM}}, \qquad (4)$$

where $\Delta p_e = -\gamma_e(\vec{\nabla} \cdot \vec{n})$ is an isotropic part of the cell normal stress (expressed by the Young–Laplace equation), $\vec{n}$ is the normal vector to the surface, and $\tilde{\boldsymbol{\sigma}}_{e\boldsymbol{V}}{}^{d\,\mathrm{CCM}}$ is the deviatoric part of the normal stress caused by CCM. The shear residual stress $\tilde{\boldsymbol{\sigma}}_{e\boldsymbol{R}\,\boldsymbol{S}}{}^{\mathrm{CCM}}$ of the epithelial cells is generated by natural convection and forced convection. The natural convection part is a consequence of the establishment of a surface tension gradient at the biointerface between migrating epithelial clusters and the surrounding epithelial cells found in a resting state, while the forced convection part is the consequence of CCM. This formulation is supported by the fact that the surface tension of active (migrating) epithelial cells is larger than the surface tension of passive (resting) epithelial cells [7]. The gradient $\vec{\nabla}\gamma_e$ guides the shear flow from the regions of lower surface tension to the regions of higher surface tension. The phenomenon represents the Marangoni effect which has been recognised within various soft matter systems. The surface tension gradient, in these systems, can be established by a change in temperature or a change in the distribution of system constituents [52]. In contrast, the surface tension gradient in multicellular systems is caused by the cellular contractility and the state of cell–cell adhesion contacts [7]. The surface tension gradient influences the shear flow by natural convection. Consequently, the cell shear residual stress caused by CCM can be expressed as

$$\vec{n} \cdot \tilde{\boldsymbol{\sigma}}_{e\boldsymbol{R}\ \boldsymbol{S}} \cdot \vec{t} = \vec{\nabla}\gamma_e \cdot \vec{t} + \vec{n} \cdot \tilde{\boldsymbol{\sigma}}_{e\boldsymbol{R}\ \boldsymbol{S}}{}^{\boldsymbol{F}} \cdot \vec{t}, \tag{5}$$

where $\vec{t}$ is the tangent vector to the surface, $\vec{\nabla}\gamma_e \cdot \vec{t}$ is the part of shear stress generated by natural convection, and $\tilde{\boldsymbol{\sigma}}_{e\boldsymbol{R}\ \boldsymbol{S}}{}^{\boldsymbol{F}}$ is the cell shear residual stress generated by the forced convection.

The viscoelastic force for the epithelial cells is equal to $\vec{\boldsymbol{F}}_{\boldsymbol{Tve}}{}^{e} = \vec{\nabla} \cdot (\tilde{\boldsymbol{\sigma}}_{e\boldsymbol{R}\boldsymbol{T}})$ (where $\tilde{\boldsymbol{\sigma}}_{e\boldsymbol{R}\boldsymbol{T}}$ is the total residual stress equal to $\tilde{\boldsymbol{\sigma}}_{e\boldsymbol{R}\boldsymbol{T}} = \tilde{\boldsymbol{\sigma}}_{e\boldsymbol{R}}{}^{\mathrm{CCM}} + \tilde{\boldsymbol{\sigma}}_{e\boldsymbol{R}}{}^{\mathrm{SD}}$, $\tilde{\boldsymbol{\sigma}}_{e\boldsymbol{R}}{}^{\mathrm{CCM}}$ is the cell residual stress (shear and normal) accumulated during CCM, and $\tilde{\boldsymbol{\sigma}}_{e\boldsymbol{R}}{}^{\mathrm{SD}}$ is the solid stress already present in the core region of two-spheroid systems) [47, 53]. The competition between these two forces induces oscillatory changes in cell velocity and the geometry of two-spheroid systems, such as oscillatory rate of neck radius change accompanied with oscillatory rate of volume and surface change [47]. These oscillatory changes of cell velocity accompanied with the relevant rheological parameters such as cell strain and corresponding cell residual stress, in the form of mechanical waves, have been also recognised during 2D CCM of epithelial monolayers [12, 15, 17] and during the cell aggregate rounding after uni-axial compression between parallel plates [47]. The force balance has been expressed by modifying the model proposed by Pajic-Lijakovic and Milivojevic as [12]

$$\langle m \rangle_e n_e(r,\tau) \frac{D\vec{v}_e(r,\tau)}{D\tau} = n_e \vec{F}_{st}^{\ e} - \vec{F}_{Tve}^{\ e}, \tag{6}$$

where τ is the time scale of hours, $\langle m \rangle_e$ is the average mass of a single epithelial cell, $\vec{v}_e$ is the epithelial cell velocity equal to $\vec{v}_e(r,\tau) = \frac{d\vec{u}_e}{d\tau}$, $\frac{D\vec{v}_e}{D\tau} = \frac{\partial \vec{v}_e}{\partial \tau} + (\vec{v}_e \cdot \vec{\nabla})\vec{v}_e$ is the material derivative [54], and $n_e(r,\tau)$ is the epithelial cell packing density.

The cell packing density change was formulated by Murray *et al.* [53] and Pajic-Lijakovic and Milivojevic [55] as

$$\frac{\partial n_e(r,\tau)}{\partial \tau} = -\vec{\nabla} \cdot \vec{J}, \tag{7}$$

where $\vec{J}$ is the flux of cells equal to $\vec{J} = \vec{J}_{conv} + \vec{J}_{cond} + \sum_i \vec{J}_i$, such that $\vec{J}_{conv} = n_e \vec{v}_e$ is the convective flux, $\vec{v}_e$ is cell velocity, $\vec{J}_{cond} = -D_{eff}\vec{\nabla}n_e$ is the conductive flux, D_{eff} is the effective diffusion coefficient, $\vec{J}_i = k_i n_e \vec{\nabla}\phi_i$ are chemotaxis fluxes such that $\phi \equiv c$ is the concentration of nutrients for the chemotaxis, the Marangoni flux such that $\phi \equiv \gamma_e$ is the surface tension of the epithelium, while k_i are the model parameters which account for various types of interactions, such as mechanical or chemical. The other type of fluxes can be neglected for the case of epithelial spheroid fusion. The Marangoni flux drive cell spreading from the region of lower surface tension (i.e., epithelial cells in resting state) to the regions of higher surface tension (i.e., migrating epithelial clusters) [55].

4.1.1. *Volumetric free energy increase caused by the work of the tissue surface tension*

Tissue surface tension exerts work on reducing the surface $W_A(\tau)$ during the fusion of two epithelial spheroids equal to

$$\frac{dW_A(\tau)}{d\tau} = -\gamma_e \frac{dA}{d\tau}, \tag{8}$$

where the rate of surface change is equal to $\frac{dA}{d\tau} = 2\pi r_N \frac{dr_N}{d\tau}$. This energy is stored within the contact between two spheroids and also within the spheroids' core regions. This process is caused by the work of CCM which is directed from the surface region to the core region of two-spheroid system. The CCM of epithelial cells induces storage of elastic energy within the core region of two-spheroid system expressed as

$$\frac{dW_A(\tau)}{d\tau} = \frac{d}{d\tau} \int_{\Delta V} \frac{1}{2} \widetilde{\sigma}_{eRV}^{CCM} : \widetilde{\varepsilon}_{eV} \, d^3r \Delta V. \tag{9}$$

It is in accordance with their rheological behaviour. Consequently, an increase in number of cells in the core region N_V accompanied with an increase in the storage energy caused by CCM lead to an increase in the volumetric free energy density $F_V(\tau)$. The resulted energy balance is expressed as

$$\frac{dF_V(\tau)}{d\tau} = \frac{d}{d\tau} \int_{\Delta V} \frac{1}{2} \widetilde{\sigma}_{eRV}^{CCM} : \widetilde{\varepsilon}_{eV} \, d^3r + \left(\frac{\partial F_V}{\partial N_V} \right)_{T_{\text{eff}}} \frac{dN_V}{d\tau}, \tag{10}$$

where N_V is the number of cells in the core region of two-spheroid system, $\left(\frac{\partial F_V}{\partial N_V} \right)_{T_{\text{eff}}}$ is the effective chemical potential of epithelial cells, and T_{eff} is the effective temperature. The concept of effective temperature has been applied for describing a rearrangement of various thermodynamic systems from glasses and sheared fluids to granular systems [56]. Pajic-Lijakovic and Milivojevic applied [33, 46] this concept to a long-time rearrangement of dense cellular systems. The effective temperature, in this case, represents a product of cell mobility and has been expressed as $(k_B T_{\text{eff}})^{1/2} \sim \langle |\vec{v}_c| \rangle$ (where $\langle |\vec{v}_c| \rangle$ is the cell average speed).

An increase in the cell compressive residual stress induces an increase in the cell packing density and can change the state of viscoelasticity, as well as the mechanism of epithelial cell migration by switching from convective through conductive (diffusion) mechanism to the damped-conductive (sub-diffusion) mechanism and reaching out the cell jamming state [57]. Three viscoelastic regimes are distinguished in this case:

(1) convective regime for the cell velocities $\vec{v}_c > 0.1 \frac{\mu m}{min}$,
(2) conductive (diffusion) regime for the cell velocities $\vec{v}_c \sim D_{\text{eff}} \frac{1}{L_{cmax}}$ (where D_{eff} is the effective diffusion coefficient

which depends on the cell packing density and corresponds to $\sim 10^{-1} \frac{\mu m^2}{min}$ [58], while L_{cmax} is the maximum velocity correlation length equal to $L_{max} \sim 150\,\mu m$ [59]) which corresponds to the velocities in the range of $\vec{v}_c \sim 10^{-3} - 10^{-2} \frac{\mu m}{min}$, and

(3) damped-conductive (sub-diffusion) regime which includes two sub-regimes, i.e., the transition and jamming sub-regimes [57].

The cell velocities $\vec{v}_c > 0.1 \frac{\mu m}{min}$ are recognised during CCM of various model systems such as (1) free expansion of MDCK and MCF-10A cell monolayers [15, 16] (2) rearrangement of confluent MDCK cell monolayers [17], and (3) cell aggregate micropipette aspiration [14]. These systems corresponds to (1) the Maxwell model (for viscoelastic liquids) for the cell velocities $\vec{v}_c \geq 1 \frac{\mu m}{min}$ and (2) the Zener model (for viscoelastic solids) for the cell velocities $0.1 \frac{\mu m}{min} < \vec{v}_c < 1 \frac{\mu m}{min}$.

In contrast to convective regime described by the Zener model, the main characteristic of conductive regime is that stress cannot relax, while cell rearrangement occurs via diffusion mechanism. The diffusion process is characterised by the linear relationship between the mean square displacement and time, i.e., $\langle r^2(\tau) \rangle \sim \tau$. The constitutive model which satisfies these two conditions is the Kelvin–Voigt model expressed as $\widetilde{\boldsymbol{\sigma}}_{ei}(r,\tau)^{\mathrm{CCM}} = G_i \widetilde{\boldsymbol{\varepsilon}}_{ei}(r,\tau) + \eta_i \dot{\widetilde{\boldsymbol{\varepsilon}}}_{ei}(r,\tau)$ $(\widetilde{\boldsymbol{\sigma}}_{ei}(r,\tau)^{\mathrm{CCM}}$ (where $\widetilde{\boldsymbol{\sigma}}_{ei}$ is the epithelial cell shear or normal stress and $\widetilde{\boldsymbol{\varepsilon}}_{ei}$ is the corresponding strain).

The cell movement in the damped-conductive regime corresponds to the sub-diffusion mechanism which is nonlinear, i.e., $\langle r^2(\tau) \rangle \sim \tau^\alpha$ (where α is the scaling parameter, i.e., the damping coefficient, which satisfies the condition $0 < \alpha < 1$). This nonlinearity in the mechanism of cell movement influences the nonlinear rheological behaviour of cell collectives which is expressed by the fractional model $\widetilde{\boldsymbol{\sigma}}_{ei}(r,\tau)^{\mathrm{CCM}} = \eta_{\alpha i} D^\alpha(\widetilde{\boldsymbol{\varepsilon}}_{ei})$ (where $D^\alpha \widetilde{\boldsymbol{\varepsilon}}(r,\tau) = \frac{d^\alpha \widetilde{\varepsilon}(r,\tau)}{d\tau^\alpha}$ is the fractional derivative and $\eta_{\alpha i}$ is the effective modulus). Caputo's definition of the fractional derivative of a function $\widetilde{\varepsilon}(r,\tau)$ was used, and it is given as $D^\alpha \widetilde{\varepsilon} = \frac{1}{\Gamma(1-\alpha)} \frac{d}{d\tau} \int_0^\tau \frac{\widetilde{\varepsilon}(r,\tau')}{(\tau-\tau')^\alpha} d\tau'$ (where $\Gamma(1-\alpha)$ is a gamma function) [60]. The transient sub-regime corresponds to a condition $\vec{v}_c \to 0$ and the parameter $\alpha = 0.5$, while for the jamming sub-regime, the cell velocity is equal to zero and the parameter α is in the range of $0 < \alpha < 0.5$. The cell packing density is approximately the same for both sub-regimes [51].

4.2. The constitutive behaviour of two cancer spheroids in contact during fusion

While the rearrangement of epithelial MCF-10A cell spheroids occurs mainly through cadherin-mediated adhesion complexes, the rearrangement of MDA-MB-157, MDA-MB-231, and MDA-MB-436 cell spheroids occurs mainly through $\beta1$ integrin-mediated adhesion complexes [7]. The CCM of these cell types corresponds to coordinated movement of cell streams and behaves as viscoelastic liquid [7,61]. The Maxwell model has been proposed to describe such kind of migration [14,33]. It is expressed as

$$\tilde{\sigma}_{ci}(r, t_s, \tau) + \tau_{Ri}\,\dot{\tilde{\sigma}}_{ci}(r, t_s, \tau) = \eta_i \dot{\tilde{\varepsilon}}_{ci}(r, \tau), \qquad (11)$$

where $i \equiv S, V, S$ is the shear change, V is the volumetric change, $\tilde{\sigma}_{ci}$ is the shear or normal stress of cancer cells, $\dot{\tilde{\sigma}}_{ci} = \frac{d\tilde{\sigma}_{ci}}{dt_s}$, η_i is the shear or volumetric viscosity, τ_{Ri} is the corresponding stress relaxation time, $\dot{\tilde{\varepsilon}}_{ci} = \frac{d\tilde{\varepsilon}_{ci}}{d\tau}$ is the strain rate, $\tilde{\varepsilon}_{ci}$ is the cancer shear or volumetric strain equal to $\tilde{\varepsilon}_{cS} = \frac{1}{2}\left(\vec{\nabla}\vec{u}_c + \vec{\nabla}\vec{u}_c^T\right)$, $\tilde{\varepsilon}_{cV} = (\vec{\nabla}\cdot\vec{u}_c)\tilde{I}$, respectively, and $\vec{u}_c$ is the cancer cell displacement field caused by CCM. Stress relaxation under constant strain rate $\dot{\tilde{\varepsilon}}_{c0i}$ per single short-time relaxation cycle can be expressed starting from the initial condition $\tilde{\sigma}_{ci}(r, t_s = 0, \tau) = \tilde{\sigma}_{c0i}$ as

$$\tilde{\sigma}_{ci}(r, t_s, \tau) = \tilde{\sigma}_{c0i}e^{-\frac{t_s}{\tau_{Ri}}} + \tilde{\sigma}_{cRi}(r, \tau)^{\text{CCM}}\left(1 - e^{-\frac{t_s}{\tau_{Ri}}}\right), \qquad (12)$$

where $\tilde{\sigma}_{cRi}(r, \tau)^{\text{CCM}}$ is the cancer cell residual stress, which is purely dissipative and equal to $\tilde{\sigma}_{cRi}(r, \tau)^{\text{CCM}} = \eta_i \dot{\tilde{\varepsilon}}_{c0i}$. The cell shear residual stress is equal to $\tilde{\sigma}_{cRS}^{\text{CCM}} \approx \tilde{\sigma}_{cRS}^{F}$ (where $\tilde{\sigma}_{cRS}^{F}$ is the shear stress that results from the forced convection). The normal residual stress of cancer cells is $\tilde{\sigma}_{RV}^{\text{CCM}} \approx \tilde{\sigma}_{cV}^{d}$ (where $\tilde{\sigma}_{cV}^{d}$ is the deviatoric part of the stress). The main characteristics of the Maxwell model is dominant elastic behaviour at short-time scale and (dissipative) viscous behaviour at long-time scale [51].

While the accumulated stress within the spheroid core region reduces movement of epithelial MCF-10A cells, it stimulates movement of cancer 4T1, MDA-MB-231, and 67NR cells [24]. Consequently, the viscoelastic force as a product of the cell residual stress distribution within the core region of two-spheroid systems acts as (1) a resistive force for the CCM of epithelial cells and (2) a driving force for the CCM of cancer cells. The viscoelastic force in this case is equal to $\vec{F}_{Tve}^{c} = \vec{\nabla} \cdot (\tilde{\sigma}_{cR}{}^{SD} - \tilde{\sigma}_{R\,ECM})$ (where $\tilde{\sigma}_{cR}{}^{SD}$ is the cancer cell solid stress, while the cell residual stress caused by CCM $\tilde{\sigma}_{cR}{}^{CCM}$ is dissipated, and $\tilde{\sigma}_{R\,ECM}$ is the residual stress accumulated within ECM) [12]. Driven by the viscoelastic force, cancer cells migrate from the core region towards the surface region of two-spheroid system. The surface tension of active (contractile) cancer cells is significantly reduced due to cell–cell repulsions [7]. Consequently, the surface tension force can be neglected. Besides the viscoelastic force, the traction force also influences movement of cancer cells. It is in accordance with the fact that cancer cells establish integrin-mediated FAs as the one of main mechanism of cell movement [7]. Strength of FAs can reduce cell movement [62]. Consequently, the cumulative effects of the dynamics of FAs arise in the form of the traction force capable of reducing cell movement. The traction force is expressed as $\rho\vec{F}_{tr}{}^{c} = \rho k \vec{u}_{ECM}$ (where k is an elastic constant of single FA, ρ is the number density of FAs, and $\vec{u}_{ECM}$ is the displacement field of ECM caused by movement of cancer cells) [53]. The movement of cancer cells is induced by the competition between these two forces, i.e., the viscoelastic force and the traction force, which leads to the oscillatory change of cell velocity and the geometry of two-spheroid systems such as the oscillatory rate of neck radius change accompanied with the oscillatory rate of volume and surface change [47]. These oscillations represent the mechanical waves, induced by CCM, which have been recognised in various cellular model systems. Corresponding force balance can be expressed by modified the model proposed by Pajic-Lijakovic and Milivojevic as [12]

$$\langle m \rangle_{c} n_{c}(r, \tau) \frac{D\vec{v}_{c}(r, \tau)}{D\tau} = \vec{F}_{Tve}{}^{c} - \rho\vec{F}_{tr}{}^{c}, \qquad (13)$$

where $\langle m \rangle_{c}$ is the average mass of a single cancer cell, $n_{c}(r, \tau)$ is the cancer cell packing density, and ρ is the local number density of FAs. Corresponding change of cancer cell packing density occurs primarily by convective flux.

4.2.1. Surface activity of cancerous cells: A decrease in the volumetric free energy density during the fusion

The scenario of the two cancer cell spheroids fusion is quite different in comparison with the fusion of epithelial spheroids. While the surface and volume decrease during the fusion of epithelial spheroids, the fusion of cancer spheroids leads to an increase in the surface and volume of two cancer spheroid system driven by the accumulated solid stress [47]. This increase leads to a decrease in the volumetric free energy density F_V of two cancer spheroid system vs. time, i.e., $\frac{dF_V}{d\tau}$. While the volumetric free energy decreases, the surface free energy increases, i.e., $\frac{dF_V}{d\tau} = -\frac{dF_A}{d\tau}$ (where F_A is the surface free energy density). A decrease in the free energy F_V represents a consequence of the energy dissipation caused by CCM of cancer cells $\dot{W}_D(\tau) = \int_{\Delta V} \frac{1}{2} \tilde{\boldsymbol{\sigma}}_{\boldsymbol{cRV}}{}^{\text{CCM}} : \dot{\tilde{\boldsymbol{\varepsilon}}}_{\boldsymbol{cV}} \, d^3 r$ and a decrease in the number of cells in the core region of two-spheroid system N_V. While the CCM of epithelial cells induces energy storage, the CCM of cancer cells is a purely diffusive process. It is in accordance with their rheological behaviour. The energy balance can be expressed as

$$\frac{dF_V}{d\tau} = -\dot{W}_D - \left(\frac{\partial F_V}{\partial N_V}\right)_{T_{\text{eff}}} \frac{dN_V}{d\tau}, \tag{14}$$

where $\dot{W}_D(\tau)$ is the energy dissipation caused by CCM of cancer cells. The main cause of establishing the different scenario in cell rearrangement during the cancer spheroid fusion in comparison with the fusion of two epithelial spheroid systems is related to a decrease in the surface tension of contractile cancer cells.

5. Conclusion

The surface activity of cancer cells is estimated by considering the simple model system, such as the fusion of two cell spheroids. While the fusion of epithelial cell spheroids, driven by the tissue surface tension, leads to a decrease in the surface and volume of two-spheroid systems, the fusion of cancer cell spheroids follows quite different scenario. The surface tension of epithelial cells exerts work on increasing the cell residual stress accumulated in the core region of two-spheroid systems, as well as the volumetric free energy density. The increase in the volumetric free energy is a product of energy storage caused by CCM and an increase in the number of cells in the core region of the two epithelial spheroid systems. While epithelial cells establish stronger E-cadherin-mediated cell–cell adhesion contacts, cancer cells form weak cell–cell adhesion contacts and β1-integrin-mediated cell–ECM adhesion contacts. Cellular contractions, significant in the spheroid surface region, generate repulsions among cancer cells which result in a decrease in the surface tension. Consequently, the surface tension of contractile cancer cells can be neglected. In the case of cancer cells, an increase in the surface and volume of two-spheroid system during fusion is driven by the solid stress accumulated within a core region of the two-spheroid system. While the accumulated stress stimulates movement of cancer cells, it reduces movement of the epithelial cells. Consequently, the solid stress directs the movement of cancer cells from the core region of two-spheroid system towards its surface. In contrast to CCM of epithelial cells, the CCM of cancer cells is a purely dissipative process at a long-time scale, described by the Maxwell model. This movement induces a decrease in the solid stress and the number of cells in the core region of two-spheroid system and on that base a decrease in the volumetric free energy density while the free energy of surface increases.

While the epithelial cells perform the volumetric cell rearrangement induced by decreasing in the surface and can undergo jamming state transition, cancer cells perform the surface rearrangement and on that base avoid the cell jamming. The origin of this interesting phenomenon lays in the ability of cancer cells to reduce the tissue surface tension and behave as surface active constituents.

Acknowledgement

This work was supported by the Ministry of Education, Science and Technological Development of the Republic of Serbia (Contract No. 451-03-68/2022-14/200135).

References

[1] A. G. Clark and D. M. Vignjevic, Models of cancer cell invasion and the rule of microenvironment, *Current Opinion in Cell Biology.* **36**, 13–22 (2015).

[2] A. Gandalovičová, T. Vomastek, D. Rosel, and J. Brábek, Cell polarity signaling in the plasticity of cancer cell invasiveness, *Oncotarget.* **7**(18), 25022–25049 (2016).

[3] H. Kubitschke, E. Blauth, P. Gottheil, S. Grosser, and J. Kaes, Jamming in embryogenesis and cancer progression, *Frontiers in Physics* (2021). doi: 10.3389/fphy.2021.666709.

[4] D. Hanahan and R. A. Weinberg, Hallmarks of cancer: The next generation, *Cell.* **144**, 646–674 (2011).

[5] M. Kalli and T. Stylianopoulos, Defining the role of solid stress and matrix stiffness in cancer cell proliferation and metastasis, *Frontiers in Oncology* (2018). doi: 10.3389/fonc.2018.00055.

[6] M. E. Dolega, M. Delarue, F. Ingremeau, J. Prost, A. Delon, and G. Cappello, Cell-like pressure sensors reveal increase of mechanical stress towards the core of multicellular spheroids under compression, *Nature Communications.* **8**, 1–9 (2017). Article number 14056.

[7] A. J. Devanny, M. B. Vancura, and L. J. Kaufman, Exploiting differential effects of actomyosin contractility to control cell sorting among breast cancer cells, *Molecular Biology of the Cell* (2021). doi: doi.org/10.1091/mbc.E21-07-0357.

[8] S. Raghuraman, A.-S. Schubert, S. Bröker, A. Jurado, A. Müller, M. Brandt, *et al.*, Pressure drives rapid burst-like coordinated cellular motion from 3D cancer aggregates, *Advanced Science.* **9**(6), e2104808 (2022).

[9] R. Z. Lin, L. F. Chou, C. C. M. Chien, and H. Y. Chang, Dynamic analysis of hepatoma spheroid formation: Roles of E-cadherin and β1-integrin, *Cell and Tissue Research.* **324**, 411–422 (2006).

[10] F. Tian, T. C. Lin, L. Wang, S. Chen, X. Chen, P. M. Yiu, *et al.*, Mechanical responses of breast cancer cells to substrates of varying stiffness revealed by single-cell measurements, *The Journal of Physical Chemistry Letters.* **11**, 7643–7649 (2021).

[11] G. Petrungaro, L. Morelli, and K. Uriu, Information flow in the presence of cell mixing and signaling delays during embryonic development, *Seminars in Cell & Developmental Biology.* **93**, 26–35 (2019).

[12]   I. Pajic-Lijakovic and M. Milivojevic, Mechanical oscillations in 2D collective cell migration: The elastic turbulence, *Frontiers in Physics* (2020). doi: 10.3389/fphy.2020.585681.

[13]   P. Marmottant, A. Mgharbel, J. Kafer, B. Audren, J. P. Rieu, J. C. Vial, *et al.*, The role of fluctuations and stress on the effective viscosity of cell aggregates, *PNAS.* **106**(41), 17271–17275 (2009).

[14]   K. Guevorkian, D. Gonzalez-Rodriguez, C. Carlier, S. Dufour, and F. Brochard-Wyart, Mechanosensitive shivering of model tissues under controlled aspiration, *PNAS.* **108**(33), 13387–13392 (2011).

[15]   X. Serra-Picamal, V. Conte, R. Vincent, E. Anon, D. T. Tambe, E. Bazellieres, *et al.*, Mechanical waves during tissue expansion, *Nature Physics.* **8**(8), 628–634 (2012).

[16]   K. D. Nnetu, M. Knorr, J. Kaes, and M. Zink, The impact of jamming on boundaries of collectively moving weak-interacting cells, *New Journal of Physics.* **14**, 115012 (2012).

[17]   J. Notbohm, S. Banerjee, K. J. C. Utuje, B. Gweon, H. Jang, Y. Park, *et al.*, Cellular contraction and polarization drive collective cellular motion, *Biophysical Journal.* **110**(12), 2729–2738 (2016).

[18]   I. Pajic-Lijakovic and M. Milivojevic, Long-time viscoelasticity of multicellular surfaces caused by collective cell migration — multi-scale modeling considerations, *Seminars in Cell & Developmental Biology.* **93**, 87–96 (2019).

[19]   E. Fabiano, J. Zhang, and C. Reinhart-King, Tissue density in the progression of breast cancer: Bedside to bench and back again, *Current Opinion in Biomedical Engineering* (2022). doi.org/10.1016/j.cobme.2022.100383.

[20]   I. Kosztin, G. Vunjak-Novakovic, and G. Forgacs, Colloquium: Modeling the dynamics of multicellular systems: Application to tissue engineering, *Reviews of Modern Physics.* **84**(4), 1791–1805 (2012).

[21]   A. Shafiee, M. McCune, G. Forgacs, and I. Kosztin, Post-deposition bioink self-assembly: A quantitative study, *Biofabrication.* **7**, 045005 (2015).

[22]   G. Dechristé, J. Fehrenbach, E. Griseti, V. Lobjois, and C. Poignar, Viscoelastic modeling of the fusion of multicellular tumor spheroids in growth phase, *Journal of Theoretical Biology.* **454,** 102–109 (2018).

[23]   S. Grosser, J. Lippoldt, L. Oswald, M. Merkel, D. M. Sussman, F. Renner, *et al.*, Cell and nucleus shape as an indicator of tissue fluidity in carcinoma, *Physical Review X.* **11**, 011033 (2021).

[24]   J. M. Tse, G. Cheng, J. A. Tyrrell, S. A. Wilcox-Adelman, Y. Boucher, R. K. Jain, *et al.*, Mechanical compression drives cancer cells toward invasive phenotype, *PNAS.* **109**(3), 911–949 (2012).

[25] B. D. Riehl, E. Kim, J. S. Lee, B. Duan, R. Yang, H. J. Donahue *et al.*, The role of fluid shear and metastatic potential in breast cancer cell migration, *The Journal of Biomechanical Engineering.* **142**, 101001 (2020).

[26] D. Mohammed, C. Y. Park, J. J. Fredberg, and D. A. Weitz, Tumorigenic mesenchymal clusters are less sensitive to moderate osmotic stresses due to low amounts of junctional E-cadherin, *Scientific Reports.* **11**, 16279 (2021).

[27] A. Guzman, R. C. Avard, A. J. Devanny, O. S. Kweon, and L. J. Kaufman, Delineating the role of membrane blebs in a hybrid mode of cancer cell invasion in three-dimensional environments, *Journal of Cell Science.* **133**, jcs236778 (2020).

[28] D. A. Rudzka, G. Spennati, D. J. McGarry, Y. H. Chim, M. Neilson, A. Ptak, *et al.*, Migration through physical constraints is enabled by MAPK induced cell softening via actin cytoskeleton re-organization, *Journal of Cell Science.* **132**, jcs224071 (2019).

[29] B. D. Riehl, E. Kim, T. Bouzid, and Y. J. Lim, The role of microenvironmental cues and mechanical loading milieus in breast cancer cell progression and metastasis, *Frontiers in Bioengineering and Biotechnology.* **8**, 608526 (2021).

[30] R. Omidvar, M. Tafazzoli-shadpour, M. A. Shokrgozar, and M. Rostami, Atomic force microscope-based single cell force spectroscopy of breast cancer cell lines: An approach for evaluating cellular invasion, *Journal of Biomechanics.* **47**, 3373–3379 (2014).

[31] M. S. Yousafzai, G. Coceano, A. Mariutti, F. Ndoye, L. Amin, J. Niemela, *et al.*, Effect of neighboring cells on cell stiffness measured by optical tweezers indentation, *Journal of Biomedical Optics.* **21**(5), 057004 (2016).

[32] S. Mondal, M. Phukan and A. Ghatak, Estimation of solid–liquid interfacial tension using curved surface of a soft solid, *PNAS.* **112**(41), 12563–12568 (2015).

[33] I. Pajic-Lijakovic and M. Milivojevic, Multiscale nature of cell rearrangement caused by collective cell migration, *European Biophysics Journal.* **50**, 1–14 (2021).

[34] T. V. Stirbat, A. Mgharbel, S. Bodennec, K. Ferri, H. C. Mertani, J. P. Rieu, *et al.*, Fine tuning of tissues' viscosity and surface tension through contractility suggests a new role for a-catenin, *PLOS One.* **8**(2), e52554 (2013).

[35] I. Pajic-Lijakovic and M. Milivojevic, Successive relaxation cycles during long-time cell aggregate rounding after uni-axial compression, *Journal of Biological Physics.* **43**, 197–209 (2017).

[36] J. C. M. Mombach, D. Robert, F. Graner, G. Gillet, G. L. Thomas, M. Idiart *et al.*, Rounding of aggregates of biological cells: Experiments and simulations, *Physica A.* **352**, 525–534 (2005).

[37] D. A. Beysens, G. Forgacs, and J. A. Glazier, Embryonic tissues are viscoelastic materials, *Canadian Journal of Physics.* **78**, 243–251 (2000).

[38] G. W. Brodland, J. Yang, and J. Sweny, Cellular interfacial and surface tensions determined from aggregate compression tests using a finite element model, *HFSP Journal.* **3**(4), 273–281 (2009).

[39] M. S. Hutson, G. W. Brodland, J. Yang, and D. Viens, Cell sorting in three dimensions: Topology, fluctuations, and fluidlike instabilities, *Physical Review Letters.* **101**, 148105 (2008).

[40] E. H. Barriga and R. Mayor, Adjustable viscoelasticity allows for efficient collective cell migration, *Seminars in Cell & Developmental Biology.* **93**, 55–68 (2019).

[41] T. S. Malinova and S. Huveneers, Sensing of cytoskeletal forces by asymmetric adherens junctions, *Trends in Cell Biology.* **28**(4), 328–341 (2018).

[42] A. Zuidema, W. Wang, and A. Sonnenberg, Crosstalk between cell adhesion complexes in regulation of mechanotransduction, *BioAssey.* **42**, 2000119 (2020).

[43] E. Warmt, S. Grosser, E. Blauth, X. Xie, H. Kubitschke, R. Stange, *et al.*, Differences in cortical contractile properties between healthy epithelial and cancerous mesenchymal cells, *New Journal of Physics* (2021). doi.org/10.1088/1367-2630/ac254e.

[44] D. Oriola, M. Marin-Riera, K. Anlas, N. Gritti, M. Matsumiya, G. Aalderink, *et al.*, Arrested coalescence of multicellular aggregates (2020). doi: https://arxiv.org/abs/2012.01455.

[45] X. Trepat, M. R. Wasserman, T. E. Angelini, E. Millet, D. A. Weitz, J. P. Butler, *et al.*, Physical forces during collective cell migration, *Nature Physics.* **5**, 426–430 (2009).

[46] I. Pajic-Lijakovic and M. Milivojevic, Jamming state transition and collective cell migration, *Journal of Biological Engineering.* **13**, 73 (2019).

[47] I. Pajic-Lijakovic and M. Milivojevic, Mechanical waves caused by collective cell migration: Generation, *European Biophysics Journal.* **51**(1), 1–13 (2022).

[48] C. Gongora, L. Candeil, N. Vezzio, V. Copois, V. Denis, C. Breil, *et al.*, Altered expression of cell proliferation-related and interferon-stimulated genes in colon cancer cells resistant to SN38, *Cancer Biology & Therapy.* **7**(6), 822–832 (2008).

[49] I. Pajic-Lijakovic and M. Milivojevic, Viscoelasticity of multicellular systems caused by collective cell migration: Dynamics at the biointerface, *European Biophysics Journal.* **49**, 253–265 (2020).

[50] I. Pajic-Lijakovic and M. Milivojevic, Collective cell migration and residual stress accumulation: Rheological consideration, *Journal of Biomechanics.* **108**, 109898 (2020).

[51] I. Pajic-Lijakovic, Chapter 2: Basic concept of viscoelasticity. In I. Pajic-Lijakovic and E. Barriga (eds.), *Viscoelasticity and Collective Cell Migration* (Academic Press, United States, 2021), p. 21.

[52] A. Karbalaei, R. Kumar, and H. J. Cho, Thermocapillarity in microfluidics—A review, *Micromachines.* **7**, 13 (2016).

[53] J. D. Murray, P. K. Maini, and R. T. Tranquillo, Mechanochemical models for generating biological pattern and form in development, *Physics Reports.* **171**(2), 59–84 (1988).

[54] R. B. Bird, W. E. Stewart, and E. N. Lightfoot, *Transport Phenomena* (John Wiley & Sons INC, New York, London, 1960), p. 84.

[55] I. Pajic-Lijakovic and M. Milivojevic, Marangoni effect and cell spreading, *European Biophysics Journal.* **51**, 419–429 (2022).

[56] J. Casas-Vazquez and D. Jou, Temperature in non-equilibrium states: A review of open problems and current proposals, *Reports on Progress in Physics.* **66**, 1937–2023 (2003).

[57] I. Pajic-Lijakovic and M. Milivojevic, Viscoelasticity and cell jamming state transition, *The European Physical Journal Plus.* **136**, 750 (2021).

[58] T. E. Angelini, E. Hannezo, X. Trepat, M. Marquez, J. J. Fredberg, and D. A. Weitz, Glass-like dynamics of collective cell migration, *PNAS.* **108**(12), 4714–4719 (2011).

[59] V. Petrolli, T. Boudou, M. Balland, and G. Cappello, Oscillations in collective cell migration. In I. Pajic-Lijakovic and E. Barriga (eds.), *Viscoelasticity and Collective Cell Migration: An Interdisciplinary Perspective across Levels of Organization* (Academic Press, US, 2021), p. 157.

[60] I. Podlubny, *Fractional Differential Equations.* Mathematics in Science and Engineering, Vol. 198 (Academic Press, London, 1999), p. 78.

[61] P. Friedl and S. Alexander, Cancer invasion and the microenvironment: Plasticity and reciprocity, *Cell.* **147**, 992–1009 (2011).

[62] S. S. Chang, A. D. Rape, S. A. Wong, W. Guo, and Y. Wang, Migration regulates cellular mechanical states, *Molecular Biology of the Cell.* **30**, 3104–3111 (2019).

Chapter 5

Modelling Cell Migration in Cancer Spread as a Response to Multi-Cue Heterogeneous Environments: A Kinetic Approach

Nadia Loy* and Martina Conte[†]

Politecnico di Torino,
Department of Mathematical Sciences "G. L. Lagrange",
Torino, Italy
*nadia.loy@polito.it
†martina.conte@polito.it

Understanding the microscopic mechanisms that influence cancer cell migration is a problem of utmost interest in cancer research, as these processes are responsible for the progression and dissemination of the tumour cells into the body. Cells perform directed motion in response to external stimuli, which they detect by sensing the environment. Precisely, cells have to sort and combine these different, and potentially competitive, stimuli, which can have both a biochemical and biophysical nature and characterise the multi-cue environment where cells move. In this chapter, we review a possible approach for the description and study of this problem, which is based on the classical kinetic equations implementing velocity-jump processes. We derive the kinetic models from the microscopic stochastic processes underlying the tactic mechanisms driving cell migration and we present three different cases of study, aimed at showing cell behaviour in response to different superposing stimuli.

1. Introduction

The initiation, progression, and metastasis of cancer are highly complex phenomena mainly due to the interaction of the cells with the external environment. In fact, the tumour microenvironment plays a fundamental role in tumour progression by means of the co-evolution of tumour cells and tumour stroma [1], which is the non-cancer cell component of the tumours' structure holding the tumour itself. The tumour stroma mainly consists of the basement membrane, fibroblasts, extracellular matrix, immune cells, and vasculature, and it plays a causative role during development, progression, and metastasis of cancer. As a consequence, the complex mechanisms of tumour progression with respect to the interactions with the external microenvironment are of the utmost interest. In particular, the key underlying process is cell migration in response to the external environment that is explored by the cell.

1.1. *Cell migration in multi-cue environments*

Cells sense the surrounding microenvironment by extending their protrusions. These measure biophysical and biochemical cues that bind to specific receptors on the cell's membrane. As a consequence, cells respond to these external stimuli by orienting their direction of motion towards specific targets and by adapting their migration strategy and speed. Specifically, it is possible to identify some factors that influence the direction of the cells and others that affect their speed. The response to directional stimuli is referred to as *taxis* and it results in the persistent migration in a certain preferential direction. An example of a biochemical cue is the concentration of soluble molecules in the extracellular space. This cue gives rise to *chemotaxis*, which is considered a *mono-directional* stimulus. Other cues generating mono-directional stimuli include electric fields (*electrotaxis*, or *galvanotaxis*), light signals (*phototaxis*), bound ligands to the substratum (*haptotaxis*), or the extracellular matrix (ECM) stiffness (*durotaxis*) [2]. In particular, the extracellular matrix, which is a major component of tumour stroma, plays a key regulator role. The ECM is characterised by a number of mechanical, biophysical, and chemical properties influencing cell migration [3,4], which is governed by the interplay between cell-generated propulsion forces, adhesion forces, and resisting forces arising from the steric hindrance properties of the matrix that influences cell adhesion and migration. As the most abundant constituent of ECM, collagen accounts for the major function of ECM, and either increased or decreased deposition of collagen can be associated with increased malignancy of a tumour [5,6]. Specifically, the alignment of the collagen fibres is shown to stimulate *contact guidance* [7,8], which is the tendency of cells to migrate by crawling on the fibres and following the directions imposed by them. Contact guidance is a *bidirectional* cue. In fact, if the fibres are not polarised, there is no preferential sense of motion along them. Concerning the speed, it generally depends on mechanical and biophysical properties of the ECM, such as stiffness, porosity, and collagen density. On a flat surface, migration speed decreases with matrix stiffness mainly due to the increased stability of focal adhesions. In a three-dimensional (3D) environment, cell migration has a biphasic nature as it is additionally impaired by the *steric hindrance* properties of the ECM that impose resisting forces to cell migration and can affect the cell's motility.

Therefore, each property of the ECM gives rise to certain cell migration responses and it is often difficult from the experimental point of view to decouple the different aspects in order to investigate the effect and role of each of them separately. However, understanding each single mechanism and its specific role in the overall dynamics is of the utmost interest. For instance, one of the most outstanding goals in the context of cancer spread and dissemination is the development of therapeutic strategies targeting specific mechanisms that play a crucial role in cancer cell invasion. Moreover, even when the cell's response to separate mechanisms is known, the cell's response to a multi-cue environment is much less understood. Some studies have shown how there can be competition or cooperation between these different stimuli. Thus, another fundamental issue concerns the way cells rank, integrate, or hierarchise them, especially when these stimuli are competing (e.g., when they are not co-aligned) [9].

1.2. *Kinetic models for cell migration*

Kinetic models are intrinsically multi-scale models. They allow starting from the microscopic description of the dynamics, including measurable parameters of the individual migration, and deriving a mesoscopic models in which cells' position and velocity, which follow the prescribed microscopic dynamics, are statistically described by a distribution function. The time evolution of this function is ruled by a kinetic transport equation with a turning operator that implements the defined microscopic dynamics. By introducing the moments of the distribution function, it is also possible to derive macroscopic formulations describing the overall dynamics of the system.

The paradigmatic dynamics of the individual migration of cells is the so-called run-and-tumble [10] that is a (generally) correlated random process in which cells alternate runs over straight lines and reorientations. Such microscopic dynamics is classically described through *velocity-jump processes* [11, 12]. These are microscopic Markovian processes that prescribe a *transition probability* T of choosing a new velocity and a *frequency of reorientation* μ, being, thus, $\frac{1}{\mu}$ the mean run time spent running on a linear tract between two consecutive reorientations. Kinetic equations implementing velocity jump processes are popularly used to model this cell migration mode called run-and-tumble.

Kinetic models implementing velocity jump processes [12] are linear transport equations that describe the evolution of a single-particle distribution function like in the Boltzmann equation [13]. Such single particle distribution gives the statistical description of the positions and velocities of the population that follows the prescribed microscopic dynamics. These models have been successfully applied to study cell migration on the ECM by contact guidance [14], binary interactions of cells migrating on a fibre network in the presence of a chemoattractant [15], tactic movement in non-locally sensed multi-cue environments [16,17], which may also include physical limits of migration [18], and in more specific studies about glioma invasion [19, 20]. Many of these papers derive the related macroscopic, usually diffusive, limits from mesoscopic settings and implement them numerically. In particular, the diffusive limit of velocity-jump processes has been deeply described in [14, 16, 21]. Moreover, kinetic equations have been proven to be very successful in modelling cell migration [14–16, 18, 22–28].

In this chapter, we present the general form of a kinetic transport equation implementing a velocity-jump process. Precisely, in the second section, we describe this equation and we show that it is possible to derive such kinetic models from microscopic stochastic processes and how to recover some of the main statistical properties of the system from the kinetic equations. Then, in the third section, we present class of models aimed at investigating the cell behaviour in response to different superposing stimuli. In all the proposed models, we take into account a non-local sensing of both cues since cells extend their protrusions in order to sense the environmental stimuli that determine the polarisation and speed of the cell. In particular, we shall present three case studies in order to describe specific phenomena: (i) chemotaxis and physical limits of migration, (ii) contact guidance and steric hindrance, and (iii) contact guidance and chemotaxis. After illustrating the specific phenomena and the processes in which they arise, we implement the individual dynamics of the cell in the microscopic model. In particular, these three cases correspond to (i) independent sensing of the cues affecting polarisation and speed, (ii) dependent sensing of the cues affecting polarisation and speed, and (iii) dependent sensing of a double directional cue affecting the polarisation. Then, the derived kinetic model will be used in order to present some numerical simulations regarding heterogeneous environments.

2. Kinetic Models for Velocity Jump Processes

2.1. *Transport kinetic equations*

A cell population may be described at a statistical level through a distribution function $p = p(t, \mathbf{x}, v, \hat{\mathbf{v}})$ parametrised by the time $t > 0$, the position $\mathbf{x} \in \Omega \subseteq \mathbb{R}^d$, the speed $v \in [0, U]$, where U is the maximal speed a cell can achieve, and the polarisation direction $\hat{\mathbf{v}} \in \mathbb{S}^{d-1}$, where $\mathbb{S}^{d-1}$ is the unit sphere boundary in $\mathbb{R}^d$. We shall denote the velocity space as $\mathcal{V} = [0, U] \times \mathbb{S}^{d-1}$. We here introduce the cell number density, or macroscopic density, as

$$\rho(t, \mathbf{x}) = \int_{\mathcal{V}} p(t, \mathbf{x}, v, \hat{\mathbf{v}}) \, dv \, d\hat{\mathbf{v}} \tag{1}$$

that is the average number of cells at location $\mathbf{x} \in \Omega$ at time $t > 0$. The kinetic model consists in the transport equation for the cell distribution function

$$\frac{\partial p}{\partial t}(t, \mathbf{x}, v, \hat{\mathbf{v}}) + \mathbf{v} \cdot \nabla p(t, \mathbf{x}, v, \hat{\mathbf{v}}) = \mathcal{J}[p](t, \mathbf{x}, v, \hat{\mathbf{v}}), \tag{2}$$

where the operator ∇ denotes the spatial gradient and the operator $\mathbf{v} \cdot \nabla$ describes the free particle drift, i.e., $\dot{\mathbf{x}} = \mathbf{v}$, where $\mathbf{v}$ is the microscopic velocity vector given by $\mathbf{v} = v\hat{\mathbf{v}}$. The term $\mathcal{J}[p](t, \mathbf{x}, v, \hat{\mathbf{v}})$, named *turning operator*, is an integral operator that describes the change in velocity which is due to interactions with the external environment that causes reorientations. In particular, in the present case, the turning operator implements a velocity-jump process in a kinetic transport equation [11, 12]. The velocity-jump process is described at the microscopic level by a Poisson process of parameter μ, that is the turning frequency, and by a transition probability T describing the choice of a new speed and direction after a reorientation. We assume that $\mu = \mu(\mathbf{x})$ may only depend on the spatial location, while the transition probability only depends on the chosen post-tumbling velocity given by the couple $(v, \hat{\mathbf{v}})$ and it may change in each spatial location $\mathbf{x} \in \Omega$. Being a transition probability, it satisfies

$$\int_V T(\mathbf{x}; v, \hat{\mathbf{v}}) \, dv d\hat{\mathbf{v}} = 1, \quad \forall \mathbf{x} \in \Omega. \tag{3}$$

The turning operator reads

$$\mathcal{J}[p](t, \mathbf{x}, v, \hat{\mathbf{v}}) = \mu(\mathbf{x}) \left(\rho(t, \mathbf{x}) T(\mathbf{x}; v, \hat{\mathbf{v}}) - p(t, \mathbf{x}, v, \hat{\mathbf{v}}) \right), \tag{4}$$

where we recognise the gain term $\mu(\mathbf{x})\rho(t, \mathbf{x})T(\mathbf{x}; v, \hat{\mathbf{v}})$ describing the fraction of cells acquiring as a new velocity $\mathbf{v} = v\hat{\mathbf{v}}$, while the term $-\mu(\mathbf{x})p(t, \mathbf{x}, v, \hat{\mathbf{v}})$ is related to cells that choose a new velocity after a re-orientation, different from the original one defined by the couple $(v, \hat{\mathbf{v}})$. As a consequence of (3), for any function T, the operator $\mathcal{J}[p]$ satisfies the property

$$\int_V \mathcal{J}[p](t, \mathbf{x}, v, \hat{\mathbf{v}}) \, dv \, d\hat{\mathbf{v}} = 0 \tag{5}$$

that expresses mass conservation for the reorientation process.

Moreover, equations (2)–(4) have to be coupled with an initial condition $p^0(\mathbf{x}, v, \hat{\mathbf{v}})$ having a fixed (normalised to 1) mass $\int_\Omega \int_V p^0(\mathbf{x}, v, \hat{\mathbf{v}}) \, dv \, d\hat{\mathbf{v}} \, d\mathbf{x} = 1$ and no-flux boundary conditions defined as

$$\int_V p(t, \mathbf{x}, v, \hat{\mathbf{v}}) \mathbf{v} \cdot \mathbf{n}(\mathbf{x}) d\hat{\mathbf{v}} \, dv = 0, \quad \forall \mathbf{x} \in \partial\Omega, \quad t > 0, \tag{6}$$

being $\mathbf{n}(\mathbf{x})$ the outward normal to the boundary at $\mathbf{x} \in \partial\Omega$. This allows obtaining conservation of the total mass in Ω for all $t > 0$ so that p is a probability density function (PDF) on $\Omega \times \mathcal{V}$ for all $t > 0$.

The modelling effort lies in the appropriate construction of the transition probability that may depend on the spatial location $\mathbf{x} \in \Omega$ as cells decide their new velocity as a consequence of a measure of the external environment. In fact, cells are capable of detecting and measuring external signals through membrane receptors located along cell protrusions that can extend over a finite radius. Information of both mechanical and chemical origins are then transduced and act as control factors for the dynamics of cells. Therefore, in the turning operator of the kinetic model, we will include the evaluation of mean fields in a neighbourhood of the reorientation position. In the following section, we shall show how to derive transition probabilities from a suitable microscopic process.

2.2. *Derivation from a microscopic stochastic process*

The kinetic model introduced in the previous section may be derived from a microscopic model describing the individual dynamics of the cells. In particular, the individual dynamics of a cell may be described by means of evolution equations for random variables taking into account the position $\mathbf{X}_t \in \Omega$, the speed $V_t \in [0, U]$, and the direction $\hat{\mathbf{V}}_t \in \mathbb{S}^{d-1}$ of a cell, whose joint distribution function is $p(t, \mathbf{X}_t = \mathbf{x}, V_t = v, \hat{\mathbf{V}}_t = \hat{v})$.

The reorientation mechanism related to the change of cell speed and direction may be described in terms of discrete in time stochastic processes [29] for the random variables V_t and $\hat{\mathbf{V}}_t$, which, during a time interval Δt, may change or not according to whether a reorientation happens or not. These dynamics may be implemented in a discrete in time random process as

$$\hat{\mathbf{V}}_{t+\Delta t} = (1 - \Sigma)\hat{\mathbf{V}}_t + \Sigma\hat{\mathbf{V}}_t',$$
$$V_{t+\Delta t} = (1 - \Sigma)V_t + \Sigma V_t', \tag{7}$$

where Σ is a Bernoulli random variable with parameter $\mu B(\mathbf{X}_t - \mathbf{Y}_t)\Delta t$, saying whether a reorientation, during which a cell changes both its direction and speed of motion, happens ($\Sigma = 1$) or not ($\Sigma = 0$). The quantity μ is the frequency of reorientation, while

B is the interaction kernel that governs the rate at which an agent in position $\mathbf{X}_t$ (in this case the cell) interacts with the surrounding environment, that is measured in $\mathbf{Y}_t$, and changes its velocity. This typically allows taking into account non-local interactions in the physical space, as this may be related to the non-local sensing that a cell performs though its protrusions. We remark that in order for Σ to be well defined, we need $\Delta t \leq 1/(\mu B(\mathbf{X}_t - \mathbf{Y}_t))$, which means that for a high frequency μ, there is a high probability of having a reorientation during a given time interval Δt. The random variables V_t' and $\hat{\mathbf{V}}_t'$ denote the new speed and direction after a reorientation. In order to recover the kinetic model (2)–(4), we must have that

$$(V_t', \hat{\mathbf{V}}_t') \sim T(\mathbf{X}_t; V_t' = v', \hat{\mathbf{V}}_t' = \hat{\mathbf{v}}'). \tag{8}$$

For the variation of the position $\mathbf{X}_t$ during a time interval Δt, we consider the kinematic relation given by

$$\mathbf{X}_{t+\Delta t} = \mathbf{X}_t + \Delta t \mathbf{V}_t. \tag{9}$$

Without intending to see the details of the formal derivation of the kinetic equation from the stochastic process (7)-(8)-(9), we mention that it relies on the evaluation of a test function φ of the observable quantities $v, \hat{\mathbf{v}}$. A limiting procedure [30] allows recovering the weak form of equations (2)–(4), that is,

$$\frac{d}{dt} \int_{\mathcal{V}} \varphi(v, \hat{\mathbf{v}}) p(t, \mathbf{x}, v, \hat{\mathbf{v}}) d\hat{\mathbf{v}} dv + \nabla_{\mathbf{x}} \cdot \int_{\mathcal{V}} \varphi(v, \hat{\mathbf{v}}) \mathbf{v} p(t, \mathbf{x}, v, \hat{\mathbf{v}}) d\hat{\mathbf{v}} \, dv$$

$$= \mu \int_{\mathcal{V}} \left[\int_{\mathcal{V}} T(\mathbf{x}; v', \hat{\mathbf{v}}') \varphi(v', \hat{\mathbf{v}}') \, d\hat{\mathbf{v}}' dv' - \varphi(v, \hat{\mathbf{v}}) \right] p(t, \mathbf{x}, v, \hat{\mathbf{v}}) d\hat{\mathbf{v}} \, dv. \tag{10}$$

2.3. *Statistical quantities*

An aggregate description for the cell population can be classically recovered through the definition of the statistical moments of the distribution function p. In particular, p is a PDF on $\Omega \times \mathcal{V}$, while for $\mathbf{x}$ fixed, the cell number density defined in (1) is not constant in time at a given location $\mathbf{x}$. Hence, in order to define statistical moments in each $\mathbf{x} \in \Omega$, we can consider the moments of the normalised population $\frac{p}{\rho}$ that is a PDF for $v, \hat{\mathbf{v}}$ for each $t > 0, \mathbf{x} \in \Omega$ fixed. Hence, we can define

- the cell mean velocity

$$\mathbf{U}(t, \mathbf{x}) = \frac{1}{\rho(t, \mathbf{x})} \int_{\mathcal{V}} p(t, \mathbf{x}, v, \hat{\mathbf{v}}) \mathbf{v} \, dv \, d\hat{\mathbf{v}}, \qquad (11)$$

- the cell variance–covariance matrix

$$\mathbb{D}(t, \mathbf{x}) = \frac{1}{\rho(t, \mathbf{x})} \int_{\mathcal{V}} p(t, \mathbf{x}, v, \hat{\mathbf{v}}) [\mathbf{v} - \mathbf{U}(t, \mathbf{x})] \otimes [\mathbf{v} - \mathbf{U}(t, \mathbf{x})] \, dv \, d\hat{\mathbf{v}}. \qquad (12)$$

Moreover, we can define the statistical moments of T that is a PDF on $\mathcal{V}$. In particular, we can define

- the mean outgoing velocity after a reorientation

$$\mathbf{U}_T(\mathbf{x}) = \int_{\mathcal{V}} T(\mathbf{x}; v, \hat{\mathbf{v}}) \mathbf{v} \, dv \, d\hat{\mathbf{v}}, \qquad (13)$$

- and the variance–covariance matrix of T

$$\mathbb{D}_T(\mathbf{x}) = \int_{\mathcal{V}} (\mathbf{v} - \mathbf{U}_T) \otimes (\mathbf{v} - \mathbf{U}_T) T(\mathbf{x}; v, \hat{\mathbf{v}}) \, dv \, d\hat{\mathbf{v}}. \qquad (14)$$

We observe that the distribution function nullifying the operator in (4) is simply

$$p(t, \mathbf{x}, v, \hat{\mathbf{v}}) = \rho(t, \mathbf{x}) T(\mathbf{x}; v, \hat{\mathbf{v}}), \qquad (15)$$

which, in general, is time dependent, but it may also be a stationary equilibrium state. As a consequence, at equilibrium, the cell population will have the average and variance–covariance matrix of T.

A relevant statistical quantity that can be defined in a reorientation process is the index of directional persistence [11]. For a microscopic velocity $\mathbf{v} = v\hat{\mathbf{v}}$ of a reorienting cell, one can define the index of directional persistence as

$$\psi_d(\mathbf{v}) = \frac{\mathbf{U}_T(\mathbf{x}) \cdot \hat{\mathbf{v}}}{|\mathbf{U}_T(\mathbf{x})|} \in [-1, 1]$$

that gives a measure of the reorientation angle for each given microscopic velocity $\hat{\mathbf{v}}$ from which a cell is reorienting, given that the average velocity of the reorientation process described by T is $\mathbf{U}_T$. In the present case, as T only depends on the post reorientation velocity, then we have that [11]

$$\mathbf{U}_T = \psi_d \hat{\mathbf{v}}.$$

Many other relevant statistical quantities may be introduced as the statistical moments of p over $\Omega \times \mathcal{V}$, such as the net displacement, the quadratic speed, and the mean squared displacement [11]. In particular, in the present setting in which T only depends on the new velocity, the evolution of the *mean squared displacement* (MSD), that is defined as

$$\mathcal{D}^2(t) := \langle ||\mathbf{x}^2|| \rangle = \int_{\mathbb{R}^n} \int_V ||\mathbf{x}||^2 p(t, \mathbf{x}, \mathbf{v}) \, d\mathbf{v} \, d\mathbf{x},$$

can be computed and it is equal to

$$\mathcal{D}^2(t) = \begin{cases} \dfrac{2S^2}{(1 - \psi_d)} \left[t - \dfrac{1}{\mu(\psi_d - 1)} \exp^{-\mu(1 - \psi_d)t} \right] & \text{if } \psi_d \neq 1, \\ S^2 t & \text{if } \psi_d = 1, \end{cases}$$

where $\mu_0 = (1 - \psi_d)\mu$ is the modified turning frequency, while $P = \frac{1}{\mu_0}$ is the persistence time on a given direction. Then, a diffusion (or motility) coefficient can be defined as $D := \frac{S^2 P}{d}$ in such a way that

$$\mathcal{D} = 2dD \left[t - \frac{1}{\mu_0}(1 - \exp^{-\mu_0 t}) \right].$$

3.   Case Studies

3.1.   *Independent cues*

3.1.1.   *Polarisation and physical limits of migration*

When migrating, the cell extends its protrusions in order to measure the cues in the external environment and decides its direction and speed of motion. From the physiological point of view, the decision process determining the new cell velocity can be split into two phases: first, the cell decides where to go and polarises and then it starts to move in that direction with a certain speed. These two processes are mainly independent and might be influenced by different chemical and mechanical cues. For example, gradients of chemical factors, ECM components, and ECM stiffness, all influence cell polarisation, while environment microstructure, availability of intracellular space and of adhesion sites, and expression of integrins, all influence cell speed. Specifically, a cell can be polarised without being able to move. This may happen, for example, in the case of cell migration on the ECM because of the presence of the so-called physical limits of migration that are linked to the presence of a too dense ECM, or, better, pores so small that a cell cannot squeeze and migrate through them. It is the case, for instance, of a cell that is encountering on its way a physical barrier, e.g., a basal membrane, and might be unable to squeeze through the fine net, but it can still extend cytoplasmic protrusions beyond the dense area [31]. In fact, cell cytoplasm is very flexible, but cell nucleus is much stiffer and its typical diameter might be larger than the ECM fibre spacing. As the pores' average size may be related to the ECM density, which we shall denote M, the mean speed may be expressed as a function of M [31]. In particular, it is found that there is an optimal matrix density M_{max} assuring the maximum possible speed and a threshold value M_{th}, which corresponds to a small pore size, that hampers the cell from moving in a certain direction [31]. Specifically, the dependence of the speed on the ECM pore size is linear, but the dependence of the density on the pore size is not [31] and the dependence of the speed on the ECM density has been shown to have a parabola-like behaviour [32].

3.1.2. *The mathematical model*

We shall consider a tactic gradient (e.g., a chemical) that affects the choice of the direction of a cell and, then, its polarisation. In particular, we shall denote

$$\mathcal{S} = \mathcal{S}(\mathbf{x}) : \Omega \longmapsto \mathbb{R}_+ \tag{16}$$

the external field affecting the taxis process, while

$$M = M(\mathbf{x}) : \Omega \longmapsto \mathbb{R}_+ \tag{17}$$

denotes the ECM density and, as mentioned in the previous paragraph, it affects the speed. As the two cues affect the polarisation and speed independently, we assume that, at the microscopic level, the stochastic process (7) is defined by $B = 1$ and

$$V_t' \sim \Psi[M(\mathbf{x})](V_t' = v'|\hat{\mathbf{v}}), \quad \hat{\mathbf{V}}_t' \sim \mathcal{B}[\mathcal{S}(\mathbf{x})](\hat{\mathbf{V}}_t' = \hat{\mathbf{v}}'), \qquad (18)$$

i.e., $\mathcal{S}$ affects the new polarisation direction $\hat{\mathbf{V}}_t'$, while Ψ affects the choice of the speed V_t' on a given direction of motion $\hat{\mathbf{v}}$. In particular, we shall consider that the choices of the direction and speed are a result of two independent non-local measures of the external fields $\mathcal{S}$ and M [18], as the cell extends its protrusions in order to sense the outer environment. In particular,

$$\mathcal{B}[\mathcal{S}(\mathbf{x})](\hat{\mathbf{v}}) := c_1(\mathbf{x}) \int_0^R \gamma_{\mathcal{S}}(\lambda)\mathcal{S}(\mathbf{x} + \lambda\hat{\mathbf{v}})d\lambda \qquad (19)$$

is a PDF that prescribes the direction of the post-reorientation velocity $\hat{\mathbf{v}}$ of a cell at position $\mathbf{x}$, c_1 being a normalisation function. In (19), the tactic cue $\mathcal{S}$ is sensed non-locally in each direction $\hat{\mathbf{v}}$ according to a sensing function $\gamma_{\mathcal{S}}$ and up to a maximum distance R from the centre of the cell, located at $\mathbf{x}$, named *sensing radius*. In particular, $\gamma_{\mathcal{S}}$ may be a Dirac delta centred in R if the cell only evaluates the information on the tip of the protrusion, while it may be a characteristic function if the cell weights uniformly the information up to the tip of the protrusion.

On the other hand,

$$\Psi[M(\mathbf{x})](v|\hat{\mathbf{v}}) := c_2(\mathbf{x}) \int_0^{R_M(\mathbf{x},\hat{\mathbf{v}})} \gamma_M(\lambda')\psi(v|M(\mathbf{x} + \lambda'\hat{\mathbf{v}}))\, d\lambda' \qquad (20)$$

is a PDF that prescribes the choice of the speed on a given direction $\hat{\mathbf{v}}$ of a cell located at $\mathbf{x}$, c_2 being a normalisation function. Here, $\psi(v|M)$ is the PDF of the possible speed v given a non-local measure of M in each direction $\hat{\mathbf{v}}$, i.e., $M(\mathbf{x} + \lambda'\hat{\mathbf{v}})$, weighted by a suitable sensing function γ_M. In particular, ψ has an average speed $\bar{v}(M)$ depending on M and a second moment D_M such that its variance is $D_M - \bar{v}(M)^2$. We shall consider a parabola-like behaviour of the speed given by [18, 32]

$$\bar{v}(M) = \bar{v}_0 + \frac{4(\bar{v}_M - \bar{v}_0)}{(M_{\text{th}} - M_0)^2}[(M - M_0)(M_{\text{th}} - M)]_+,$$

where M_{th} is the threshold value of the ECM density above which cells are not able to migrate as pores are too narrow, while $\bar{v}_M$ is the maximum speed possible achieved for $M_{max} = \frac{1}{2}(M_{th} + M_0)$. The value M_0 is the minimal value of ECM density allowing cells to migrate at a minimal speed $\bar{v}_0$. In (20), the quantity $R_M(\mathbf{x}, \hat{\mathbf{v}})$ is a modified sensing radius for the sensing function γ_M of the ECM density M that allows including physical limits of migration due to the ECM itself. This modified sensing radius is defined by assuming that a cell cannot measure the external cue M in a physical region that cannot be reached, namely in which the possible average speed vanishes. In particular, the ECM density M_{th} represents this physical limit and we shall consider the non-constant sensing radius defined by [18]

$$R_M(\mathbf{x}, \hat{\mathbf{v}}) = \begin{cases} R & \text{if } M(\mathbf{x} + \lambda\hat{\mathbf{v}}) \le M_{th} \quad \forall\lambda \in [0, R], \\ \inf\{\lambda \in [0, R] : M(\mathbf{x} + \lambda\hat{\mathbf{v}}) > M_{th}\} & \text{otherwise.} \end{cases}$$

(21)

In this case, a kinetic model (2)–(4) can be derived and the transition probability implementing the prescribed microscopic dynamics is [16, 18]

$$T[\mathcal{S}, M] = c(\mathbf{x})B[\mathcal{S}(\mathbf{x})]\hat{\mathbf{v}}\Psi[M(\mathbf{x})](v|\hat{\mathbf{v}}).$$

(22)

The latter has been shown to be able to describe physical limits of migration, thanks to the fact that the transition probability is actually an independent factorisation of a transition probability ($\mathcal{B}$) for the choice of the direction and of a transition probability (Ψ) for the choice of the speed.

3.1.3. *Numerical simulations*

As a title of example, we show a numerical simulation of the model (2)–(4) with (22)-(19)-(20)-(21). In particular, we consider a chemoattractant given by

$$\mathcal{S}(x, y) = \frac{m_{\mathcal{S}}}{\sqrt{2\pi\sigma_{\mathcal{S}}^2}}e^{-\frac{((x,y)-(x_{\mathcal{S}},y_{\mathcal{S}}))^2}{2\sigma_{\mathcal{S}}^2}},$$

(23)

with $(x_S, y_S) = (4, 4)$, $m_S = 10$, $\sigma_S^2 = 0.1$. The ECM density has an analogous profile

$$M(x, y) = \frac{m_M}{\sqrt{2\pi\sigma_M^2}} e^{-\frac{((x,y)-(x_M,y_M))^2}{2\sigma_M^2}}, \tag{24}$$

with $m_M = 1.2$, $\sigma_M^2 = 0.4$, and $(x_M, y_M) = (2.5, 2.5)$. As a threshold value for the ECM, we choose $M_{\text{th}} = 0.8$. The initial condition for the cell population is a Gaussian

$$\rho_0(x, y) = r_0 e^{-\frac{((x,y)-(x_0,y_0))^2}{2\sigma_0^2}}, \tag{25}$$

with $(x_0, y_0) = (1.5, 1.5)$, $r_0 = 0.5$, and $\sigma_0^2 = 0.2$. The maximum sensing radius is $R = 0.3$. In Fig. 1, we can observe that cells are attracted by the chemoattractant and move in the direction of the increasing gradient of S, but they encounter a too high ECM density in the centre of the domain through which cells cannot migrate, being $M_{\text{th}} = 0.8$. As a consequence, they are slowed down, but they manage to migrate in the favourable tactic direction imposed by S thanks to the positive sensing radius that manages to reach regions outside the too high ECM density. Then, in order to migrate in the direction of the increasing gradient of S, the cells surround the too dense region in the centre of the domain.

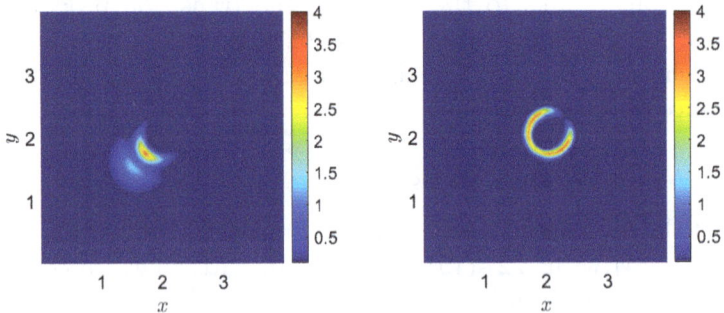

Fig. 1. Case study 1 (independent cues): Chemotaxis and physical limits of migration on the ECM. Cells start from $(1.5, 1.5)$ and migrate in the direction of the increasing gradient imposed by S that is located in $(4, 4)$. The ECM in the centre of the domain blocks the cells, which surround the region, where M is above M_{th}.

3.2. Dependent cues

3.2.1. The role of the ECM in breast cancer dissemination

Cell–ECM interactions have a prominent role in the development and dissemination of breast cancer cells because the stromal matrix surrounding tumours may be highly linearised as compared to the ECM of normal epithelial tissue thus leading to an enhanced invasiveness [33–36]. Provenzano [34] introduces the concept of tumour-associated collagen signatures (TACS), referring to an environmentally elevated collagen density and collagen fibre reorganisation, that are used to stage mammary carcinoma tumour progression levels. Specifically, TACS-1 denotes the presence of dense collagen without specific alignment, TACS-2 are collagen fibres stretched around the tumour that likely arose from stretching of the stroma due to tumour growth, and TACS-3 identify collagen fibres aligned normally to the tumour boundary regions that display an irregular shape, which is indicative of local tumour growth and invasion. Therefore, the study of cell response to a locally aligned matrix is of utmost interest, as it could suggest therapeutic strategies to target stromal invasion. The ECM, through its multiple biophysical and biochemical cues, has other effects in the dissemination of tumour cancer cells. Most of all, it is known that collagen-dense breast tissue increases also the risk of breast carcinoma, although the relationship between collagen density and tumourigenesis is not well understood [37]. In particular, steric hindrance related to collagen density has a great effect on MDA-MB 231 breast cancer cells in 3D collagen gels [38]. As already mentioned in the previous section, the effect of collagen density mainly concerns the speed of cells. In particular, regarding MDA-MB 231 breast cancer cells, it has been shown that increasing matrix density leads to reduced mean squared displacements and cell speeds (both mean and effective velocity) [39]. Therefore, the interplay between contact guidance and steric hindrance plays a significant role in breast cancer progression and dissemination. Provenzano, in particular, puts the evidence on the fundamental role of these two aspects in his works [34, 37]. Nevertheless, a systematic study of the coupling of these two aspects has not been well investigated. This is mainly related to the difficulty of building experimental settings in which the two mechanisms can be studied together as purely superposing effects, for instance, because the alignment of the fibres alters the porosity at the microscopic scale [40].

3.2.2. *The mathematical model*

We now want to describe cell migration on the ECM and, in particular, the two mechanisms: *contact guidance*, which concerns the choice of the direction and depends on the fibrous structure of the ECM, and *steric hindrance*, which affects cell speed and is regulated by the density of the ECM itself. Therefore, we introduce the distribution function of the ECM fibres $m = m(\mathbf{x}, \hat{\mathbf{v}}), \hat{\mathbf{v}} \in \mathbb{S}^{d-1}$, describing the statistical distribution of the fibres identified by their direction $\hat{\mathbf{v}} \in \mathbb{S}^{d-1}$ in each point of the physical space $\mathbf{x} \in \Omega \subset \mathbb{R}^d$. The macroscopic density of the ECM is defined at each point $\mathbf{x} \in \Omega$ by

$$M(\mathbf{x}) := \int_{\mathbb{S}^{d-1}} m(\mathbf{x}, \hat{\mathbf{v}}) \, d\hat{\mathbf{v}}. \tag{26}$$

Hence, the distribution

$$q(\mathbf{x}, \hat{\mathbf{v}}) := \frac{m(\mathbf{x}, \hat{\mathbf{v}})}{M(\mathbf{x})} \tag{27}$$

is, for each $\mathbf{x} \in \Omega$, the PDF describing the statistical distribution of the directions of the fibres at $\mathbf{x} \in \Omega$. In particular, as the fibres are not polarised, we assume that q (and therefore m) is even as a function of $\hat{\mathbf{v}}, \forall \mathbf{x} \in \Omega$, which implies that the average direction of the fibres vanishes

$$\mathbb{E}_q := \int_{\mathbb{S}^{d-1}} q(\mathbf{x}, \hat{\mathbf{v}}) \hat{\mathbf{v}} \, d\hat{\mathbf{v}} = \mathbf{0}.$$

In order to describe the microscopic dynamics of the cell, we shall consider transition probabilities as PDF of the random variables V_t' and $\hat{\mathbf{V}}_t'$ given by [30]

$$V_t' \sim \psi(V_t' | M(\mathbf{Y}_t)), \quad \hat{\mathbf{V}}_t' = \hat{\mathbf{V}}_t^m \sim m(\mathbf{Y}_t, \hat{\mathbf{V}}_t^m). \tag{28}$$

Again, $\psi = \psi(v|M)$ is a PDF of the speeds, conditioned by the ECM density M, and it has an average speed $\bar{v}(M)$ depending on M and a second moment D_M such that its variance is $D_M - \bar{v}(M)^2$. In particular, the sensing radius will affect the support of the interaction kernel given by

$$B(\mathbf{y} - \mathbf{x}) = \delta(\mathbf{y} - (\mathbf{x} + \lambda\hat{\mathbf{v}}^m))\gamma(\lambda), \tag{29}$$

where $\gamma(\lambda)$ is a sensitivity function having compact support in $[0, R_M(t, \mathbf{x}, \hat{\mathbf{v}}^m)]$ and δ is the Kronecker delta. This models the fact that a cell in $\mathbf{x}$ measures the information given by m in each position $\mathbf{y} = \mathbf{x} + \lambda\hat{\mathbf{v}}^m$, i.e., along each direction $\hat{\mathbf{v}}^m$, with $\lambda \in [0, R_M(t, \mathbf{x}, \hat{\mathbf{v}}^m)]$, and the information is weighted according to γ, that, again, is a sensing function that may be a Dirac delta or a Heaviside function. This allows deriving a kinetic model (2)–(4) with transition probability given by [30]

$$T[m](\mathbf{x}; v, \hat{\mathbf{v}}) = \int_0^{R_M(\mathbf{x},\hat{\mathbf{v}})} \frac{m(\mathbf{x} + \lambda\hat{\mathbf{v}}, \hat{\mathbf{v}})}{\bar{M}(\mathbf{x})} \psi(v|M(\mathbf{x} + \lambda\hat{\mathbf{v}}))\gamma(\lambda)\, d\lambda \tag{30}$$

and turning frequency at the population level given by $\eta = \mu\bar{M}$, being

$$\bar{M}(\mathbf{x}) = \int_{\mathbb{S}^{d-1}} \int_0^{R_M(\mathbf{x},\hat{\mathbf{v}})} m(\mathbf{x} + \lambda\hat{\mathbf{v}}, \hat{\mathbf{v}})\gamma(\lambda)d\lambda\, d\hat{\mathbf{v}}$$

that is an average of the ECM density over the measured neighbourhood, where the information is weighted by γ.

3.2.3. *Numerical simulations*

In this section, we present some numerical simulations of the microscopic model (7)-(9)-(28) and of the kinetic model (2)-(4)-(30). We represent the fibre structure with a bimodal von Mises distribution, with given concentration parameter $k > 0$ and preferential direction of migration θ_q:

$$q(\theta) = \frac{1}{4\pi I_0(k)} \left(\exp\left[k\cos(\theta - \theta_q)\right] + \exp\left[-k\cos(\theta - \theta_q)\right]\right). \tag{31}$$

The PDF of the speed will be given by

$$\psi(v|M) = \frac{1}{2\pi I_0(k_\psi)} \exp\left[k_\psi \cos\left(2\pi\frac{v - \bar{v}(M)}{U}\right)\right], \tag{32}$$

where k_ψ is the concentration parameter and $I_0(k_\psi)$ is the Bessel function of order 0, where we impose the experimentally measured value of the mean speed $\bar{v}(M)$ for the different values of the matrix density M. In particular, we shall consider two different experimental settings and comparisons of the experimental results and the outcomes of experiments *in silico* that we perform by running simulations of the microscopic model (7)-(9)-(28) that we integrate with a Monte Carlo scheme [30] and of the kinetic model that we integrate with a finite difference scheme [16]. In the first experimental setting [39], we consider a domain $\Omega = [-150, 150] \times [-150, 150] \, \mu m^2$ with 10^4 cells moving with maximum speed $U = 0.4 \, (\mu m/min)$. We impose the measured average speed of cells migrating over three different ECM densities 2.5 mg/mL, 4 mg/mL, and 6 mg/mL and having corresponding average speeds given by $\bar{v}(M) = [0.1696, 0.104, 0.063] \frac{\mu m}{min}$. Choosing $\mu = 1.8 \cdot 10^{-2} \, (1/min)$, which corresponds to a frequency of about 1 (1/hr), the mean squared displacements of the cells in the three experimental settings defined by the three different values of M are recovered (see Fig. 2(a)) [30]. In the same work, we manage to recover not only the same behaviour in the cell tracking but also the same effective speed measured experimentally.

In the second experimental setting [41], the authors investigate how the ECM density affects cancer cells' escape and invasion, using a microfluidic-based strategy (similar to the experiments in [39]) on human breast cancer cells within a type I collagen gel. In particular, the movement of 400 cancer cells, under the action of an interstitial flow, through the collagen for two different collagen densities has been tracked over a period of 16 days, showing how lower collagen concentration promotes a faster tumour escape towards an empty cavity.

In order to mimic the same experimental results [41], we consider a domain $\Omega = [0, 1000] \times [0, 600] \, \mu m^2$. On the left side of the domain, between $x = 0$ and $x = 600 \, \mu m$, we locate 400 cells of radius $R = 15 \, \mu m$, while on the right side, we consider the empty cavity at a distance of $171 \, \mu m$ or $180 \, \mu m$, in the case M = 2.5 mg/mL or M = 3.9 mg/mL, respectively, from the tumour cells. In the two cases, the experimental mean speed reported in [41] are 0.0166 and 0.0137 $\mu m/min$. We have performed the same *in silico* experiments by running numerical simulations of both the microscopic model (7)-(9)-(28) (with $B = 1$ as we are on a spatially homogeneous setting) with 400 cells and the kinetic model (2)-(4)-(33), with ψ given by (32) and q being the uni-modal von Mises distribution with $\theta_q = 0$.

This choice of q mimics the presence of an oriented interstitial flow. We set $k = 0.5$ in order to recover the experimental results reported in [41]. In particular, running n simulations for $N = 400$ cells with $n = 73$ for $M = 2.5\,\text{mg/mL}$ and $n = 55$ for $M = 3.9\,\text{mg/mL}$ of the microscopic model and calculating for each of them the distance between the cavity and the tumour cells at 2, 4, 6, 8, and 10 days and considering the median of the obtained values allows recovering a very good agreement with experimental results [30]. In Fig. 2(b), we report the integration of the kinetic model for two different values of M. We remark that for the lower value of ECM density ($M = 2.5\,\text{mg/mL}$), the distance decreases more fastly with respect to the one relative to migration on the denser ECM ($M = 3.9\,\text{mg/mL}$).

From the point of view of heterogeneous environments, the kinetic model (2)-(4)-(33) allows describing interfaces between regions with different fiber alignment and ECM density. In particular, in a setting in which the interface separates a region with ECM density above M_{th}, that hamper cells from moving, and a region where the ECM density is below M_{th}, trapped cells initially located in the region where $M > M_{\text{th}}$ manage to escape the too dense region thanks to the non-locality [30].

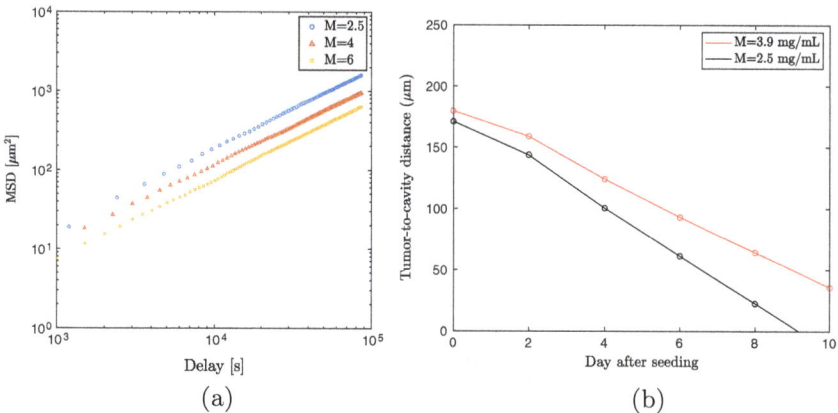

(a)   (b)

Fig. 2. Contact guidance and steric hindrance. In (a), we present a comparison with the experimental results concerning steric hindrance and, specifically, we show the mean squared displacement of three *in silico* experiments on three different ECM densities [39]. In (b), we present the solution of the kinetic model (2)-(4)-(33) with two different ECM densities corresponding to the experimental mean speed reported in [41] that are 0.0166 and 0.0137 μm/min.

3.3.   Double directional cues

3.3.1.   Chemotaxis and contact guidance

In tumour spread and metastasis formation, cancer cells that are surrounded by the stroma follow the aligned fibres at the tumour–stroma interface in order to reach blood and lymphatic vessels [42–44]. Chemotactic gradients may accelerate and enhance these processes [2, 45]. In breast cancer, increased fibrillar collagen in the mammary stroma directly regulates the three-dimensional mechanical microenvironment of mammary epithelial cells, influencing proliferation and phenotype. Collagen surrounding normal epithelial structures in breast tissue is typically curly and smooth. However, parallel with tumour development, collagen progressively thickens, linearises, and stiffens which promotes metastasis by fostering cells migration into ECM. Indeed, intravital imaging shows that breast cancer cells and leukocytes migrate rapidly along collagen fibres. Moreover, the stromal fibroblasts can regulate epithelial cells in part through secretion of specific soluble growth factors and chemokines. For instance, TGF-β has been associated with reactive stroma, fibrosis, and epithelial cell invasion [44, 44]. As a consequence, the interplay between chemotaxis and contact guidance is of the utmost interest. At the microscopic individual level, it has been shown experimentally that chemical gradients and fibre alignment have been shown to be additive when the cues are co-aligned, while contact guidance dominates when the chemical gradient and the direction of alignment of the fibres are perpendicular [46].

3.3.2.   The mathematical model

We now want to describe a microscopic dynamics in which the cell polarises as a consequence of a double directional cue: contact guidance and chemotaxis. We then consider a distribution of fibres (27), while, for what concerns chemotaxis, we consider a chemoattractant defined in (16). The cell extends its protrusions and senses in each direction $\hat{\mathbf{v}}$ and senses both quantities

$$\mathcal{S}(\mathbf{x} + \lambda\hat{\mathbf{v}}), \quad q(\mathbf{x} + \lambda\hat{\mathbf{v}}, \hat{\mathbf{v}}), \quad \forall \mathbf{x} \in \Omega, \quad \forall \hat{\mathbf{v}} \in \mathbb{S}^{d-1}, \quad \lambda \leq R,$$

in order to decide its direction of motion. In particular, in the description of the stochastic microscopic dynamics, we choose

$$\hat{\mathbf{V}}'_t \sim \mathcal{S}(y)\, q(y, \hat{\mathbf{v}}')$$

with B, again, given by (29).

As a consequence, we obtain the model (2)–(4) with the transition probability $T = T[q, \mathcal{S}]$:

$$T[q, \mathcal{S}](\mathbf{x}, v, \hat{\mathbf{v}}) = c(\mathbf{x}) \int_{\mathbb{R}_+} \gamma(\lambda) \mathcal{S}(\mathbf{x} + \lambda \hat{\mathbf{v}})\, q(\mathbf{x} + \lambda \hat{\mathbf{v}}, \hat{\mathbf{v}}) d\lambda\, \psi(v). \quad (33)$$

Here, there is no cue affecting the PDF of the speed $\psi(v)$. The latter transition probability (33) allows describing the fact that co-aligned fibres (inducing contact guidance) and chemotaxis cooperate, while in case of perpendicular cues (fibres perpendicular to the direction in which the gradient of $\mathcal{S}$ increases), the fibre alignment dominates the dynamics [17].

3.3.3. *Numerical simulations*

As the model (2)-(4)-(33) allows reproducing the microscopic dynamics regulated by the superposition of contact guidance and chemotaxis, in this section, we propose two sets of simulations allowing investigation of cell motion on a spatially heterogeneous environment in the presence of both a fibre network and a chemoattractant. We now consider a domain Ω divided in several regions that are characterised by different average directions of the fibres. In particular, we shall consider a sensing function given by $\gamma = H(R - \lambda)$.

As a first scenario, we shall consider the domain schematised in Fig. 3(a). The fibre distribution q is given by a von Mises distribution with θ_q illustrated by the linear tracts in each sub-domain, while in the whole domain, we have $k(x, y) = 50$. The initial condition of the cells is represented in Fig. 3(c), with initial density $r_0 = 0.1$, while the chemoattractant has a Gaussian profile (23) centred in $(x_\mathcal{S}, y_\mathcal{S}) = (4, 4)$, with $m_\mathcal{S} = 10$ and $\sigma_\mathcal{S}^2 = 0.5$, as shown in Fig. 3(b). We observe that cells do not migrate collectively towards the chemoattractant, but they divide into two main separated clusters (see Figs. 3(d)–(f)): in fact, although the sensing radius $R = 0.8$ is quite large, the cells that are closer to the left boundary remain

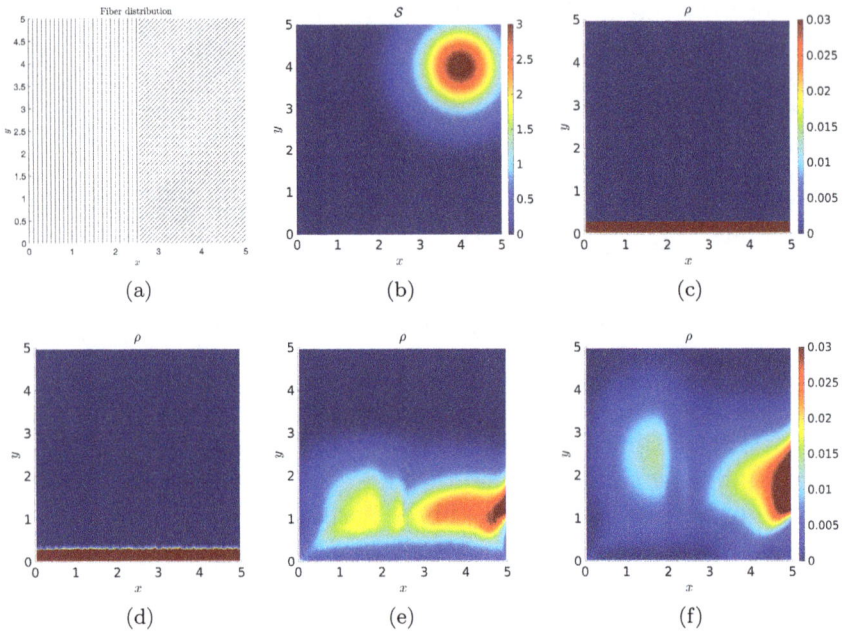

Fig. 3. Migration of cells in an heterogenous domain as illustrated in (a). The sensing radius of the cells is $R = 0.8$. The chemoattractant (b) is (23) with $m_{\mathcal{S}} = 10$ and $\sigma_{\mathcal{S}}^2 = 0.5$. The initial cell profile (c) evolves in time as illustrated in (d)–(f).

trapped in the first sub-domain, showing a loss of adhesion with the rest of the cell population. As shown in Fig. 3, even though the cells that are in the left sub-domain horizontally align to the chemoattractant, the high degree of alignment of the fibre does not allow them to escape this region, even for large times. As a second scenario, we shall consider the domain represented in Fig. 4(a); in each sub-domain, θ_q is represented by the direction illustrated by the black lines, while the parameter $k(x, y) = 50$. The initial condition of the cell population is (25) with $(x_0, y_0) = (4, 0.5)$, while the chemoattractant has a Gaussian profile (23) centred in $(x_{\mathcal{S}}, y_{\mathcal{S}}) = (2, 4.5)$ with $m_{\mathcal{S}} = 10$ and $\sigma_{\mathcal{S}}^2 = 0.05$. We observe that cells do not migrate directly towards the chemoattractant as they sense the heterogeneous fibrous environment and, consequently, adapt their migration to it. In particular, cells that are able to reach and sense the isotropic sub-domain where the fibres are uniformly distributed (defined by $1 \leq x \leq 3$ and $0 \leq y \leq 3$) go

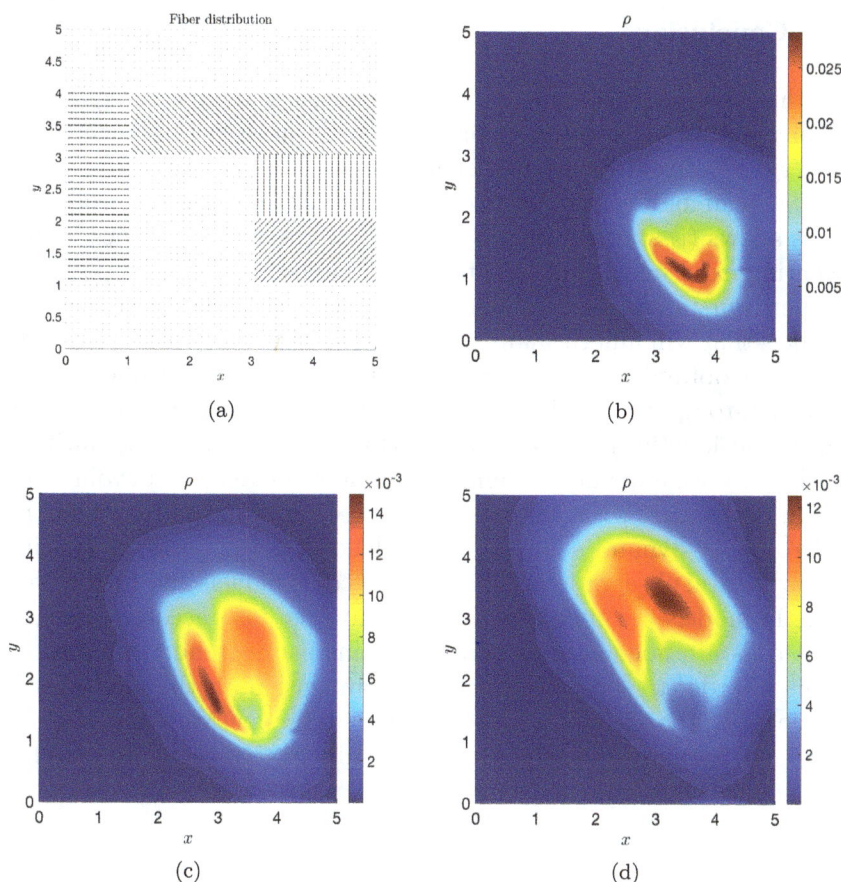

Fig. 4. Migration of cell in an heterogenous domain as illustrated in (a). The sensing radius of the cells is $R = 0.7$. The chemoattractant is (23) with $m_\mathcal{S} = 10$ and $\sigma_\mathcal{S}^2 = 0.05$. The initial cell profile evolves in time as illustrated in (b)–(d).

in this direction imposed by the gradient of the chemoattractant. On the other hand, in the sub-domain $3 \leq x \leq 5$ and $1 \leq y \leq 2$, they follow the direction of fibre alignment, that is, $\pi/4$, perpendicular to the favourable direction imposed by $\mathcal{S}$. However, the sensing radius $R = 0.7$ allows the cells that are closer to the right boundary to escape quite fast the disadvantageous (in terms of preferential direction) sub-domains and, following first the direction $\pi/2$ in $2 \leq y \leq 3$ and, then, $3\pi/4$ in $3 \leq y \leq 4$, to reach the chemoattractant.

4. Conclusion

In this chapter, we have reviewed the classical kinetic equations
implementing velocity-jump processes that have been shown to be
a very effective tool to model cell migration. In particular, such
models can be derived from discrete in time stochastic processes.
This allows (i) starting from a detailed microscopic dynamics implementing experimental observations, (ii) having a numerical platform
to perform *in silico* experiments, (iii) formally deriving mesoscopic
models that will inherit many of the details of the microscopic model,
and (iv) obtaining a full statistical description of the microscopic
model through the statistical distribution of the cell population. As
such, the kinetic model allows describing the aggregate quantities,
such as average quantities, and obtaining their temporal evolution.

In particular, we have presented three case studies in which the
microscopic dynamics has been modelled on the basis of specific
experimental observations. These microscopic models and the derived
kinetic models are non-local in order to take into account the fact
that cells are not material points but, instead, extend their protrusions in order to sense the microenvironment. Both the microscopic
models and the kinetic model are integrated numerically and used in
order to compare with experimental results or to investigate possible
heterogeneous multi-cue environments.

References

[1] F. Min, Y. Jingping, P. Chunwei, and Y. Yan Li, Collagen as a double-
      edged sword in tumor progression, *Tumor Biology.* **35**, 2871–2882.
[2] L. Lara and I. Schneider, Directed cell migration in multi-cue
      environments, *Integrative Biology.* **5**(11), 1306–1323 (2013).
[3] M. Paszek, N. Zahir, K. Johnson, J. Lakins, G. Rozenberg, and
      A. Gefen, *et al.*, Tensional homeostasis and the malignant phenotype,
      Cancer Cell. **8**, 241–254 (2005).
[4] D. Butcher, T. Alliston, and V. Weaver, A tense situation: Forcing
      tumour progression, *Nature Reviews Cancer.* **9**, 108–122 (2009).
[5] K. R. Levental, H. Yu, L. Kass, J. N. Lakins, M. Egeblad, J. T. Erler,
      et al., Matrix crosslinking forces tumor progression by enhancing
      integrin signaling, *Cell.* **139**, 891–906 (2009).
[6] S. A. Arnold, L. B. Rivera, A. F. Miller, J. G. Carbon, S. P. Dineen,
      Y. Xie, *et al.*, Lack of host sparc enhances vascular function and

tumor spread in an orthotopic murine model of pancreatic carcinoma, *Disease Models & Mechanisms.* **3**, 57–72 (2010).

[7]   P. Friedl and E.-B. Brocker, The biology of cell locomotion within three dimensional extracellular matrix, *Cellular and Molecular Life Sciences.* **57**, 41–64 (2000).

[8]   P. Friedl, Prespecification and plasticity: Shifting mechanisms of cell migration, *Current Opinion in Cell Biology.* **16**, 14–23 (2004).

[9]   A. M. Rajnicek, L. E. Foubister, and C. D. McCaig, Prioritising guidance cues: Directional migration induced by substratum contours and electrical gradients is controlled by a rho/cdc42 switch, *Developmental Biology* **312**(1), 448–460 (2007).

[10] H. C. Berg, *Random Walks in Biology*, revised edn. (Princeton University Press, 1983).

[11] H. G. Othmer, S. R. Dunbar, and W. Alt, Models of dispersal in biological systems, *Journal of Mathematical Biology* **26**(3), 263–298 (1988).

[12] D. W. Stroock, Some stochastic processes which arise from a model of the motion of a bacterium, *Zeitschrift für Wahrscheinlichkeitstheorie und verwandte Gebiete.* **28**(4), 305–315 (1974).

[13] C. Cercignani, *The Boltzmann Equation and Its Applications* (Springer, New York, 1987).

[14] T. Hillen, M5 mesoscopic and macroscopic models for mesenchymal motion, *Journal of Mathematical Biology.* **53**(4), 585–616 (2006).

[15] A. Chauviere, T. Hillen, and L. Preziosi, Modeling cell movement in anisotropic and heterogeneous network tissues, *Networks and Heterogeneous Media.* **2**(2), 333–351 (2007).

[16] N. Loy and L. Preziosi, Kinetic models with non-local sensing determining cell polarization and speed according to independent cues, *Journal of Mathematical Biology.* **80**, 373–421 (2020).

[17] M. Conte and N. Loy, Multi-cue kinetic model with non-local sensing for cell migration on a fibers network with chemotaxis, *Bullettin of Mathematical Biology.* **84**(42), 1–46 (2022).

[18] N. Loy and L. Preziosi, Modelling physical limits of migration by a kinetic model with non-local sensing, *Journal of Mathematical Biology.* **80**, 1759–1801 (2020).

[19] C. Engwer, C. Stinner, and C. Surulescu, On a structured multiscale model for acid-mediated tumor invasion: The effects of adhesion and proliferation, *Mathematical Models and Methods in Applied Sciences.* **27**, 1355–1390 (2017).

[20] M. Conte, L. Gerardo-Giorda, and M. Groppi, Glioma invasion and its interplay with nervous tissue and therapy: A multiscale model, *Journal of Theoretical Biology.* **486**, 110088 (2020).

[21] T. Hillen and H. G. Othmer, The diffusion limit of transport equations derived from velocity-jump processes, *SIAM Journal of Applied Mathematics.* **61**, 751–775 (2000).

[22] V. Calvez, G. Raoul, and C. Schmeiser, Confinement by biased velocity jumps: Aggregation of escherichia coli, *Kinetic and Related Models.* **8**(4), 651–666 (2015).

[23] F. A. C. C. Chalub, P. A. Markowich, B. Perthame, and C. Schmeiser, Kinetic models for chemotaxis and their drift-diffusion limits, *Monatshefte für Mathematik.* **142**(1), 123–141 (2004).

[24] A. Chauviere, T. Hillen, and L. Preziosi, Modeling the motion of a cell population in the extracellular matrix, *Discrete and Continuous Dynamical Systems - B.* **2007** (Supplemental volume), 250–259 (2007).

[25] F. Filbet, P. Laurencot, and B. Perthame, Derivation of hyperbolic models for chemosensitive movement, *Journal of Mathematical Biology.* **50**, 189–207 (2005).

[26] F. Filbet and K. Yang, Numerical simulation of kinetic models for chemotaxis, *SIAM Journal on Scientific Computing, Society for Industrial and Applied Mathematics.* **36**(3), B348–B366 (2014).

[27] N. Loy, T. Hillen, and K. Painter, Direction dependent turning leads to anisotropic diffusion and persistence, *European Journal of Applied Mathematics* (2021).

[28] N. Loy and L. Preziosi, Stability of a non-local kinetic model for cell migration with density dependent orientation bias, *Kinetic and Related Models.* **13**(5), 1007–1027 (2020).

[29] L. Pareschi and G. Toscani, *Interacting Multiagent Systems: Kinetic Equations and Monte Carlo Methods* (Oxford University Press, Oxford, 2013).

[30] M. Conte and N. Loy, A non-local kinetic model for cell migration: A study of the interplay between contact guidance and steric hindrance, *SIAM Journal on Applied Mathematics.* S429–S451 (2023).

[31] K. Wolf, M. Te Lindert, M. Krause, S. Alexander, J. Te Riet, A. L. Willis, *et al.*, Physical limits of cell migration: Control by ECM space and nuclear deformation and tuning by proteolysis and traction force, *The Journal of Cell Biology.* **201**, 1069–1084 (2013).

[32] G. Charras and E. Sahai, Physical influences of the extracellular environment on cell migration, *Nature Reviews.* **15**, 813–824 (2014).

[33] W. Han, S. Chen, W. Yuan, Q. Fan, J. Tian, X. Wang, *et al.*, Oriented collagen fibers direct tumor cell intravasation, *Proceedings of the National Academy of Sciences.* **113**(40), 11208–11213 (2016).

[34] P. Provenzano, K. Eliceir, J. Campbell, D. Inman, J. White, and P. Keely, Collagen reorganization at the tumor-stromal interface facilitates local invasion, *BMC Medicine.* **4**(1), 1–15 (2006).

[35] A. Ray, R. Morford, N. Ghaderi, D. Odde, and P. Provenzano, Dynamics of 3d carcinoma cell invasion into aligned collagen, *Integrative Biology.* **10**, 100–112 (2018).

[36] A. Ray, Z. Slama, R. Morford, S. Madden, and P. Provenzano, Enhanced directional migration of cancer stem cells in 3d aligned collagen matrices, *Biophysical Journal.* **112**(5), 1023–1036 (2017).

[37] P. Provenzano, D. Inman, K. Eliceiri, J. Knittel, L. Yan, C. Rueden, *et al.*, Collagen density promotes mammary tumor initiation and progression, *BMC Medicine.* **6**(1), 1–15 (2008).

[38] M. Condor, C. Mark, R. Gerum, N. Grummel, A. Bauer, J. M. Garcia Aznar, *et al.*, Breast cancer cells adapt contractile forces to overcome steric hindrance, *Biophysical Journal.* **116**, 1305–1312 (2019).

[39] J. Plou, Y. Juste-Lanas, V. Olivares, C. delAmo, C. Borau, and J. Garcia-Aznar, From individual to collective 3D cancer dissemination: Roles of collagen concentration and TGF-β, *Scientific Reports.* **8**(1), 12723 (2018).

[40] P. Taufalele, J. Vanderburgh, A. Munoz, M. Zanotelli, and C. Reinhart-King, Fiber alignment drives changes in architectural and mechanical features in collagen matrices, *PLoS One.* **14**, e0216537 (2019).

[41] J. Tien, U. Ghani, Y. Dance, A. Seibel, M. Karakan, K. Ekinci, *et al.*, Matrix pore size governs escape of human breast cancer cells from a microtumor to an empty cavity, *Iscience.* **23**(11), 101673 (2020).

[42] P. Steeg, Targeting metastasis, *Nature Reviews Cancer* **16**, 201–218 (2016).

[43] P. Provenzano, K. Eliceiri, J. Campbell, *et al.*, Collagen reorganization at the tumor-stromal interface facilitates local invasion, *BMC Medicine.* **4**(1), 38 (2006).

[44] P. Provenzano, K. Eliceiri, and P. Keely, Shining new light on 3d cell motility and the metastatic process, *Trends in Cell Biology.* **19**(11), 638–648 (2009).

[45] B. A. Bromberek, P. A. J. Enever, D. I. Shreiber, M. D. Caldwell, and R. T. Tranquillo, Macrophages influence a competition of contact guidance and chemotaxis for fibroblast alignment in a fibrin gel coculture assay, *Experimental Cell Research* **275**(2), 230–242 (2002).

[46] H. Sundararaghavan, R. Saunders, D. Hammer, and J. Burdick, Fiber alignment directs cell motility over chemotactic gradients, *Biotechnology and Bioengineering* **110**(4), 1249–1254 (2013).

Chapter 6

Multi-Scale Mathematical Modelling and Simulations of Chemo-Viro-Therapies for Cancer

Andrei Ciprian Macarie and Dumitru Trucu*

*Division of Mathematics, School of Science and Engineering,
University of Dundee, Dundee, UK*
**trucu@maths.dundee.ac.uk*

Oncolytic viruses (OVs) have gained increasing attention in cancer research due to their immunotherapeutic potential and low side effect profile. However, OVs have been typically used so far as monotherapy and that resulted in limited efficacy. To address this issue, OVs are increasingly being combined with chemotherapies. In this chapter, we develop a multi-scale mathematical model to study the interactions between tumour cells, chemovirotherapy, and the extracellular matrix (ECM). Our model shows that either monotherapy is less effective than the combination therapy, which is consistent with experimental results.

1. Introduction

Oncolytic viruses have the ability to recognise, infect, and destroy tumour cells while generating an immune response to combat future cancer recurrences [1]. While the general goal of the use of OVs is to achieve a systemic immune response, which usually takes several months, the use of highly genotoxic (i.e., DNA damage) regimens (such as chemotherapy) in combination with oncolytic therapy has recently become of significant interest [2]. Known in short as *chemovirotherapy*, such a combination of therapies results in a reduced cytotoxic (i.e., toxic to cells) effect on healthy cells and the overall toxicity associated with chemotherapies, as fewer doses of the chemotherapeutic (or simply *chemo*) agent are used [3]. Different synergistic effects may occur depending on which chemotherapeutic agent and virus are used. An example of this would be the combination of oncolytic adenovirus and the chemo agent called Temozolomide (TMZ), which results in increase in autophagy and the killing of immunogenic cells. This therapy has also been shown to be less risky and safer [1,4].

Chemovirotherapy has been tested experimentally and clinically in several cancers, including breast, head, and neck squamous cell, lung, colon, oesophageal, gastric, liver, prostate, pancreatic adenocarcinoma, and glioblastoma [1,3,5–7]. However, despite all the advances in chemovirotherapies recorded so far, the mechanism of the combination effect of chemotherapeutics and OVs, the choice of the right agents and viruses, dosage and delivery methods are still unclear, suggesting that more research is needed on the synergistic effects and interactions between these two therapies [1,2,6].

As rightly portrayed by Nguyen *et al.* [8], in this *war against cancer*, the OVs are proposed as *fighters* that are sent into battle against *the target* represented here by the cancer cells, while the chemotherapeutic drugs stand for the chemical warfare. To achieve success in this "war", it is essential to identify the best strategies, given the strengths and weaknesses of the "forces sent in" (i.e., OVs, drugs and immune cells) considered not only individually but also collectively, as well as their level of interaction while in action. For this, various action scenarios need to be considered, and in this context, mathematical modelling and the subsequent analysis enable a robust platform for their development. Accounting on key dynamic characteristics of both the tumour cells, OVs, and chemo drugs, as well as their interactions, through mathematical modelling we aim to decipher the mechanisms that will ultimately enable strategies for optimal combined treatment. In this context, the past few decades have seen increasing efforts to develop more complex and sophisticated mathematical models of viro- and chemo-therapies for cancer treatment [9–11]. At the same time, significant progress has been made in developing multi-scale moving-boundary modelling and computational frameworks for tumour growth [12, 13]. The combination of these modelling approaches has paved the way for the work that is discussed in this chapter.

One of the first spatio-temporal mathematical models of chemovirotherapy treatment for cancer was presented by Malinzi *et al.* [10]. Their model built on previous works by Tian [14] and Malinzi *et al.* [9], which introduced ODEs approaches for virotherapy treatment with virus burst size and a mathematical model describing the tumour-immune-virus dynamics, respectively. These early works concluded that the virus burst size and infection rates are key to the success of virotherapy treatment and that chemovirotherapy treatment is more effective than either monotherapies [9, 10]. More recent works developed spatio-temporal multi-scale models to capture the dynamics of OV–cancer interactions that spans across several spatial and temporal scales. In this context, Alzahrani *et al.* [13] presented a novel multi-scale moving-boundary model describing the interactions between tissue-scale (macro-scale) cancer cells, extracellular matrix (ECM), oncolytic virus (OV), and cell-scale tumour invasive edge uPA micro-dynamics. Their results showed that tumour control can be achieved, but possible relapses are possible, hence complete tumour elimination is a challenge [13].

In this chapter, we build upon the work proposed in [12, 13] to develop and analyse a chemovirotherapy model that includes uninfected and infected tumour cells, an OV, a chemo drug, and the density of the ECM. The objective is to analyse the spatio-temporal distribution and interactions of the tumour cells with the OV, the chemo drug, and the ECM, and determine the parameters that will generate positive outcomes for cancer containment when the chemovirotherapy treatment is applied.

2.   Multi-Scale Mathematical Model Construction

In this section, we build the mathematical model according to multiple assumptions based on several relevant previous papers [10, 12, 13]. We focus on addressing the spatio-temporal evolution of an avascular solid tumour, starting with the exploration of the the macro-scale collective dynamics and then continuing with the modelling description of the micro-scale proteolytic activity that takes place at the invasive edge.

2.1. *The macro-dynamics*

To explore the multi-scale interactions between tumour cells, an OV, and a chemo drug, we assume that the coupled complex dynamics take place on a growing tumour spatial domain $\Omega(t)$ that expands within an environmental tissue domain $Y \in \mathbb{R}^2$ over a time period $[0, T_f]$ (i.e., $t \in [0, T_f]$). The dynamics that we consider here includes a density of uninfected tumour cells, $u(x,t)$, a density of infected tumour cells, $i(x,t)$, a density of the OV, $v(x,t)$, a density of the chemo agent/drug, $c(x,t)$, and the extracellular matrix (ECM) density denoted here by $e(x,t)$. In the presence of proliferation, during their local random and directed motility, both cells populations will interact with the viral particles density (which will also exercise a spatio-temporal transport within the tumour region) while being exposed to a diffusive chemotherapeutic process.

Considering first the macro-scale, at any given spatio-temporal macro-node $(x,t) \in \Omega(t) \times \{t\}$, $t \in [0, T_f]$, the cancer cells population $u(x,t)$ is infected by the OV $v(x,t)$, giving rise to an infected cell population $i(x,t)$. Moreover, the tumour environment is subjected to a chemo drug $c(x,t)$, which is administered intratumourally. Therefore, the tumour cells die due to both the virus and the chemotherapy cytotoxicity and this way get eliminated from the total tumour mass that we denoted here by $(u + i)(x,t)$. All of these interactions are happening in the presence of the macro-scale ECM density $e(x,t)$, which is degraded by the cancer cells and the chemo drug.

Uninfected tumour cells — $u(x,t)$: For the population of uninfected tumour cells, we assume that the cancer cells exercise both a random motility, at a constant diffusion rate $D_u > 0$, and a directed movement against ECM gradients towards higher ECM levels (i.e., "a haptotactic movement") with a constant haptotactic coefficient $\eta_u > 0$. Furthermore, cancer cells are assumed to proliferate logistically at a rate $\alpha_u > 0$, decay at a rate $\beta > 0$ due to the virus infection, and experience lysis in response to the chemo drug at a rate $\delta_u > 0$. The interactions of the uninfected cancer cells with both virus and the chemo agent are explored here via terms of Michaelis–Menten form to account for saturation, where $K_u > 0$ and $K_c > 0$ are constants related to lysis rates at which both the virus and the chemo drug are half-maximal, respectively, similarly to [10]. Therefore, the governing dynamics for the uninfected tumour cells is given by the following equation:

$$\frac{\partial u}{\partial t} = D_u \Delta u - \eta_u \nabla \cdot (u \nabla e) + \alpha_u u (1 - u) - \frac{\beta u v}{K_u + u} - \frac{\delta_u u c}{K_c + c}. \quad (1)$$

Infected tumour cells — $i(x, t)$: Similarly, for the infected tumour cells, we assume both random motility, with constant diffusion rate $D_i > 0$, and directed haptotactic movement towards higher ECM levels with haptotactic coefficient $\eta_i > 0$. This cell population is further expanded through the permanent supply of newly infected cancer cells (i.e., the cells from the uninfected cancer cells that get infected with the virus at rate $\beta > 0$) and finally experience lysis due to the chemo drug at a rate $\delta_i > 0$, as well as death due to the virus at rate $\delta > 0$. Again, here the exposure to the chemo agent is explored through a term of Michaelis–Menten form, with the same constant $K_c > 0$ as for the uninfected cells. Therefore, the dynamics of the infected cancer cells is given by

$$\frac{\partial i}{\partial t} = D_i \Delta i - \eta_i \nabla \cdot (i \nabla e) + \frac{\beta u v}{K_u + u} - \frac{\delta_i u c}{K_c + c} - \delta i. \quad (2)$$

Oncolytic virus — $v(x, t)$: The OV is assumed to move randomly, with diffusion constant $D_v > 0$, as well as towards higher ECM levels with haptotactic coefficient $\eta_v > 0$. The virus replicates inside the infected cells, and new viral particles (i.e., "virions") are released at a rate $b > 0$ (which is also known under the name of *burst size*). The larger the burst size b, the higher is the number of new virions released. Further, while the virus dies naturally at a rate $\delta_v > 0$, the population of free virus particles is also reduced when the virus infects the previously uninfected cancer cells at a rate $\beta > 0$. Finally, the virus intake within the tumour microenvironment is explored here through a positive term $g_v^p(x,t)$ that is spatio-temporally distributed and is taken to be

$$g_v^p(x,t) = \sum_{i=1}^{p} \rho_g(i)\gamma_{t_i}(t) \cdot v(x,0), \qquad (3)$$

where $v(x,0)$ is the initial viral condition described in (17) and $\gamma_{t^*}(t)$ is

$$\gamma_{t^*}(t) = \begin{cases} \exp\left(\dfrac{1}{\theta^2} - \dfrac{1}{\theta^2 - |t - t^*|^2}\right), & t \in [t^*, t^* + \theta), \\ 0, & t > t^* + \theta, \end{cases} \qquad (4)$$

where $t^* \in \{t_i \,|\, i = 1, p\}$ are the times of viral injections and the injection effect basic time length is given by $0 < \theta < \min\{|t_i - t_j| \,|\, i, j = 0, p \text{ with } i \neq j\}$. Finally, $\rho_g : \{1, \ldots, N_{\max}\} \to \{0, 1\}$ is a switch variable that is set to 1 when we administer the viral therapy in a given interval $[t_i, t_{i+1})$ and to zero when the OV therapy is off in that time period. Thus, the governing equation for the viral dynamics is as follows:

$$\frac{\partial v}{\partial t} = D_v \Delta v - \eta_v \nabla \cdot (v \nabla e) + bi - \frac{\beta u v}{K_u + u} - \delta_v v + g_v^p(x,t). \qquad (5)$$

Chemotherapeutic drug density — $c(x,t)$: Similar to [10], we assume that the chemo delivery process is of a reaction–diffusion type. Thus, the chemo agent is assumed here to diffuse at a constant rate $D_c > 0$ while naturally decaying at rate $\lambda > 0$. Finally, the chemo agent is administered to the tumour according to a time-dependent scheduling explored here via function $g_c(x,t)$ whose particular form will be specified in accordance with the case considered. Hence chemotherapy delivery process is governed by the following equation:

$$\frac{\partial c}{\partial t} = D_c \Delta c + g_c(x,t) - \lambda c. \qquad (6)$$

Extracellular matrix — $e(x,t)$: While the ECM does not exercise any spatial movement, this is continuously degraded by the uninfected and infected cancer cells in the environment at the rate $\sigma_u > 0$ and $\sigma_i > 0$, respectively; this is also remodelled logistically (i.e., regrows until the tissue carrying capacity is reached) at a rate $\alpha_e > 0$.

Finally, the ECM is also assumed to be degraded by the chemo agent at rate $\sigma_c > 0$. Therefore, the ECM dynamics is governed by

$$\frac{\partial e}{\partial t} = -e(\sigma_u u + \sigma_i i + \sigma_c c) + \alpha_e e(1 - e - u - i)^+, \tag{7}$$

where $(\cdots)^+$ represents as usual the positive part of the expression $(\cdots)$.

2.2. Micro-scale dynamics and its top-down and bottom-up links to macro-scale

At micro-scale, we consider the leading edge proteolytic dynamics of the urokinase plasminogen activator, called simply the uPA System, which in brief aggregates the coupled dynamics of three major molecular components (species):

- urokinase plasminogen activator (uPA),
- plasminogen activator inhibitor (PAI-1),
- plasmin.

While all the coupled dynamics of the uPA System components is influenced directly by the macro-dynamics taking place on $\Omega(t)$, this enzymatic system acts within a cell-scale (micro-scale) neighbourhood of the invasive edge of the tumour, i.e., on a micro-scale envelope of the tumour interface

$$\mathbf{B}(\partial\Omega(t), \epsilon) := \bigcup_{x \in \partial\Omega(t)} \mathbf{B}_{\|\cdot\|_\infty}(x, \epsilon),$$

of micro-scale radius $\epsilon > 0$, where a cross-boundary local enzymatic transport takes place. This causes degradation of the neighbouring peritumoural ECM distribution that it meets, and this way creates room for further tumour progression.

As detailed in [12, 13], in order to explore the uPA System proteolytic interfacial dynamics, it is convenient to decouple this in a bundle of micro-dynamic processes taking place on the bundle of overlapping micro-scale domains that constitute the interfacial neighbourhood $\mathbf{B}(\partial\Omega(t), \epsilon)$. Thus, let's denote

$$\epsilon Y(x) := \mathbf{B}_{\|\cdot\|_\infty}(x, \epsilon), \quad \forall x \in \partial\Omega,$$

and ignoring for notation convenience the barycenter x, as in [12], each such ϵY will be referred to as ϵ-*micro-domain* (and due to the topology enabled by $\|\cdot\|_\infty$, we note that in 2D each micro-domain ϵY is in fact a rectangle of size 2ϵ). In this context, on each boundary micro-domain ϵY, over a small time span $\Delta t > 0$, the activity of the uPA system is given by the local micro-scale spatio-temporal coupled transport at $(y, \tau) \in \epsilon Y \times [0, \Delta t]$ of the micro-scale molecular densities of uPA, PAI-1, and plasmin that are denoted here by $a(y, \tau)$, $p(y, \tau)$, and $m(y, \tau)$, respectively.

The boundary micro-dynamics: As explained in detail in [13], at any $(y, \tau) \in \epsilon Y \times [0, \Delta t]$, a source of uPA denoted as $f_{uPA}^{\epsilon Y}(y, \tau)$ is induced non-locally from the cancer cells macro-dynamics. Furthermore, once secreted, the uPA binds to the available cell-surface uPAR receptors (i.e., dedicated receptors for uPA), while some of the uPA is inactivated by binding to inhibitor PAI-1. At the same time, for the inhibitor PAI-1, a second influence of the macro-dynamics within the micro-scale activity arises through the removal of the inhibitor PAI-1 via indiscriminate binding to surrounding ECM, process that was modelled in [13] in the form of another non-local term denoted as $f_{PAI-1}^{\epsilon Y}(y, \tau)$. Finally, plasmin is activated from its inactive form of plasminogen (that is available in ECM) both directly by the uPA as well as indirectly through the PAI-1 removal caused by PAI-1 binding to surrounding ECM.

Therefore, the dynamics of the tumour invasive edge proteolytic micro-processes can be mathematically described as follows. While per unit time the uPA is assumed to exercise random movement with constant diffusion rate $D_a > 0$, this is produced non-locally by the macro-scale cancer cells distribution at a rate $\psi_{12} > 0$ (thereby establishing a first macro-scale to micro-scale top-down link in this model). In addition, the uPA bounds available uPAR receptors at a rate $\psi_{13} > 0$ and at the same time is inhibited by PAI-1 density $p(\cdot, \cdot)$ at a rate $\psi_{11} > 0$. Hence, the uPA dynamics is governed by

$$\frac{\partial a}{\partial \tau} = D_a \Delta h_1 - \psi_{11} a p + (\psi_{12} - \psi_{13} u) f_{uPA}^{\epsilon Y}(y, \tau), \qquad (8)$$

where $f_{uPA}^{\epsilon Y}(y, \tau)$ represents the uPA source at the micro-scale node $(y, \tau) \in \epsilon Y \times [0, \Delta t]$ induced non-locally from the macro-scale cancer cells dynamics, whose exact expression with full details is given in [13].

Further, while the inhibitor PAI-1 density spatial transport per unit time is dictated by random movement with diffusion coefficient $D_p > 0$, its production is accomplished through plasmin activation at a rate $\psi_{23} > 0$. Further, the PAI-1 is removed from the system through binding to the uPA at a rate $\psi_{21} > 0$, as well as through indiscriminate binding to the surrounding macro-scale ECM density at a rate $\psi_{22} > 0$ (thereby establishing a second notable macro-scale to micro-scale top-down link). Hence, the governing equation for PAI-1 is given by

$$\frac{\partial p}{\partial \tau} = D_p \Delta p - \psi_{21} a p - \psi_{22} p f^{\epsilon Y}_{PAI-1}(y, \tau) + \psi_{23} m, \qquad (9)$$

where $f^{\epsilon Y}_{PAI-1}$ is the PAI-1 removal non-local effect induced at micro-scale from the macro-scale by the surrounding macroscopic density of ECM, whose exact expression with full details are again given in [13].

Finally, the density change per unit time of plasmin is given by local diffusion with diffusion coefficient $D_m > 0$, natural decay at a rate $\psi_{33} > 0$ and production due to both direct plasminogen activation through uPA binding to uPAR at a rate $\psi_{31} > 0$, and binding of PAI-1 to the surrounding ECM at a rate $\psi_{32} > 0$. Hence, plasmin's dynamics is governed by

$$\frac{\partial m}{\partial \tau} = D_m \Delta m + \psi_{31} a f^{\epsilon Y}_{uPA}(y, \tau) + \psi_{32} p f^{\epsilon Y}_{PAI-1}(y, \tau) - \psi_{33} m. \quad (10)$$

Brief overview of top-down and bottom-up links between macro-scale and micro-scale: As discussed already earlier, the macro-scale dynamics critically contribute to the emergence of the proteolytic boundary micro-dynamics by providing both the source for the uPA and major avenue for the removal of PAI-1 inhibitor via the non-local operators $f^{\epsilon Y}_{uPA}$ and $f^{\epsilon Y}_{PAI-1}$, respectively, thereby establishing a strong top-down link. However, a major connection of critical importance in the reverse direction is also established. Indeed, as established in [12], proteolytic activity carried out during the micro-dynamics (by plasmin in this case) degrades the surrounding peritumoural ECM. As shown with full details in [12], the pattern of significant degradation of ECM caused by the micro-dynamics allows for a multi-scale mathematical description of the emergent boundary velocity field that defines the law for the macro-scale tumour boundary movement. Therefore, a bottom-up link between micro- and macro-scale is this way established, through which the proteolytic dynamics at micro-scale dictates the changes in tumour of boundary morphology at macro-scale [12].

Finally, from a semi-discretised time perspective enabled by an uniformly split of the macro-scale time interval $[0, T_f]$ in a collection of small intervals $\{[k\Delta t, (k + 1)\Delta t]\}_{k=0, k_{\max}}$, the macro-dynamics that takes place on $\Omega(k\Delta t)$ over the time period $[k\Delta t, (k + 1)\Delta t]$ taken together with the micro-dynamics that it induces via the top-down links on each of the boundary micro-domains $\epsilon Y \in \mathbf{B}$ $(\partial\Omega(k\Delta t), \epsilon)$ (over the corresponding micro-scale time period $[0, \Delta t]$) is for convenience referred to as *stage k* of this coupled two-scale dynamics. In this context, as detailed in [12, 13], the bundle of boundary micro-dynamics from stage k determines the law for the relocation of $\partial\Omega(k\Delta t)$ (i.e., by prescribing the precise direction and displacement magnitude for the relocation of each of the points on $\partial\Omega(k\Delta t)$), progressing this way the stage k tumour domain $\Omega(k\Delta t)$ into the newly obtained domain $\Omega((k + 1)\Delta t)$ that is defined by the relocated tumour boundary, on which the overall tumour dynamics continues with stage $k + 1$.

2.3. *Summary of the full model equations at both macro- and micro-scales*

In summary, the macro-scale dynamics is given by

$$\begin{cases} \dfrac{\partial u}{\partial t} = D_u \Delta u - \eta_u \nabla \cdot (u\nabla e) + \alpha_u u(1 - u) - \dfrac{\beta uv}{K_u + u} - \dfrac{\delta_u uc}{K_c + c}, \\[2ex] \dfrac{\partial i}{\partial t} = D_i \Delta i - \eta_i \nabla \cdot (i\nabla e) + \dfrac{\beta uv}{K_u + u} - \dfrac{\delta_i uc}{K_c + c} - \delta i, \\[2ex] \dfrac{\partial v}{\partial t} = D_v \Delta v - \eta_v \nabla \cdot (v\nabla e) + bi - \dfrac{\beta uv}{K_u + u} - \delta_v v + g_v^p(x, t), \\[2ex] \dfrac{\partial c}{\partial t} = D_c \Delta c + g_c(x, t) - \lambda c, \\[2ex] \dfrac{\partial e}{\partial t} = -e(\sigma_u u + \sigma_i i + \sigma_c c) + \alpha_e e(1 - e - u - i), \end{cases}$$

$$(11)$$

while the micro-scale is given as

$$
\begin{cases}
\dfrac{\partial a}{\partial \tau} = D_a \Delta h_1 - \psi_{11} ap + (\psi_{12} - \psi_{13} u) f_{uPA}^{\epsilon Y}(y, \tau), \\[2ex]
\dfrac{\partial p}{\partial \tau} = D_p \Delta p - \psi_{21} ap - \psi_{22} p f_{PAI-1}^{\epsilon Y}(y, \tau) + \psi_{23} m, \\[2ex]
\dfrac{\partial m}{\partial \tau} = D_m \Delta m + \psi_{31} a f_{uPA}^{\epsilon Y}(y, \tau) + \psi_{32} p f_{PAI-1}^{\epsilon Y}(y, \tau) - \psi_{33} m.
\end{cases}
\tag{12}
$$

3. Simulation Scenarios and Results

In this section, we explore computationally several scenarios for chemovirotherapy that a growing tumour is exposed to, aiming to highlight differences and potential treatment avenues for controlling cancer progression. Each scenario is organised as follows: a brief explanation of the scenario postulated, followed by the chosen values of the parameters, and finally, the results are showed and discussed. In the simulations considered in the following, unless otherwise specified, we use the baseline parameter values from Table A.1 for macro-dynamics, and those from Table A.2 for the micro-dynamics.

Finally, the associated numerical implementation of this multi-scale moving boundary framework uses a finite difference method approach at macro-scale (involving central differences and midpoint approximations) and a finite element method at micro-scale (involving square meshes and bilinear shape functions on each micro-domain ϵY), see [12, 13] for further details.

3.1. *Initial conditions*

Unless otherwise specified, for the baseline set of initial conditions, for both cancer cells populations ECM and OV, we use here those considered previously in [13], while for the chemotherapy (that was not considered in [13]), we consider null conditions. All these baseline initial conditions are shown in Fig. 1 and are mathematically given as follows:

- For uninfected cancer cells,

$$
u(x, 0) = w(x, (4, 4)), \quad x \in Y,
\tag{13}
$$

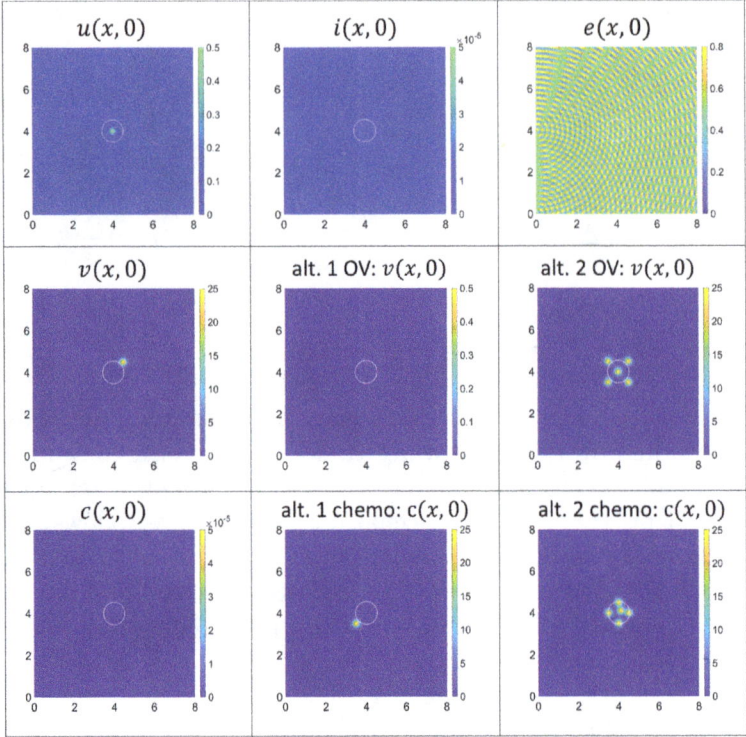

Fig. 1. First row and first column of pictures in this figure show the baseline initial conditions for the model's variables, while the rest of the pictures shows alternative initial conditions that we consider for the OV and chemo agent.

where for $\forall x \in Y$, the function $w(x, \cdot): Y \to \mathbb{R}_+$ is given by

$$w(x, y) := \frac{\left(\exp\left(-\frac{\|x-y\|_2^2}{\sqrt{\Delta x \Delta y}} \right) - \exp(-28.125) \right) \phi(x, y)}{2}, \quad (14)$$

where $\phi(x, y) := (\chi_{B(y, 0.5-\gamma)} * \psi_\gamma)(x)$, for any $y \in Y$. Finally, here ψ_γ is the usual mollifier of radius γ, with $0 < \gamma << \epsilon/6$ whose expression is given in Appendix A.1.

- For infected cancer cells,

$$i(x, 0) = 0. \quad (15)$$

- For the ECM,

$$e(x, 0) = \frac{1 + 0.3 \sin(4\pi \| x \|_2) + \sin(4\pi \| (4, 0) - x \|_2)}{2}. \quad (16)$$

- For the OV,

$$v(x, 0) = w(x, (4.5, 4.5)), \quad x \in Y. \tag{17}$$

- For the chemo drug,

$$c(x, 0) = 0. \tag{18}$$

Furthermore, in some of the simulations, we will also consider the following alternative scenarios for the initial conditions for OV and chemo agent, namely:

- alternative scenarios for OV initial conditions:
  - alternative scenario 1 for OV:

$$v(x, 0) = 0, \tag{19}$$

  - alternative scenario 2 for OV:

$$v(x, 0) = \sum_{i=1}^{5} w(x, y_i), \tag{20}$$

  where $y_1 := (4.5, 4.5)$, $y_2 := (4.5, 3.5)$, $y_3 := (3.5, 3.5)$, $y_4 := (3.5, 4.5)$, and $y_5 := (4, 4)$, with $w(x, \cdot)$ given in (14),
- alternative scenarios for chemo agent initial conditions:
  - alternative scenario 1 for chemo agent:

$$c(x, 0) = w(x, (3.5, 3.5)), \tag{21}$$

  with $w(x, \cdot)$ given in (14),
  - alternative scenario 2 for chemo agent:

$$c(x, 0) = \sum_{i=1}^{5} w(x, z_i), \tag{22}$$

  where $z_1 := (4, 3.5)$, $z_2 := (4.5, 4)$, $z_3 := (4.1, 4.1)$, $z_4 := (4, 4.5)$, and $z_5 := (3.5, 4)$, with $w(x, \cdot)$ given in (14).

3.2. *Scenario 1: Virus only*

In a first scenario, to asses the effectiveness of the virotherapy in terms of tumour containment and reduction, we consider this as a monotherapy (i.e., this is administered alone via the delivery function $g_v^p(x,t)$ given in (3) with $\rho_g \equiv 1$, $p = N_{\max}$, and $t_i = i\Delta t$), in the absence of any chemo therapy (i.e., $g_c(x,t) = 0$). Here we use the baseline initial conditions given in (13)–(18), with the following modified parameter values: $D_c = 0$, $\delta_u = 0$, $K_u = 1$, $\delta_i = 0$, $\sigma_c = 0$, and $\lambda = 0$. The numerical simulation for this scenario shown in Fig. 2 reveals that as the time progresses, the virus density increases throughout the tumour, infecting the tumour and following its spatio-temporal distribution. The density of uninfected cells is reduced, and the amount of infected cells increases. However, the morphology of the tumour does not change significantly, and the tumour continues to expand. Even though the virus infects most of the tumour, it does not reduce the overall tumour density. This is because the virus is not able to kill enough tumour cells to compensate for the growth of the tumour.

The results of this simulation suggest that virotherapy alone is not an effective treatment for cancer. In order to be effective, virotherapy would need to be combined with other therapies, such as chemotherapy.

3.3. *Scenario 2: Chemotherapy only*

Aiming now to explore the perspectives of chemotherapy administered as a monotherapy, we alter here the baseline initial conditions given in (13)–(18) by replacing the following: (1) the initial condition for OV with the first alternative considered in (19), and (2) the initial condition for the chemo agent with the alternative considered in (21). Furthermore, we also alter several parameters as follows: $K_u = 1$, $\delta_u = 2.08 \cdot 10^{-4}$, $\delta_i = 2.5 \cdot 10^{-4}$, $\lambda = 0.17375$, and $\sigma_c = 0.075$. As we are simulating chemotherapy alone and no OV is administered (i.e., $\rho_g \equiv 0$ in (3)), no infected cancer cell population emerges in within the dynamics. The simulation obtained in this scenario, which are shown in Fig. 3, indicates that the bulk of the tumour density remains in the centre of the domain throughout its evolution. However, the tumour still expands towards higher ECM gradients. The overall density is higher when compared to the previous scenario. The morphology of the tumour is quite different in comparison to Scenario 1, with finger-like ramifications of the tumour.

These results suggest that also chemotherapy alone is not an effective treatment for cancer. The tumour is able to grow despite

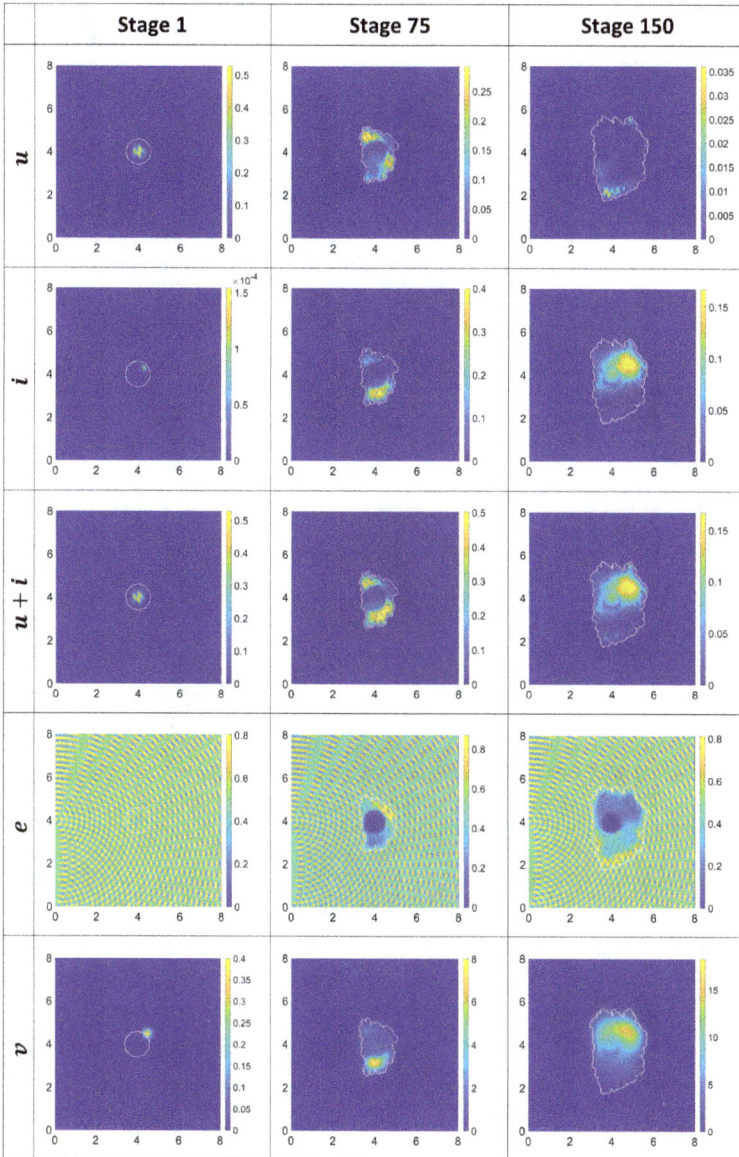

Fig. 2. Results from Scenario 1 at three macro–micro stages (1, 75 and 150), showing (u) uninfected cancer cells density, (i) infected cancer cells density, $(u + i)$ total cancer cells density, (e) ECM density, and (v) virus density.

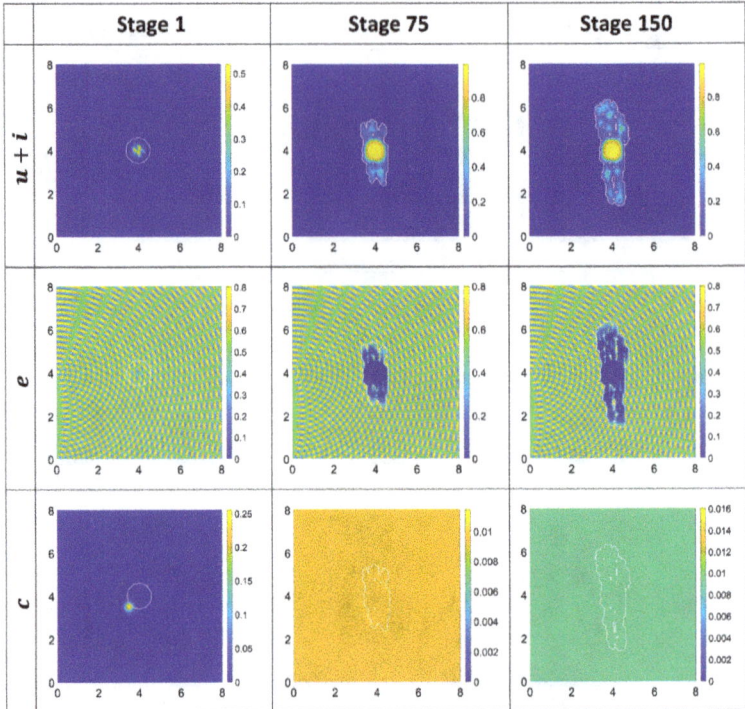

Fig. 3. Results from Scenario 2 at three macro–micro stages (1, 75 and 150), showing $(u + i)$ total cancer cells density, (e) ECM density, and (c) chemo drug density.

the presence of chemotherapy, and the morphology of the tumour changes in a way that suggests that the tumour is becoming more aggressive. This is likely due to the fact that chemotherapy kills some tumour cells, but it also damages the tumour microenvironment, which can create conditions that favour the expansion of the tumour cells. Therefore, this simulation suggests that chemotherapy would need to be combined with other therapies in order to be effective, and for this, a prime candidate would be indeed the oncolytic virus therapy.

3.4. *Scenario 3: Virus first and then chemotherapy*

In this scenario, in the presence of the same set of parameters as in Scenario 2 and assuming the baseline initial conditions (13)–(18), we explore the situation when the OV is administered first via the viral delivery function $g_v^p(x,t)$ given in (3), with $\rho_g \equiv 1$, $p = N_{max}$, and $t_i = i\Delta t$. Then, after 5 macro–micro stages, we start administering also the chemo drug according to the chemo delivery function $g_c(x,t)$ given by

$$g_c(x,t) := \sum_{i=5}^{N_{max}} \gamma_{t_i}(t)c(x,0)$$

with $\gamma_{t_i}(t)$ being the scheduling function given in (4) and $t_i := i\Delta t$ for any $i = 1 \ldots N_{max}$, where $N_{max} = [T_f/\Delta t]$.

From the simulation for this scenario, shown in Fig. 4, we observe that the total tumour density fluctuated several times and relapsed in several occasions. The tumour was almost eradicated at a certain moment, but then it relapsed. This leads to the conclusion that this combination of viral and chemo therapy has the potential to have a synergistic effect. Further, we would also like to note that the morphology of the tumour is similar to the viral monotherapy treatment (considered in Scenario 1). Finally, similar to the previous scenarios, the choices of values and initial conditions did not lead to the containment or suppress the tumour. This suggests that more elaborate strategies of the treatment are needed.

3.5. *Scenario 4: Chemotherapy first and then virus*

In this scenario, assuming again the same parameter set as in Scenario 2, we investigate the administration of the chemo drug first, with the baseline initial condition given in (13)–(18) altered as follows: (1) for the OV, we consider alternative 1 initial condition given in (19), and (2) for the chemo agent, we consider alternative 1 initial condition given in (21). Furthermore, the chemotherapy is applied now from stage 1, and so mathematically, preserving the notations established so far, this is given by the chemo delivery function $g_c(x,t)$ defined as

$$g_c(x,t) := \sum_{i=1}^{N_{max}} \gamma_{t_i}(t)c(x,0), \tag{23}$$

where $t_i := i\Delta t$, for all $i = 1, \ldots, N_{max}$. However, the OV is incorporated only after five stages via the viral delivery function $g_v^p(x,t)$

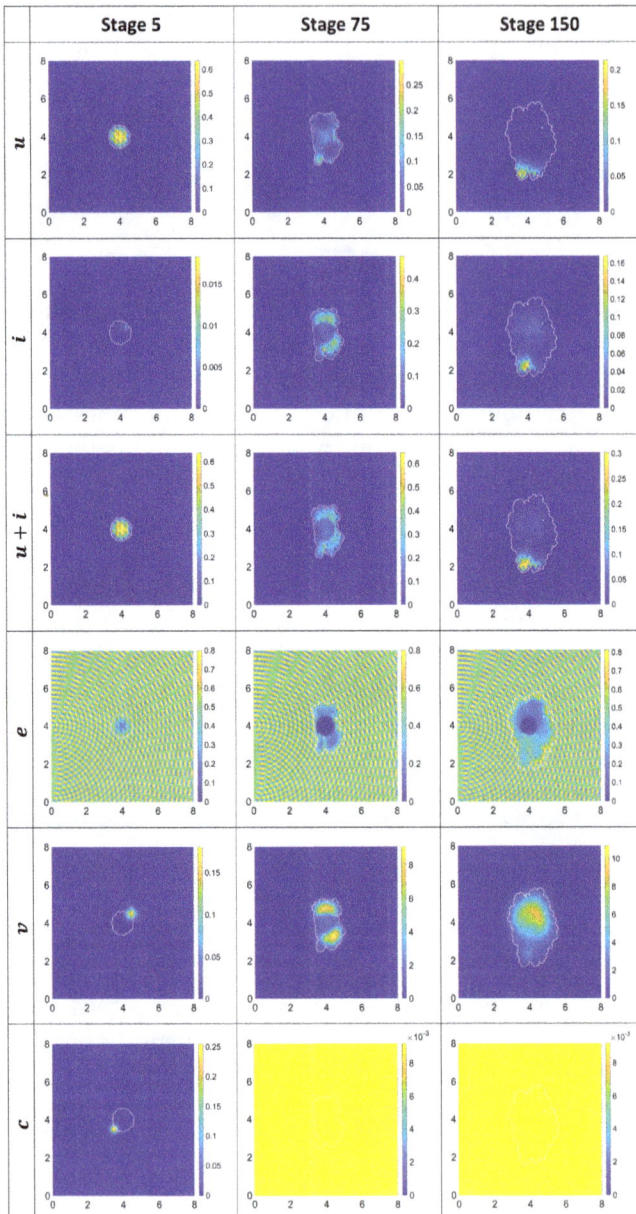

Fig. 4. Results from Scenario 3 at three macro-micro stages (5, 75 and 150), showing (u) uninfected cancer cells density, (i) infected cancer cells density, $(u + i)$ total cancer cells density, (e) ECM density, (v) virus density, and (c) chemo drug density.

given in (3) for $p = N_{max}$ and

$$\rho_g(i) = \begin{cases} 0, & i = 1, \ldots, 4, \\ 1, & i \geq 5, \end{cases}$$

$$\text{with} \quad t_i = i\Delta t, \quad i \geq 5.$$

As observed from the results presented in Fig. 5, the outcomes of this treatment strategy are similar to the ones obtained in Scenario 3, with the exception of a higher density for the infected cells and virus. This indicates that the virus was able to survive longer and infect more cells. This simulation also indicates that the tumour was almost eradicated but then it relapsed in two main occasions. The morphology of the tumour is similar to the one in Scenario 3. Moreover, the total amount of tumour cells was higher, as well. Finally, with the chosen values and initial conditions, administering the chemotherapy first and then the OV therapy leads to a slightly worse overall tumour. This suggests that the chemo drug may have damaged the tumour microenvironment in a way that made it more difficult for the virus to be effective.

3.6. Scenario 5: Combined therapies with constant drug infusion

In this section, we explore the perspective of a modified combination of viral and chemo therapies in which besides the viral therapy administered as in Scenario 3, the chemo agent is assumed to be delivered at constant level (both in space and time), i.e., $g_c(x, t) = 10$ for all $(x, t) \in Y \times [0, T]$. This is started in the presence of baseline initial conditions (given in (13)–(18)) that have been altered by replacing the initial condition for the chemo agent with the alternative 1 initial condition proposed in (21). Finally, the parameter set is maintained again as in Scenario 2.

The simulation results for this case presented in Fig. 6 show total containment of the tumour. The morphology of the tumour barely changes throughout the N_{max} macro–micro computational stages, which indicates an efficient tumour containment under this strategy.

This simulation also indicates that the tumour was almost eradicated but with a small relapse. This suggests that the combination

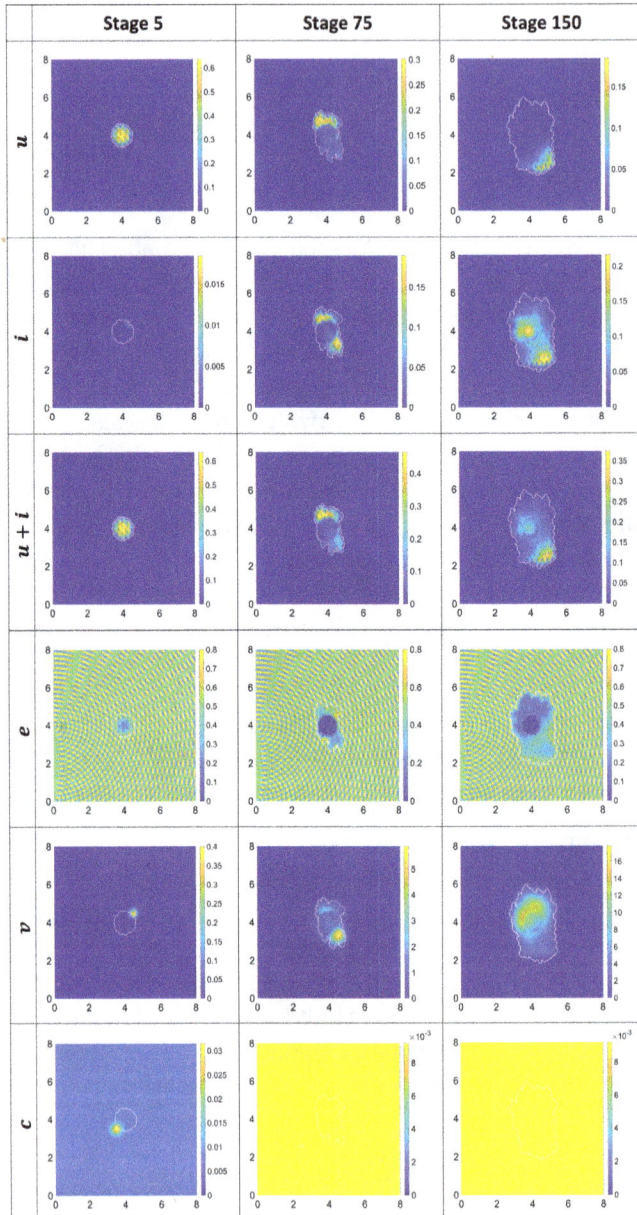

Fig. 5. Results from Scenario 4 at three macro–micro stages (5, 75 and 150), showing (u) uninfected cancer cells density, (i) infected cancer cells density, ($u + i$) total cancer cells density, (e) ECM density, (v) virus density, and (c) chemo drug density.

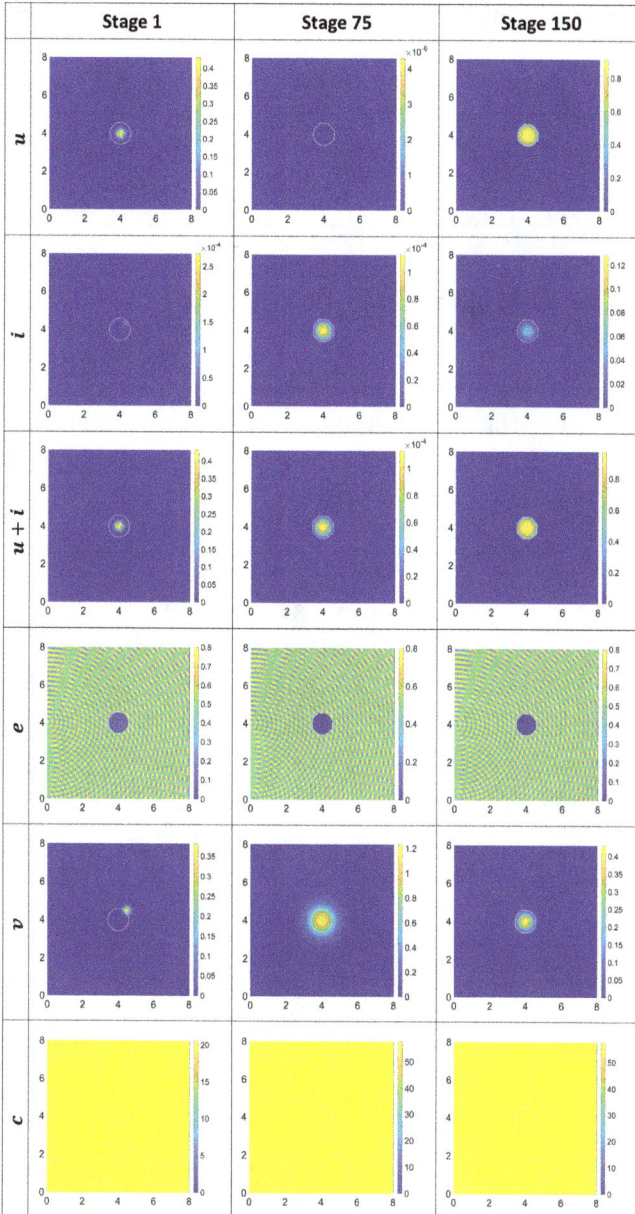

Fig. 6. Results from Scenario 5 at three macro–micro stages (1, 75 and 150), showing (u) uninfected cancer cells density, (i) infected cancer cells density, ($u + i$) total cancer cells density, (e) ECM density, (v) virus density, and (c) chemo drug density.

of chemotherapy and virotherapy can be effective in killing tumour cells, but it may not be able to completely eradicate the tumour.

With the chosen values and initial conditions, this scenario shows the potential of combining these two therapies to achieve fairly efficient containment and suppression of the tumour. However, one drawback from this scenario is that it would be too toxic to apply in real-life scenarios, as we are constantly administering the chemo drug.

3.7. Scenario 6: Combined therapies administered at the same time

Maintaining precisely the same initial conditions as in Scenario 5 while considering the same parameter set as in Scenario 2, here we explore the potential of a combined chemovirotherapy in which both the OV and the chemo agent follow the same delivery scheduling that is given by

$$g_c(x,t) := \sum_{i=1}^{N_{\max}} \gamma_{t_i}(t)c(x,0),$$

$$g_v^p(x,t) := \sum_{i=1}^{N_{\max}} \gamma_{t_i}(t)v(x,0), \tag{24}$$

where $t_i := i\Delta t$, for all $i = 1,\ldots,N_{\max}$. The results for this scenario are present in Fig. 7 and show on one hand a similar evolution for the tumour morphology to ones seen in Scenarios 1, 3, and 4. On the other hand, these simulation results also reveal that the outcomes of this treatment are similar to the ones from Scenarios 3 and 4, with the exception of higher densities for uninfected and infected cells and total tumour mass $(u + i)(x,t)$. Finally, with the chosen parameter values, the simulation does not show an efficient tumour containment.

3.8. Scenario 7: Combined therapies with improved parameter values

In this scenario, we explore the administration of both the chemo drug and the OV at the same time distributions (i.e., eventually at a variety of chosen macro–micro stages but both deliveries of OV and

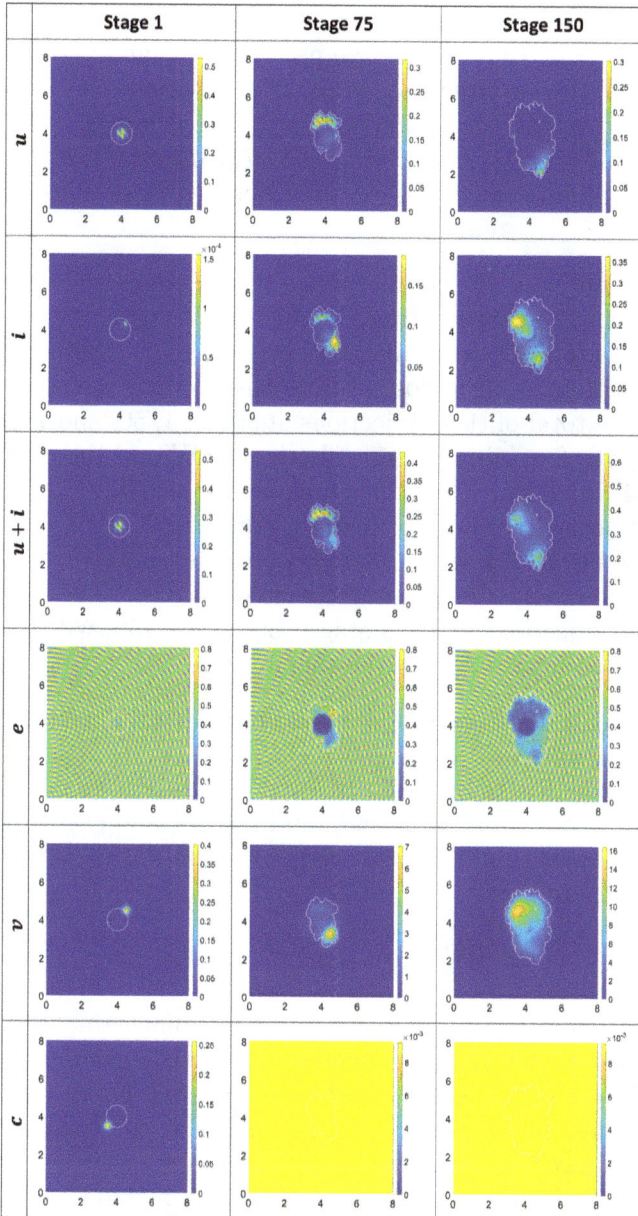

Fig. 7. Results from Scenario 6 at three macro–micro stages (1, 75 and 150), showing (u) uninfected cancer cells density, (i) infected cancer cells density, ($u + i$) total cancer cells density, (e) ECM density, (v) virus density, and (c) chemo drug density.

chemo occurring simultaneously during the selected stages) and same spatial locations. Here we use the parameters that showed improved tumour suppression from the variety of simulations that we ran (not shown here), namely $5 \cdot \beta$, $\alpha_u/5$, $2 \cdot \sigma_u$, $2 \cdot \sigma_I$, $b = 3$, $\delta/4$, $K_u = 1$, $\delta_u = 2.08 \cdot 10^{-4}$, $\delta_i = 2.5 \cdot 10^{-4}$, $\lambda = 0.17375/2$ and $2 \cdot \sigma_c$. For a better understanding, we proposed six different cases for this scenario, namely:

- **Case 1**: only one injection at stage 1 with one initial dose of both the OV and the chemo drug,
- **Case 2**: a total of three injections at stages 1, 50, and 100, respectively, with one initial dose of both the OV and the chemo drug,
- **Case 3**: a total of three injections at stages 1, 50, and 100, respectively, with five initial doses of both the OV and the chemo drug,
- **Case 4**: injections every 10 stages but stage 150, with one initial dose of both the OV and the chemo drug,
- **Case 5**: injections every 10 stages but stage 150, with five initial doses of both the OV and the chemo drug,
- **Case 6**: injections every 5 stages but stage 150, with five initial doses of both the OV and the chemo drug.

To keep the discussion short, we will only show the results obtained from cases 1 and 6.

Figure 8 shows the results for case 1 when we assume the same initial conditions from Scenario 5, and the OV and chemo injections are administered simultaneously right at the initiation of the process, i.e., are delivered by

$$g_v^p(x,t) = \gamma_0(t)v(x,0) \quad \text{and} \quad g_c(x,t) = \gamma_0(t)c(x,0).$$

We observe that the tumour in this case is much smaller and with more compact morphology when compared to Scenarios 1–4 and 6 but still larger than the one observed in Scenario 5. Furthermore, we observe smaller densities across all stages with the exception of the ECM simulations by comparison to all previous scenarios, indicating at first a better treatment. However, we can conclude here that only one dose is not enough to suppress the tumour.

Cases 2–5 show signs of improvement in treatment outcomes as the number of injections increases, as well as the initial doses administered. However, though the tumour is not suppressed, the

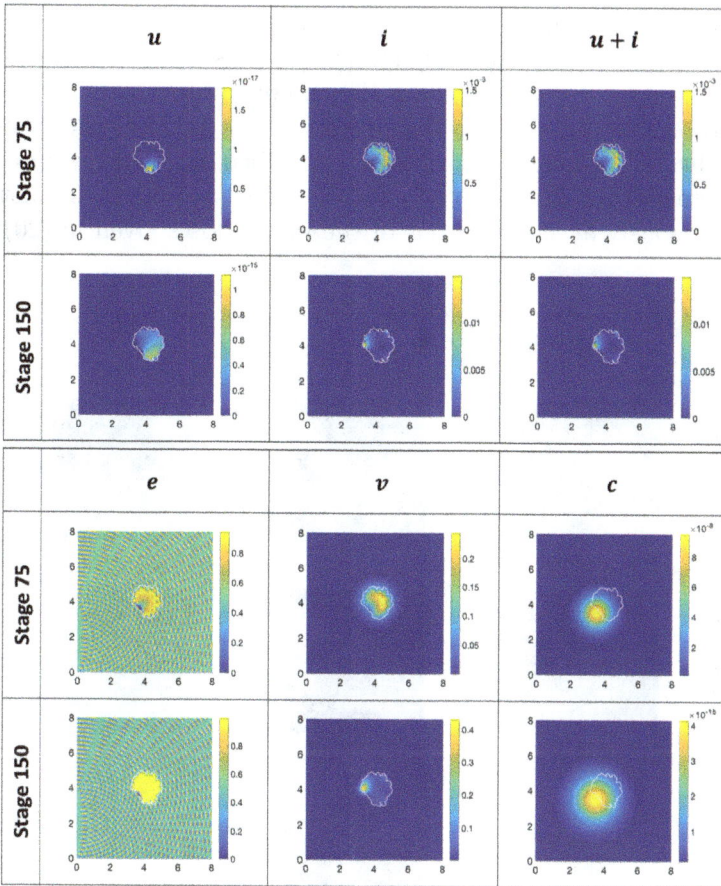

Fig. 8. Results of the simulations from case 1, Scenario 7, at macro–micro stages 75 and 150, showing (u) uninfected cancer cells density, (i) infected cancer cells density, ($u + i$) total cancer cells density, (e) ECM density, (v) virus density, and (c) chemo drug density.

waiting time for relapse is monotonically increasing with regard to the number of simultaneous injections. The morphology of these cases is quite similar, but getting more compact and smaller as we increase the number of simultaneous injections uniformly distributed in time of OV and chemo dosage (i.e., more frequent exposure to such injections). This suggests that administering multiple doses of these agents can lead to a further reduction in tumour size, but it is not enough to completely eradicate the tumour.

Furthermore, from the results in cases 2–5 (not shown or detailed here), administering these injections at the same locations but at different stages does not contain the tumour properly.

Figure 9 presents results from case 6 which explores the situation when the OV and chemo injections are carried out at every 5 macro–micro stages over the period of a total of 150 stages and administered simultaneously at the locations of the initial doses given in (20) and

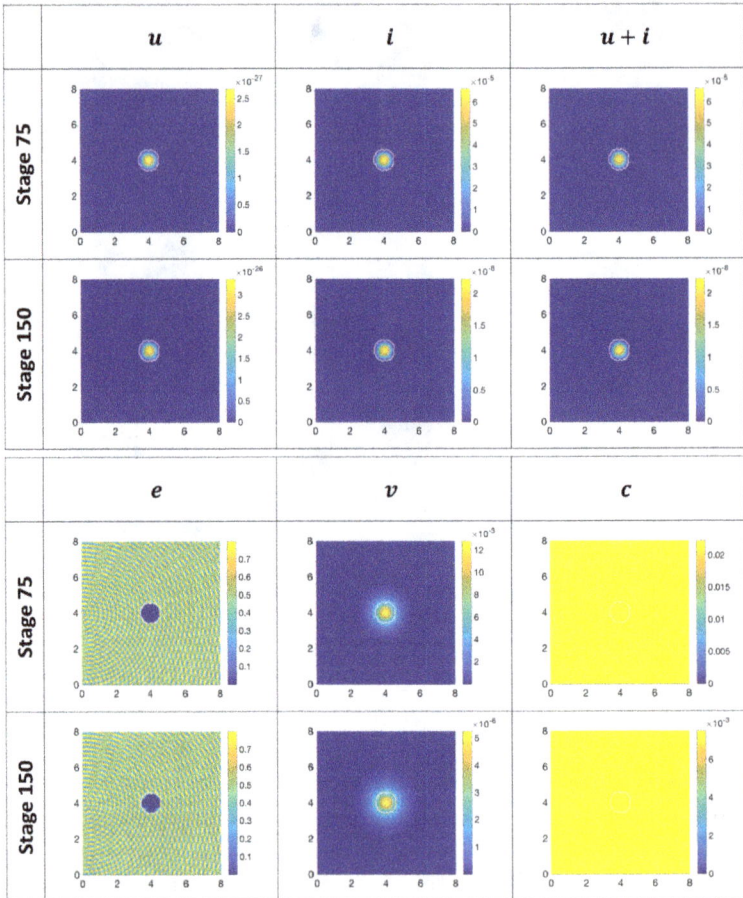

Fig. 9. Results of the simulations from case 6, Scenario 7, at macro–micro stages 75 and 150, showing (u) uninfected cancer cells density, (i) infected cancer cells density, ($u + i$) total cancer cells density, (e) ECM density, (v) virus density, and (c) chemo drug density.

(22), respectively. Thus, the OV and chemo agent delivery functions are mathematically very similar to the ones given in (24), namely in this case these are given by

$$g_c(x,t) := \sum_{i=1}^{[N_{\max}/5]} \gamma_{t_i}(t)c(x,0),$$

$$g_v^p(x,t) := \sum_{i=1}^{[N_{\max}/5]} \gamma_{t_i}(t)v(x,0),$$

(25)

where $t_i := 5(i-1)\Delta t$, for all $i = 1, \ldots, [N_{\max}/5]$.

The tumour morphology observed in case 6 is slightly more compact when compared with the previous five cases within the current scenario. The difference is that the bulk of the tumour's density is located at the centre of the tissue domain. This is due to injecting every five stages around the location of the initial conditions, which converge to the centre of the domain. Moreover, the relapses found in the previous cases also happen in this case but later and more abruptly. The densities are also similar with the exception of higher densities for $i(x,t)$, $(u+i)(x,t)$, $v(x,t)$, and a smaller ECM density. Case 6 shows a slightly more improved morphology, with slower relapse times and lastly the smallest total tumour mass of all cases. We conclude that we obtain a better tumour suppression when we administer initial OV and chemo doses at two groups of five uniformly spatially distributed locations (that do not necessarily coincide) and then increase the number of simultaneous injections (uniformly distributed over time) at the same locations (as the initial doses).

4.   Conclusions and Discussion

In this chapter, we developed a mathematical model of spatio-temporal dynamics of chemovirotherapy treatment to cancer. The multi-scale moving boundary framework proposed by [12], later used by [13] for oncolytic virotherapy, was modified and used in this chapter to describe the interactions between the tissue-scale (macro-scale) cancer cells (uninfected and infected) populations, ECM, OV, and chemo drug, in the presence of the cell-scale tumour invasive edge uPA System micro-dynamics.

We considered seven main scenarios at macro-scale, each representing different treatment options, virotherapy, chemotherapy, as well as several spatio-temporal combinations of viral and chemo therapy.

Scenario 1 and 2 (virotherapy and chemotherapy as monotherapies, respectively) do not contain the tumour effectively, as shown in Figs. 2 and 3, respectively. In Scenario 1, the virus seems to properly infect the tumour but it does not suppress it. Furthermore, in Scenario 2, the tumour exhibited fingering and elongated infiltration with no signs of tumour suppression nor containment.

Scenarios 3 and 4 (virus first then chemo, chemo first then virus, respectively) show similar morphologies to Scenario 1, but the densities of the tumour are smaller, with higher tumour mass in Scenario 4, exhibiting some improvement but do not contain the tumour either with the baseline values, as shown in Figs. 4 and 5, respectively.

Scenario 5 (combined therapies with constant chemo drug infusion) shows total tumour containment, suggesting that the combined therapy is much more effective than either monotherapies, which is in agreement with previous clinical and experimental studies [2, 3, 5–7, 15], and mathematical studies [10–13] on virotherapy and chemovirotherapy. Note that the tumour is contained due to the constant administration of the chemo drug, which is not a realistic approach as it is highly toxic.

Scenario 6 (combined therapies with chemo and OV delivery functions $g_c(x, t)$ and $g_v^p(x, t)$, respectively) does not show an effective tumour containment, which is why we performed different parameter variations, based on the findings by [10, 13] to obtain an effective combined therapy. We specifically experimented on the following: infected cancer cells death rate δ; infection rate β; ECM degradation rates σ_u, σ_i, and σ_c; virus burst size b; drug lysis rates δ_u and δ_i; tumour growth rate α_u; and the initial doses of both agents (the OV and chemo drug).

The experiments on the previously stated parameters led us to successful therapeutical cases, with improved tumour suppression scenarios for the following parameter changes with respect to the baseline values: (a) reduced infected cell death rate, (b) increased viral infection rate, (c) increased ECM degradation rates, (d) increased virus burst size, (e) smaller uninfected growth rate, and (f) introducing the spatial distribution of initial virus and drug doses. These experiments are not shown in this chapter.

Scenario 7 shows the different cases when spatio-temporal injections of both the chemo drug and the OV are administered. We concluded that the best cases are when we inject both the chemo drug and the OV at least every five stages with five initial doses for both agents.

In conclusion, combining the best parameters and the spatio-temporal injections every five stages with five initial doses for both agents led to a much better tumour suppression and control, indicating that the combination of both therapies is much more effective, and containment is possible if the treatment is not stopped, situation that is not realistic as this becomes highly toxic over time. Hence, further research is needed to determine the right time to stop treatment as well as the optimal time of delivery of doses at appropriate spatial locations.

A.1. Appendix A

The mollifier $\psi_\gamma : \mathbb{R}^2 \to \mathbb{R}_+$ used in Section 3 is given by

$$\psi_\gamma(x) = \begin{cases} \exp\left(\dfrac{1}{\gamma^2} - \dfrac{1}{\gamma^2 - \|x\|_2^2}\right), & x \in \mathbf{B}(0,\gamma), \\ 0, & x \in \mathbb{R}^2 \setminus \mathbf{B}(0,\gamma). \end{cases}$$

A.2. Appendix B

Here we include the tables with the baseline values for the parameters considered for our model at both macro- and micro-scales. Furthermore, any other choice in the parameter values (i.e., beyond the ones included in these tables) is explained as appropriate in the text.

Table A.1. The baseline parameter values for the macro-dynamics.

Parameters	Values	References
Y	$[0,8] \times [0,8]$ environmental tissue domain	[13]
D_u	0.00675	[13]
D_i	0.0054	[13]
D_v	0.0036	[13]
D_c	0.0067	Estimated
η_u	$2.85 \cdot 10^{-2}$	[13]
η_i	$2.85 \cdot 10^{-2}$	[13]
η_v	$2.85 \cdot 10^{-3}$	[13]
α_u	0.25	[13]
α_e	0.015	[13]
β	$79 \cdot 10^{-3}$	[13]
δ_u	0.005	[10]
K_u	10^5	[10]
K_c	10^5	[10]
δ_i	0.006	[10]
δ	0.05	[13]
b	2	[13]
δ_v	0.025	[13]
σ_u	0.15	[13]
σ_i	0.075	[13]
σ_c	$[0.075 - 0.15]$	Estimated
λ	4.17	[10]
ϵ	$2 \cdot \Delta x$ (size of the micro-scale)	Estimated
$N_{\max}$	150 (number of macro–micro stages)	Estimated

Table A.2. The baseline parameter values for the micro-dynamics.

Parameters	Values	References
D_a	2.5×10^{-3}	[13]
D_p	3.5×10^{-3}	[13]
D_m	4.91×10^{-3}	[13]
ψ_{11}	0.75	[13]
ψ_{12}	0.215	[13]
ψ_{13}	0.3	[13]
ψ_{21}	0.75	[13]
ψ_{22}	0.55	[13]
ψ_{23}	0.5	[13]
ψ_{31}	0.11	[13]
ψ_{32}	0.75	[13]
ψ_{33}	0.5	[13]

References

[1] J. S. Apolonio, V. L. de Souza Gonçalves, M. L. C. Santos, M. S. Luz, J. V. S. Souza, S. L. R. Pinheiro, *et al.*, Oncolytic virus therapy in cancer: A current review, *World Journal of Virology.* **10**(5), 229–255 (2021). doi: 10.5501/wjv.v10.i5.229.

[2] E. Binz and U. M. Lauer, Chemovirotherapy: Combining chemotherapeutic treatment with oncolytic virotherapy, *Oncolytic Virotherapy.* **4**, 39 (2015).

[3] C.-J. Tai, C.-H. Liu, Y.-C. Pan, S. H. Wong, C.-J. Tai, C. D. Richardson, *et al.*, Chemovirotherapeutic treatment using camptothecin enhances oncolytic measles virus-mediated killing of breast cancer cells, *Scientific Reports.* **9**(1), 1–13 (2019).

[4] I. Liikanen, L. Ahtiainen, M. L. Hirvinen, S. Bramante, V. Cerullo, P. Nokisalmi, *et al.*, Oncolytic adenovirus with temozolomide induces autophagy and antitumor immune responses in cancer patients, *Molecular Therapy: The Journal of the American Society of Gene Therapy.* **21**(6), 1212–1223 (2013). doi: 10.1038/mt.2013.51.

[5] K. Zaoui, S. Bossow, C. Grossardt, M. Leber, C. Springfeld, P. Plinkert, *et al.*, Chemovirotherapy for head and neck squamous cell carcinoma with EGFR-targeted and cd/uprt-armed oncolytic measles virus, *Cancer Gene Therapy.* **19**(3), 181–191 (2012).

[6] T. Fujiwara, S. Kagawa, H. Kishimoto, Y. Endo, M. Hioki, Y. Ikeda, *et al.*, Enhanced antitumor efficacy of telomerase-selective oncolytic adenoviral agent obp-401 with docetaxel: Preclinical evaluation of chemovirotherapy, *International Journal of Cancer.* **119**(2), 432–440 (2006).

[7] E. Binz, S. Berchtold, J. Beil, M. Schell, C. Geisler, I. Smirnow, *et al.*, Chemovirotherapy of pancreatic adenocarcinoma by combining oncolytic vaccinia virus glv-1h68 with nab-paclitaxel plus gemcitabine, *Molecular Therapy-Oncolytics.* **6**, 10–21 (2017).

[8] A. Nguyen, L. Ho, and Y. Wan, Chemotherapy and oncolytic virotherapy: Advanced tactics in the war against cancer, *Frontiers in Oncology.* **4**, 145 (2014).

[9] J. Malinzi, P. Sibanda, and H. Mambili-Mamboundou, Analysis of virotherapy in solid tumor invasion, *Mathematical Biosciences.* **263**, 102–110 (2015).

[10] J. Malinzi, A. Eladdadi, and P. Sibanda, Modelling the spatiotemporal dynamics of chemovirotherapy cancer treatment, *Journal of Biological Dynamics.* **11**(1), 244–274 (2017).

[11] J. Malinzi, Mathematical analysis of a mathematical model of chemovirotherapy: Effect of drug infusion method, *Computational and Mathematical Methods in Medicine.* **2019** (2019).

[12]   D. Trucu, P. Lin, M. A. J. Chaplain, and Y. Wang, A multi-scale moving boundary model arising in cancer invasion, *Multi-scale Modeling & Simulation.* **11**(1), 309–335 (2013).

[13]   T. Alzahrani, R. Eftimie, and D. Trucu, Multi-scale modelling of cancer response to oncolytic viral therapy, *Mathematical Biosciences.* **310**, 76–95 (2019).

[14]   J. P. Tian, The replicability of oncolytic virus: defining conditions in tumor virotherapy, *Mathematical Biosciences & Engineering.* **8**(3), 841 (2011).

[15]   J. G. Gomez-Gutierrez, J. Nitz, R. Sharma, S. L. Wechman, E. Riedinger, E. Martinez-Jaramillo, *et al.*, Combined therapy of oncolytic adenovirus and temozolomide enhances lung cancer virotherapy in vitro and in vivo, *Virology.* **487**, 249–259 (2016).

Chapter 7

Spatio-Temporal-Structural Approaches in Cancer and Immunity Focussed on Oncolytic Viral Therapies

Arran Hodgkinson[*,‡] and **Dumitru Trucu**[†,§]

[*]*School of Mathematics and Physics, Queen's University Belfast, Belfast, Northern Ireland, UK*
[†]*Division of Mathematics, School of Science and Engineering, University of Dundee, Dundee, UK*
[‡]*arran.hodgkinson@qub.ac.uk*
[§]*trucu@maths.dundee.ac.uk*

Although much progress has been made in the targeted treatment of cancer cells, for which mathematical modelling has played an active role, resistance phenomena continue to confound success in this field. Within this context, oncolytic viruses have demonstrated promising outcomes by targeting cancerous cells *in situ*, but interacting negatively with the innate immune interferon (IFN) response, which acts to reduce viral replication and persistence. Building on existing work in spatio-temporal-structural modelling, we take the case of IFN-mediated, temporally local, acquired resistance to oncolytic viral (OV) therapies for use in oncology. Building a spatio-temporal-structural model of the cell-scale dynamics of OV uptake and IFN-based innate immune signalling, within its spatial context, we study and compare two scenarios: one in which cells are incapable of mounting such an immune response and one in which they are capable. In the former case, the cancer cell population proceeds asymptotically towards zero, with the OV multiplying within the cell and causing almost complete lysis among the population. In the latter case, the onset of infection causes IFN to be secreted from infected cells and, upon binding to neighbouring cells, causes the shutdown of the cells' replicative structures and protects sufficient numbers of cells from OV lysis to allow a regrowth of the population or (resistance phenomena). In all, the heterogeneity and correlated behaviours modelled through spatio-temporal-structural modelling techniques allows for distributed dynamics among a cell population and, in so doing, demonstrates predictive potential beyond its immediate uses and into more complex biological phenomena.

1.   Introduction

As increasing numbers of targeted and generalised cancer therapies are produced by the research community and pharmaceutical industry, the problem of innate and acquired resistance continues to confound a definitive response to cancer. In this context, identifying more flexible modelling approaches able to integrate cell population spatio-temporal dynamics coupled with key cell signalling pathways and interactions with the immune system, both in the absence and presence of external pathogens (such as onlcolytic viruses), remains central to gaining a deeper understanding of the entire cancer development and treatment process. To that end, spatio-temporal-structural modelling approaches introduced in the pioneering works [1,2] offer an elegant and robust avenue for aggregating and capturing mathematically all these complex cell population dynamics. Indeed, the relatively recent introduction of spatio-temporal-structural modelling frameworks for mathematical biology, beginning with Domschke *et al.* [1], has allowed for the simultaneous and coevolutionary spatial and structural processes to be modelled in coordination. Thus, one can follow the evolution of a single population, or sub-population, in a system of spatial and functional (or phenotypic) system of coordinates, just as one would expect to be able to track a single cell. Moreover, the explicit numerical and analytic treatment of spatio-temporal-structural systems [3] has facilitated its extrapolation into the study of oncological and immunological processes.

1.1. *Biological responses to viruses and pathogens*

Biological tissues are complex aggregates of individual cells, each with differing lineages, epigenetics, phenotypes, and spatial environments. In order to coordinate behaviour, then, cells contain biochemical structures which can communicate their current state and alert cells in their immediate and more distant vicinity to allow for their concomitant response to these chemical messengers. This is particularly crucial in the tissue-wide response to the presence of a pathogenic intrusion in the form of a biological or viral infection, where large groups of cells and, eventually, the organism as a whole, must coordinate a response [4]. A specific example lies in the detection, amplification, and communication of a precursor signal which eventually leads to the recruitment of T-cells to the site of infection [5].

The immune system comprises all of the cells, throughout the body, and refers to their specific, coordinated response to a pathogen. In particular, cells throughout the body express membrane receptors capable of dynamically changing their conformational state in response to chemokines [5] or cytokines [6] released into their microenvironment.

In several ways, this mechanism is similar to quorum-sensing in bacterial cells [7], where cells will amplify chemical signalling molecules to indicate their biochemical response to and agreement with the initial signal, thus conveying the signal to further spatial locations. This effect is similarly observed in developmental biology, where responsive signals are secreted to achieve a tissue-wide patterning [8,9]. Others have referred to systems of secretion and sensation [10,11] or sensing and reciprocating systems [2], though we shall use the neutral term 'molecular stimulus amplification' (MSA) in order to emphasise the amplification component of the process or the term 'molecular stimulus amplifiers' (MSAs) to refer to the system's constituents. One characteristic feature of these systems is biomolecular thresholding, which allows the signal to decay when the stimulus is sufficiently diminished [12].

This ability for cells to interpret and amplify a molecular signal is a critical component of the local immune system, allowing signals to be locally amplified and globally received. The interferon (IFN) amplification is one such pathway involved in the innate immune response (IIR) to pathogenic infection.

1.2. The IFN response

With particular significance in the response to pathogenic viruses, the majority of human cells produce the immune ligand, IFN in response to the uptake of pathogenic materials from their environment. Not only is this an MSA but has particular relevance to the function of oncolytic viruses (OVs) since, upon detection, the IFN molecule down-regulates the synthesis of genetic materials, such as viruses, achieving the biological function of retarding pathogenicity.

The sub-families of IFN molecules are delineated on the basis of their function and affinity for their respective, membrane-bound receptors. As such, the 13 IFNα sub-classes of molecules are of low affinity and the unique IFNβ sub-class of molecules is of high affinity, while the receptors for each type are identical. In order to activate the cell's downstream anti-pathogenic activity, IFNα or IFNβ must bind to both IFNα/β receptor 1 (IFNAR1) or 2 (IFNAR2), which presents itself on the surface of the target cell. In particular, IFNAR2 exhibits a 10-fold higher association rate to IFN molecules than does IFNAR1, while it is the association of IFNAR1 and IFNAR2, caused by the binding of an extra-cellular IFN ligand, which activates downstream anti-pathogenic signalling [13, 14].

The downstream pathway is then activated upon the co-phosphorylation of the intra-cellular, JAK1 signalling complex of INFAR2 by the tyk2 signalling complex of IFNAR1 [15]. These co-phosphorylated complexes, in turn, phosphorylate the STAT1 and STAT2 transcription factors to initiate the intra-cellular JAK–STAT pathway. This pathway is completed upon the binding of STAT1 and STAT2 to the IFN regulatory (transcription) factor (IRF)-9, the complex of which is known as IFN-stimulated gene factor (ISGF)-3 [15, 16], which may then enter the nucleus [17] and further activate the production of anti-pathogenic proteins and transcription factors known as IFN-stimulated genes (ISGs) [15, 16].

In particular, the ISGs IRF-7 and IRF-3 are capable of binding one another, to form the IRF-7-3 molecular complex, and promoting the transcription of the *IFNα* and *IFNβ* genes themselves [18]. This positive feedback loop will serve to amplify the IFN signal not only for the Jak-Stat activated cell but also in its nearest neighbours and further afield. This process is, however, attenuated through the transcription of the ISG known as USP18, which competitively binds IFNAR2, displacing JAK1 and deactivating, or down-regulating, the JAK–STAT pathway, as a whole [19]. This effect has been confirmed in studies which verified that USP18-bound IFNAR2 was less effective at activating the IRF7 transcription factor [20–22].

Of significance to OV therapies, several ISGs include genes directly down-regulating viral replication in the cell. For example, the down-regulation or deletion of ISG15 [23], ISG54, or ISG56 [24] have all been shown to permit an increased susceptibility to infection by viruses. Through a similar mechanism to ISG54 and ISG56, the protein kinase R (PKR) has been shown to phosphorylate the eukaryotic translational initiation factor 2 (eIF2α), encouraging its recycling [25] and effectively inhibiting its initiation of viral translation. The full spectrum of IFN-initiated responses to viral replication is neither fully understood nor enumerated, but IFN is known to play a major role in interrupting and halting viral replication [26].

The IFN response, therefore, constitutes an important initial response to the uptake of a pathogen by the cell, shutting down critical pathways of infection and signalling the danger of pathogenic uptake to nearby cells. The positive and negative feedback loops included within this IFN response allows both for a rapid potentiation and amplification of an initial signal, upon pathogenic uptake, as well as a modulation of the signal in the absence of a continuing threat. This local immune response becomes critical, particularly in the case of oncolytic viral (OV) therapies, wherein cancer cells interpret the therapy as a foreign pathogen.

1.3. *Oncolytic viral therapies for cancer*

OVs were engineered in response to the loss of immune responses observed in established cancerous tumours and designed to preferentially enter cancer cells, over healthy cells, and lyse the tissue, before themselves being eradicated by the host's immune system [27, 28].

OVs are known to exert a substantial toll on the surrounding tissue, lysing healthy cells as well as cancer cells, and several studies have attempted to quantify this using a cost–benefit analysis-type approach [29]. As exemplified in early clinical trials using

OV therapies, OVs show promising perspectives for the treatment of cancer *in situ* [30], but resistance continues to be a major concern for OVs [31]. This is despite the fact that OVs have demonstrated success even where the cancer has demonstrated resistance to targeted therapies [32,33]. At least in the case of M1 viruses, OV therapy has been shown to overcome cancer-mediated immune checkpoint inhibition and reactivate anti-cancer T-cells [34]. Cancer resistance to OV therapies has spawned its own field of research, which attempts to use innovative therapies, such as pre-emptive [35], inhibitory [36,37], protein-based [38–40], or bacterial [41] therapies, to overcome this resistance and resensitise the tumour to OVs.

Although the adaptive immune system has been flagged as a potential mediator of resistance to repeated therapy, levels of OV-specific antibodies appear not to correlate with OV success or lysis rates [42]. In innate immunity, cancer cells interact with natural killer (NK) T-cells by down-regulating their major histocompatibility complex (which communicates that the cells are harmonious with the body's immune ecosystem) and causing infected cancer cells to be targeted and removed. In practice, this should eradicate the virus prior to the cell population's lysis, but NK cells have been shown to have a positive effect on the overall success of OV therapies [43,44]. Immunosuppressive cytokines, such as IL-10 or TGFβ, released by OV-infected cancer cells may also play a role in active immune resistance [45] though the effect of the immune system on the success of OV therapies is, as yet, inconclusive.

1.4. Phenomenology and modelling of therapeutic resistance in cancer

Cancer cells, within the context of the whole tumour, are known to exhibit varying phenotypes in response to treatment [46] and, simultaneously, to exhibit differential behaviours on the basis of their spatial environment [47]. Moreover, each of these identified sub-populations exhibit unique survival strategies and will, necessarily, interact with one another on the basis of their complementarity, or otherwise [48].

Complex cancer cell population behaviours, such as drug resistance, were also mathematically treated with the spatio-temporal-structural modelling framework, namely through other approaches including the following: continuous (temporal and spatial) [49–53];

phenotypically discretised populations [54]; discrete or stochastic populations [55–60]. Waclaw *et al.* have effectively utilised spatial models of cancer cell dynamics, in a discrete structural context, to investigate the effect of spatial cell exchange mechanisms on biological heterogeneity [61, 62], though they used a reductive discretisation for describing the complex dynamics of structural heterogeneity within the cancer population. Researchers have, similarly, employed non-spatial, structured population, partial differential equation (PDE) models to analytically investigate the effect on phenotypic heterogeneity of exposing cancer to hypothetical cancer treatments [63,64]. Spatial heterogeneity with respect to hypoxia has been explored in one study in OV therapy for solid tumours [65] but did not explore resistance phenomena. In the particular modern case of OVs, several pathways of resistance have already been identified, often relating to the activation of the innate immune system [66]. Further, in a different study, resistance to Adenovirus OV therapy was found to correlate strongly with a significant up-regulation of IFN signalling pathways and their downstream targets [67]. Huff *et al.* [68] found that resistance to their OV therapy was mediated by APOBEC3 in an IFN-β-related manner. Similarly, silencing the IRF-7 gene, critical to the formation of the IRF-7-3 transcription factor complex which amplifies the IFN signal, has been shown to confer additional sensitivity to OVs in the context of lung cancer [69]. This evidence demonstrates a critical role for the immune IFN signalling pathway in conferring systematic resistance to various OV therapies and motivates further exploration of this important mechanism.

The first model to explore the simultaneous effects of spatial and structural heterogeneity on the phenomenology of resistance in cancer analysing the particular dynamics leading to heterogeneously acquired, systemic resistance to targeted therapies in solid tumours was proposed in [70]. This model was further extended [71] and applied to single-cell sequencing data [72] from *in vivo* primary derived xenograft (PDX) melanoma tumours. The authors found that spatial heterogeneity could yield a protected niche of sensitive cells, surrounded by a layer of metabolically resistant cells, allowing the sensitive core of the tumour to continue growing even as the tumour presents as resistant overall [71]. This spatio-temporal-structural approach shows significant promise for understanding the interplay between spatial and biochemical heterogeneity in cancer resistance.

We have previously explored the contribution of spatial heterogeneity to the outcome of infection and IFN signalling, in the initial,
local response to a pathogen [2]. Here, we attempt to combine this
work on the spatio-temporal-structural modelling of IFN dynamics
with similar models of cancer resistance to understand the dynamics
of IFN-mediated resistance to OV therapies.

2. A Model to Explore IFN-Interrupted Oncolytic Viral Therapy

In order to model a tumour growing under experimental conditions,
within a spatially heterogeneous and controlled environment, we consider only three primary quantities of interest:

(1) The tumour cell population, which we shall denote c, responds
to a virus by allowing its internal replication and producing IFN,
which may, in turn, be bound and lead to anti-viral cellular
responses. This tumour cell population, in the absence of inter-
ference, exhibits proliferation and diffusive, or random, motion
through the implicit growth medium.
(2) The quantity of oncolytic virions in the extracellular environment, or growth medium, shall be denoted v and is contributed
to through cellular lysis, while diffusing through the growth
medium.
(3) The quantity of unbound, extracellular IFN molecules shall be
denoted m and is produced by infected or sufficiently bound
cells, whilst diffusing through the growth medium. The virion
and IFN populations shall be subjected to independent, natural
degradative processes.

In order to understand the dynamics of the OV, in the context
of the tumour, as well as the response of the cancer cells, this problem is fundamentally posed in terms of a spatio-temporal system
of PDEs. To accurately constitute the dynamics within the tumour
cell population, however, we require a description of the population's
evolution in terms of its internal viral load (IVL), denoted u, and its
fractional, surface–ligand binding (FSLB) of IFN, denoted β.

Therefore, let $\mathcal{I} := [0, T]$ be an arbitrary time interval, with
$T > 0$, upon which the experiment is to take place and let $\mathcal{D} :=
[-X, X]^d$ be a bounded spatial domain of dimension $d \in \{1, 2, 3\}$,

where $X \in (0, \infty)$. Then, $t \in \mathcal{I}$ and $x \in \mathcal{D}$ are independent temporal and spatial variables, respectively. Next, considering the cancer cell population in particular, let $\mathcal{V} := [0, U]^u$ be an IVL, with some maximum viral load $U \in (0, \infty)$, and $\mathcal{B} := [0, 1]^b$ be an FSLB domain, where $b \in \mathbb{Z}_+$ is the number of structurally distinct molecules available for binding. For the purposes of this study, we take $b = 1$. As defined above, $u \in \mathcal{V}$ and $\beta \in \mathcal{B}$ are taken to be independent IVL and extra-cellular FSLB, respectively.

2.1. Derivation of a spatio-temporal-structural framework

This derivation follows closely the analysis of Hodgkinson *et al.* [2] and gives rise to a flexible spatio-temporal-structural system of PDEs which may be characterised for analogous problems to those of immediate concern here. That is, any problem wherein a pathogenic load, u, and surface–ligand binding are of primary concern to the dynamics of a population of cells may be characterised within the framework here derived, while the extension of this system may be achieved by the extrapolation of the steps taken herein.

Let us consider a cell population defined in time, space, IVL, and FSLB is defined as $c : \mathcal{I} \times \mathcal{D} \times \mathcal{V} \times \mathcal{B} \to \mathbb{R}_+$, and let F, G, and H be arbitrarily chosen compact sets in $\mathcal{D}$, $\mathcal{V}$, and $\mathcal{B}$ (say, for instance, intervals in d, u, and b dimensions), respectively. Then, the total mass of cells in the subspace $F \times G \times H$, at a given time t, is given by

$$\hat{c}(t) = \int_H \int_G \int_F c(t, x, u, \beta) \, dx \, du \, d\beta. \tag{1}$$

Then, the change in the total mass of cells in $F \times G \times H$ per unit time is given by accounting for the overall fluxes across the spatial and structural boundaries, $\partial(F \times G \times H)$, alongside the total source of cells on $F \times G \times H$, and so we have

$$\frac{d\hat{c}}{dt} = \int_H \int_G \int_F \hat{S}(t, x, u, \beta) \, dx \, du \, d\beta$$

$$- \int_H \int_G \int_{\partial F} \hat{\Xi}(t, x, u, \beta) \cdot \mathfrak{n}(x) \, d\sigma_{d-1}(x) \, du \, d\beta$$

$$- \int_F \int_H \int_{\partial G} \hat{U}(t, x, u, \beta) \cdot \mathfrak{n}(u) \, d\sigma_{u-1}(u) \, d\beta \, dx$$

$$- \int_G \int_F \int_{\partial H} \hat{B}(t, x, u, \beta) \cdot \mathfrak{n}(\beta) \, d\sigma_{b-1}(\beta) \, dx \, du, \qquad (2)$$

where $\hat{S}$, $\hat{\Xi}$, $\hat{U}$, and $\hat{B}$ are fluxes in total mass, space, IVL, and FSLB and where σ_{d-1}, σ_{u-1}, and σ_{b-1} are surface measures on $\partial\mathcal{D}$, $\partial\mathcal{V}$, $\partial\mathcal{B}$, respectively. Here, for simplicity, we use here the unified notation $\mathfrak{n}(\cdot)$ to denote the normal vector on the boundary of the relevant space at the indicated point.

Further, assuming that $\hat{F}$, $\hat{G}$, and $\hat{H}$ are smooth enough, i.e., they are at least in the class of continuously differentiable vector fields, $\mathcal{C}^1$, one can use Stokes' theorem to express this in terms of the total divergence of the respective fields as

$$\frac{d\hat{c}}{dt} = \int_H \int_G \int_F \hat{S}(t, x, u, \beta) \, dx \, du \, d\beta$$

$$- \int_H \int_G \int_F \nabla_x \cdot \hat{\Xi}(t, x, u, \beta) \, dx \, du \, d\beta$$

$$- \int_F \int_H \int_G \nabla_u \cdot \hat{U}(t, x, u, \beta) \, du \, d\beta \, dx$$

$$- \int_G \int_F \int_H \nabla_\beta \cdot \hat{B}(t, x, u, \beta) \, d\beta \, dx \, du. \qquad (3)$$

Next, using Lebesgue's dominated convergence theorem, one can move the time derivative inside the integral for $\hat{c}$, such that

$$\int_H \int_G \int_F \frac{\partial \hat{c}}{\partial t} \, dx \, du \, d\beta = \int_H \int_G \int_F \hat{S}(t, x, u, \beta) \, dx \, du \, d\beta$$

$$- \int_H \int_G \int_F \nabla_x \cdot \hat{\Xi}(t, x, u, \beta) \, dx \, du \, d\beta$$

$$- \int_F \int_H \int_G \nabla_u \cdot \hat{U}(t, x, u, \beta) \, du \, d\beta \, dx$$

$$- \int_G \int_F \int_H \nabla_\beta \cdot \hat{B}(t, x, u, \beta) \, d\beta \, dx \, du. \qquad (4)$$

The definite integral on $F \times G \times H$ can be rewritten on the real space $\mathbb{R}^{d+u+b}$, using the indicator function $\mathbf{1}$ to retain the appropriate subregion, as

$$\int_{\mathbb{R}^{d+u+b}} \left[\frac{\partial \hat{c}}{\partial t}\right] \mathbf{1}_{F \times G \times H}(x, u, \beta) \, dx \, du \, d\beta$$

$$= \int_{\mathbb{R}^{d+u+b}} \left[\hat{S}(t, x, u, \beta)\right] \mathbf{1}_{F \times G \times H}(x, u, \beta) \, dx \, du \, d\beta$$

$$- \int_{\mathbb{R}^{d+u+b}} \left[\nabla_x \cdot \hat{\Xi}(t, x, u, \beta)\right] \mathbf{1}_{F \times G \times H}(x, u, \beta) \, dx \, du \, d\beta$$

$$- \int_{\mathbb{R}^{d+u+b}} \left[\nabla_u \cdot \hat{U}(t, x, u, \beta)\right] \mathbf{1}_{F \times G \times H}(x, u, \beta) \, du \, d\beta \, dx$$

$$- \int_{\mathbb{R}^{d+u+b}} \left[\nabla_\beta \cdot \hat{B}(t, x, u, \beta)\right] \mathbf{1}_{F \times G \times H}(x, u, \beta) \, d\beta \, dx \, du. \quad (5)$$

Given F, G, and H are compact with piecewise smooth boundaries, then $\{F \times G \times H \mid F, G, H \text{ compact subsets in } \mathcal{D} \times \mathcal{V} \times \mathcal{B}, \text{ respectively}\}$ is a family of generators for the associated Borelian σ-algebra on $\mathcal{D} \times \mathcal{V} \times \mathcal{B}$, and as a consequence, we can write the above in terms of indicator functions on any arbitrary subspace, $A \subseteq \mathcal{D} \times \mathcal{V} \times \mathcal{B}$,

$$\int_{\mathbb{R}^{d+u+b}} \left[\frac{\partial \hat{c}}{\partial t}\right] \mathbf{1}_A(x, u, \beta) \, dx \, du \, d\beta$$

$$= \int_{\mathbb{R}^{d+u+b}} \left[\hat{S}(t, x, u, \beta)\right] \mathbf{1}_A(x, u, \beta) \, dx \, du \, d\beta$$

$$- \int_{\mathbb{R}^{d+u+b}} \left[\nabla_x \cdot \hat{\Xi}(t, x, u, \beta)\right] \mathbf{1}_A(x, u, \beta) \, dx \, du \, d\beta$$

$$- \int_{\mathbb{R}^{d+u+b}} \left[\nabla_u \cdot \hat{U}(t, x, u, \beta)\right] \mathbf{1}_A(x, u, \beta) \, du \, d\beta \, dx$$

$$- \int_{\mathbb{R}^{d+u+b}} \left[\nabla_\beta \cdot \hat{B}(t, x, u, \beta)\right] \mathbf{1}_A(x, u, \beta) \, d\beta \, dx \, du. \quad (6)$$

Furthermore, since the above equality holds true for any Borellian set A, then we have that the same equality holds true for any simple function ν (i.e., we can replace 1_A with ν), and so we have

$$\int_{\mathbb{R}^{d+u+b}} \left[\frac{\partial \hat{c}}{\partial t}\right] \nu(x, u, \beta) \, dx \, du \, d\beta$$

$$= \int_{\mathbb{R}^{d+u+b}} \left[\hat{S}(t, x, u, \beta)\right] \nu(x, u, \beta) \, dx \, du \, d\beta$$

$$- \int_{\mathbb{R}^{d+u+b}} \left[\nabla_x \cdot \hat{\Xi}(t, x, u, \beta)\right] \nu(x, u, \beta) \, dx \, du \, d\beta$$

$$- \int_{\mathbb{R}^{d+u+b}} \left[\nabla_u \cdot \hat{U}(t, x, u, \beta)\right] \nu(x, u, \beta) \, du \, d\beta \, dx$$

$$- \int_{\mathbb{R}^{d+u+b}} \left[\nabla_\beta \cdot \hat{B}(t, x, u, \beta)\right] \nu(x, u, \beta) \, d\beta \, dx \, du. \tag{7}$$

Moreover, since the set of simple functions is dense in $\mathcal{L}^1$ within the family of test functions $\mathcal{C}^\infty$, we note that the above equation also holds true for any test function $\phi \in \mathcal{C}^\infty$, $\nu(t, x, u, \beta)$ (i.e., we can replace ν with ϕ), which finally enables us to obtain the following PDE:

$$\frac{\partial}{\partial t} c(t, x, u, \beta) = \hat{S}(t, x, u, \beta) - \nabla_x \cdot \hat{\Xi}(t, x, u, \beta)$$

$$- \nabla_x \cdot \hat{U}(t, x, u, \beta) - \nabla_x \cdot \hat{B}(t, x, u, \beta). \tag{8}$$

Recall that $\hat{S}$, $\hat{\Xi}$, $\hat{U}$, and $\hat{B}$ are vector fields defining the respective fluxes of the cellular population, c, in total mass, space, IVL, and FSLB.

2.2. Model phenomenology

As a minimal model, we explore the dynamics of three primary species:

(1) **The cancer cell population, $\hat{c}$:** $\mathcal{I} \times \mathcal{D} \times \mathcal{V} \times \mathcal{B} \to \mathbb{R}_+$, which evolves in time, space, IVL and FSLB. This gives us the ability to observe the concurrent influence on each of these dimensions of difference over time, alongside their specific interactions, resulting in the death or survival of the tumour cell population.
(2) **The molecular IFN population, $\hat{m}$:** $\mathcal{I} \times \mathcal{D} \to \mathbb{R}_+$, is assumed to evolve in time and space, alone, and is produced by the cellular population, in response to pathogenic uptake.

(3) **The OV population, $\hat{v}$:** $\mathcal{I} \times \mathcal{D} \to \mathbb{R}_+$, is the primary pathogen in this system, replicating within cancer cells and evoking a molecular IFN response.

2.2.1. *Cancer cell dynamics*

To simplify the model, in this first instance, we conceive the spatial dynamics as taking place within a Petri dish or other *in vitro* medium (such as a tumour spheroid), such that the spatial flux term can be given by homogeneous diffusive dynamics

$$\hat{\Xi}(t, x, u, \beta) = -D_c \nabla_x \hat{c}(t, x, u, \beta), \tag{9}$$

with the diffusion rate D_c. Here, diffusion represents the stochastic motion of cells which are unaccounted for by causal dynamics.

In the case of IVL flux, this is mediated by the influx of extracellular OVs into the cell; the replication of OVs, which have previously entered the cell; and the stochastic components of viral replication (i.e., the randomness in the rate of this process due either to accelerated replication or viral degradation). The uptake of extracellular OVs into the host cell is assumed to be proportional to the mass of OVs outside the cell, v, and an intrinsic uptake rate for the system, χ_v. Meanwhile, the internal OV replication rate is given by χ_u and is proportional to the available mass of internal OV, u. Viral uptake and replication are assumed to be arrested upon sufficient activation of the JAK–STAT pathway, represented only through upstream IFN FSLB, β, in this model. The form of this arrest and its relation to FSLB is given by the sigmoidal function $\sigma_v : \mathcal{B} \to [0, 1]$. Given that random replicative or degradative processes are assumed to occur with a rate D_u, proportional to the mass of OV, u, within the cell, we obtain

$$\hat{U}(t, x, u, \beta) = \sigma_v(\beta)\Big(\chi_v \hat{v}(t, x) + \chi_u u \hat{c}(t, x, u, \beta)$$

$$- D_u u \nabla u \hat{c}(t, x, u, \beta)\Big). \tag{10}$$

In practice, the sigmoidal function on cellular viral load, $\sigma_v(\cdot)$, is given by

$$\sigma_v(\beta) = \left(1 + \exp\left(q_\beta(\beta - \frac{1}{2})\right)\right)^{-1}. \tag{11}$$

The flux in FSLB, then, is simply proportional to the extracellular mass of available ligands, m, and is assumed to occur with a rate χ_m. This binding rate is further limited by the availability of surface receptors upon the target cell which, considering that FSLB is assumed to be fractional, is given simply by $(1 - \beta)$, such that

$$\hat{B}(t, x, u, \beta) = \chi_m \hat{m}(t, x)(1 - \beta) \; \hat{c}(t, x, u, \beta). \tag{12}$$

The source term is meaningfully thought of in terms of a mitosis term and a viral lysis term: the mitosis term is assumed to be logistic, with the carrying capacity of cells given by K_c, and the rate of mitosis given by α_c. The destruction, or lysis, of cells is assumed to occur only through virally mediated processes and upon reaching sufficient levels of IVL. The degradation rate, itself, is given by ξ_c, while the probability density function (PDF), or likelihood of lysis function, is given by $\ell : \mathcal{V} \to [0, 1]$ and is normalised on the domain $\mathcal{V}$, such that

$$\hat{S}(t, x, u, \beta) = \alpha_c \left(1 - \frac{1}{K_c} \hat{c}(t, x, u, \beta) \right) \hat{c}(t, x, u, \beta)$$
$$- \xi_c \ell(u) \; \hat{c}(t, x, u, \beta). \tag{13}$$

In practice, the exponential function on cellular viral load, $\ell(\cdot)$, is given by

$$\ell(u) = R_u \exp \left(r_u(u - K_u) \right), \tag{14}$$

where R_u is a constant of normalisation for $\ell(u)$.

2.2.2. IFN molecular dynamics

The dynamics of the IFN molecule is separable into spatial, binding, and source dynamics: The spatial dynamics of the IFN molecule population are assumed to be exclusively diffusive, relying on no local extracellular currents for molecular motility, with a rate D_m. The binding dynamics are given by the structural $(\mathcal{V} \times \mathcal{B})$ integral over the cellular binding flux term, $\hat{B}(t, x, u, \beta)$, modulated by a conversion term, K_m, between the fractional binding of the cellular binding domain and the true number of molecules required for saturation. This conversion factor can be thought of as a carrying capacity for the surface receptors of a given cell in the population. Finally, the source dynamics of the IFN molecules are governed by the activity of the cell population, as a function $\sigma_m : \mathcal{B} \to [0, 1]$ of cellular binding, multiplied by the production rate, α_m. We assume the natural degradation of the IFN ligands at a rate ξ_m. These relations are mathematically denoted by

$$\frac{\partial}{\partial t}\hat{m}(t, x) = D_m \nabla_x^2 \hat{m}(t, x) - K_m \chi_m \hat{m}(t, x) \int_{\mathcal{B}} (1 - \beta) \int_{\mathcal{V}} c \, du \, d\beta$$

$$+ \alpha_m \int_{\mathcal{B}} \int_{\mathcal{V}} \frac{1}{2} \Big(\sigma_m(u) + \beta \Big) \, \hat{c}(t, x, u, \beta) \, du \, d\beta$$

$$- \xi_m \hat{m}(t, x). \tag{15}$$

In practice, the sigmoidal function on cellular viral load, σ_m, is given by

$$\sigma_m(u) = \Big(1 + \exp \Big(q_u (\frac{1}{2} K_u - u) \Big) \Big)^{-1}. \tag{16}$$

2.2.3. *Extracellular OV dynamics*

The dynamics of the OV are, likewise, separable into spatial, infective, lytic, and degradative dynamics: the spatial dynamics are assumed to be exclusively diffusive, with a rate D_v. The infective uptake of the virus to the cellular population is given by the structural $(\mathcal{V} \times \mathcal{B})$ integral over the uptake term of the IVL flux, $\hat{U}(t, x, u, \beta)$, given explicitly by

$$\hat{U}(t, x, u, \beta) = \chi_v \sigma_v(\beta) \hat{v}(t, x) \hat{c}(t, x, u, \beta). \tag{17}$$

The lytic dynamics, describing the lysis of the cell caused by the build-up of pathogenic viral material in the cell, and the resultant release of virions into the extracellular space are given by the degradative rate of the cellular population, in $\hat{S}(t, x, u, \beta)$, multiplied by the particular viral occupation of the degraded cells, u. A source term, given by the Dirac delta distribution in time centred around t_{dose}, $\delta_t(t - t_{\text{dose}})$, allows for the OV dose of $v_{\text{dose}}(x) > 0$ to be given at $t > 0$ while the natural degradation of virions occurs with a rate

ξ_v, such that

$$\frac{\partial}{\partial t} v(t,x) = D_v \nabla_x^2 \hat{v}(t,x) - \chi_v \hat{v}(t,x) \int_B \sigma_v(\beta) \int_V \hat{c}(t,x,u,\beta)\, du\, d\beta$$

$$+ \xi_c \int_V \ell(u) u \int_B \hat{c}(t,x,u,\beta)\, d\beta\, du$$

$$+ v_{\mathrm{dose}}(x)\delta_t(t - t_{\mathrm{dose}}) - \xi_v \hat{v}(t,x). \tag{18}$$

2.3. *Model summary*

We use the notational convenience of $c := \hat{c}(t,x,u,\beta)$, $m := \hat{m}(t,x)$ and $v := \hat{v}(t,x)$ to summarise the above-delineated system of PDEs as

$$\frac{\partial}{\partial t} c = D_c \nabla_x^2 c - \nabla_u \cdot \sigma_v(\beta) \left[\left(\chi_v v + \chi_u u \right) c - D_u u \nabla_u c \right]$$

$$+ \chi_m m \nabla_\beta \cdot (1 - \beta)c + \alpha_c c \left(1 - \frac{c}{K_c} \right) - \xi_c \ell(u)c,$$

$$\frac{\partial}{\partial t} m = D_m \nabla_x^2 m - K_m \chi_m m \int_B (1 - \beta) \int_V c\, du\, d\beta$$

$$+ \alpha_m \int_B \int_V \frac{1}{2} \left(\sigma_m(u) + \beta \right) c\, du\, d\beta - \xi_m m,$$

$$\frac{\partial}{\partial t} v = D_v \nabla_x^2 v + \int_B \int_V \left[\xi_c \ell(u) u - \chi_v \sigma_v(\beta) v \right] c\, du\, d\beta$$

$$+ v_{\mathrm{dose}}(x)\delta_t(t - t_{\mathrm{dose}}) - \xi_v v. \tag{19}$$

3. Results of Simulation

Simulated solutions are given for the initial value problem (IVP) given by the system of PDEs (19), with the parameters given in Table 1, and with initial conditions given by

$$c(0, x, u, \beta) := K_c c_0^*, \quad \text{with} \quad c_0^* \propto \mathcal{N}_{x,u,\beta}(\mu_x, s_x, \mu_u, s_u, \mu_\beta, s_\beta),$$

$$m(0, x) := 0,$$

Table 1. Table of parameters for the simulation of (19).

Rate description	Symbol	Value	Units
Random motion of cells	D_c	10^{-3}	$\text{cm}^2\ \text{day}^{-1}$
Random OV load	D_u	10^4	virus day^{-1}
Cellular OV uptake	χ_v	10^{-5}	virus day^{-1}
Intra-cellular viral replication	χ_u	2.0	virus day^{-1}
Cellular binding of IFN	χ_m	10^{-8}	mol day^{-1}
Cellular mitosis	α_c	0.1	day^{-1}
Cellular carrying capacity	K_c	10^6	cell
Cellular degradation by OV	ξ_c	0.5	day^{-1}
Cellular OV capacity	K_u	10^6	virus
Diffusion of IFN	D_m	10^{-2}	$\text{cm}^2\ \text{day}^{-1}$
IFN production	α_m	10^3	$\text{mol (cell day)}^{-1}$
IFN capacity	K_m	10^2	virus
Natural degradation of IFN	ξ_m	1.0	day^{-1}
Diffusion of OV	D_v	10^{-2}	$\text{cm}^2\ \text{day}^{-1}$
Natural degradation of OV	ξ_v	0.5	day^{-1}
OV dose	K_v	10^9	virus
Sigmoidal sharpness	q_β	16	—
Sigmoidal sharpness	q_u	2×10^{-5}	—
Exponential steepness	r_u	3×10^{-5}	—
Time of OV dose	t_{dose}	2.0	day

$$v(0, x) := 0,$$

$$v_{\text{dose}} := K_v v_0^*, \quad \text{with} \quad v_0^* \propto \mathcal{N}_x(\mu_v, s_v), \tag{20}$$

where $\mathcal{N}_{x,u,\beta}(\mu_x, s_x, \mu_u, s_u, \mu_\beta, s_\beta)$ is the normal distribution in (x, u, β) with means $\mu_x = 0$, $\mu_u = 0$, and $\mu_\beta = 0$ and standard deviations $s_x = 1/\sqrt{50}$, $s_u = 10^{-3}$, $s_\beta = 10^{-3}$, respectively, and likewise for $\mathcal{N}_x(\cdot, \cdot)$ with $\mu_v = 0$ and $s_v = 1/\sqrt{50}$. In all cases, MatLab has been used for the generation of numerical results using a finite differences approximation scheme, in space and structure, and a Mac-Cormack predictor–corrector scheme for temporal integration.

In particular, we present two sets of solutions: first for a cancer under OV treatment in the absence of an IIR and the second for a cancer alongside an IIR. In the case where the cancer is simulated without an accompanying IIR to the effects of the OV, the parameter value $\alpha_m = 0$ is used, giving rise to the solution $m(t, x) := 0$, $\forall t \in \mathcal{I}$. Moreover, by integrating each of the quantities c, m, and v over (x, u, β), we provide a comparison between the respective populations of cancer, IFN, and extra-cellular OV in each case. Finally, by integrating the cancer population across (x, u, β), we are able to give a comparative response of the cancer cells, in terms of their centre of mass (COM) in viral uptake and IFN binding, across time. In order to make the appreciation of the spatial and structural results for all populations, in each case, we present the overall comparative results first sequentially.

3.1. *Comparative results for cancer without or alongside IIR*

The comparative results are given for the simulation of (19) without (Fig. 1, top) or alongside (Fig. 1, bottom) an IIR as a fold change of the total population obtained as an integral across (x, u, β) for c, m, and v. The fold change is with respect to $\int_B \int_V \int_D c_0 \, dx \, du \, d\beta$ in the cancer population, c, to $\max_{t \in \mathcal{I}}(m)$ in the IFN population, and to K_m in the OV population.

First, note that, due to the parameter choice of $\alpha_m = 0$, the IFN population does not increase from m_0 in the case without an IIR, whereas it does increase in the alternate case. Second, note that in the case exploring OV dynamics alongside an IIR (Fig. 1, top), the peak extracellular OV mass is elevated in comparison to the case without an IIR (Fig. 1, bottom). Despite this increase in the peak OV mass, the population cultured alongside an IIR develops resistance to the OV treatment and begins to regrow at $t \approx 10$, reaching its initial population at $t \approx 30$.

Next, we observe the dynamics in the COM of the cancer cell population, c, in (β, u) as a function of time. Due to the absence of environmental IFN, the COM in the IFN binding domain, β, does not diverge from $\beta = 0$ in the case excluding an IIR (Fig. 2, top). On the other hand, within the OV uptake domain, u, the cancer cell population sees a shift in its COM towards $u = 1$ as the OV dose is given and the OV population begins to increase, while it sees a retrogressive shift towards $u = 0$ as the cell population dies and the OV population recedes asymptotically to $v = 0$. In the case observed alongside an IIR (Fig. 2, bottom), the COM in binding, β, sees a monotonic increase, beginning shortly after the initial dose of OV therapy, v. In the OV uptake domain, u, this population sees a similar

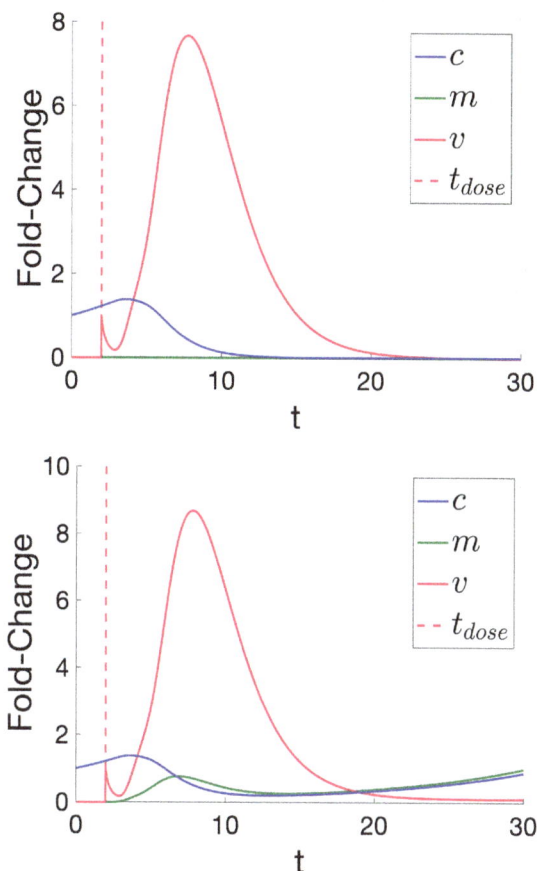

Fig. 1. Simulated results for (19) given in terms of fold-change in cancer, c; IFN, m; and OV, v, populations across time, either without (top, achieved using $\alpha_m = 0$) or alongside (bottom) an IIR.

increase to its comparator, though reaching its initial turning point as the COM in β passes $\frac{1}{2}$ and subsequently converging asymptotically to $u = \frac{1}{2}$. This steady state for the COM in OV uptake is caused by a combination of the protective effect of the IIR, or IFN binding, alongside the diffusive dynamics of the population in u. This will be observed yet more clearly in the distributed dynamics (Section 3.3).

Next, we observe the spatio-temporal-structural dynamics of the cancer cell population, c, experiments without and alongside an IIR in order to understand the effects of heterogeneity on outcomes.

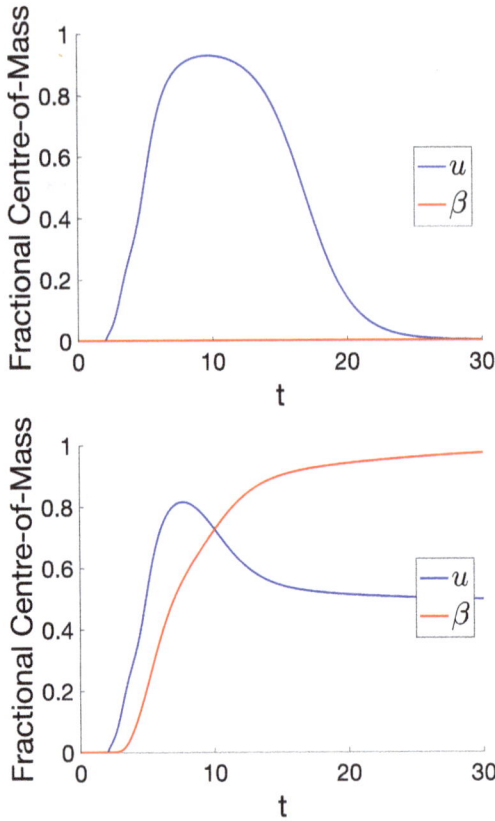

Fig. 2. Simulated results for (19) given in terms of the fractional COM for the cancer cell population, c, in viral load, u, and IFN binding, β, across time, either without (top, achieved using $\alpha_m = 0$) or alongside (bottom) an IIR.

3.2. *Results for cancer without IIR*

Beginning with the spatio-structural cancer cell population without an IIR, the results are given only in terms of space (Fig. 3) since the absence of IFN in the system leads only to linear dynamics in the structure. Observe, in this case, that even after the initial OV dose is given, at $t = 2$, the cancer cell population continues to grow until its turning point at $t = 4$ (Fig. 3), as observed in the total mass results (Fig. 1, top). Meanwhile, the OV population continues to grow until $t = 8$ (Fig. 3), sustaining the increase in OV uptake (Fig. 2, top) and cell death rate, before the OV, too, begins to decrease and

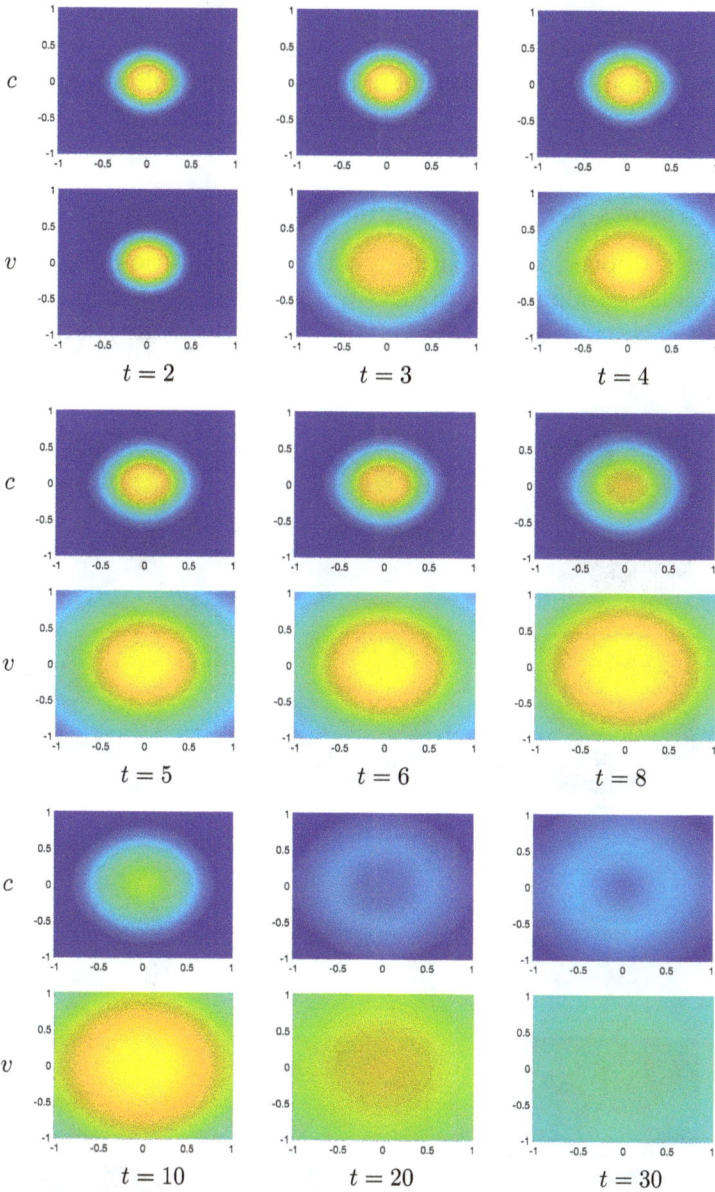

Fig. 3. Simulated results for (19) given in space for the cancer, c, and OV, v, populations and $t \in \{2, 3, 4, 5, 6, 8, 10, 20, 30\}$ without an IIR achieved using $\alpha_m = 0$.

homogenise across the domain (Fig. 3) as a result of spatially diffusive processes. This yields a travelling wave solution in the spatial cancer cell population, which is further subjected to spatial homogenisation as $t \to \infty$.

3.3.   *Results for cancer alongside IIR*

In order to move to the spatio-structural presentation of the cancer cell population alongside an IIR, we give four population distributions at each time point (Figs. 4–6): respectively the spatial cancer

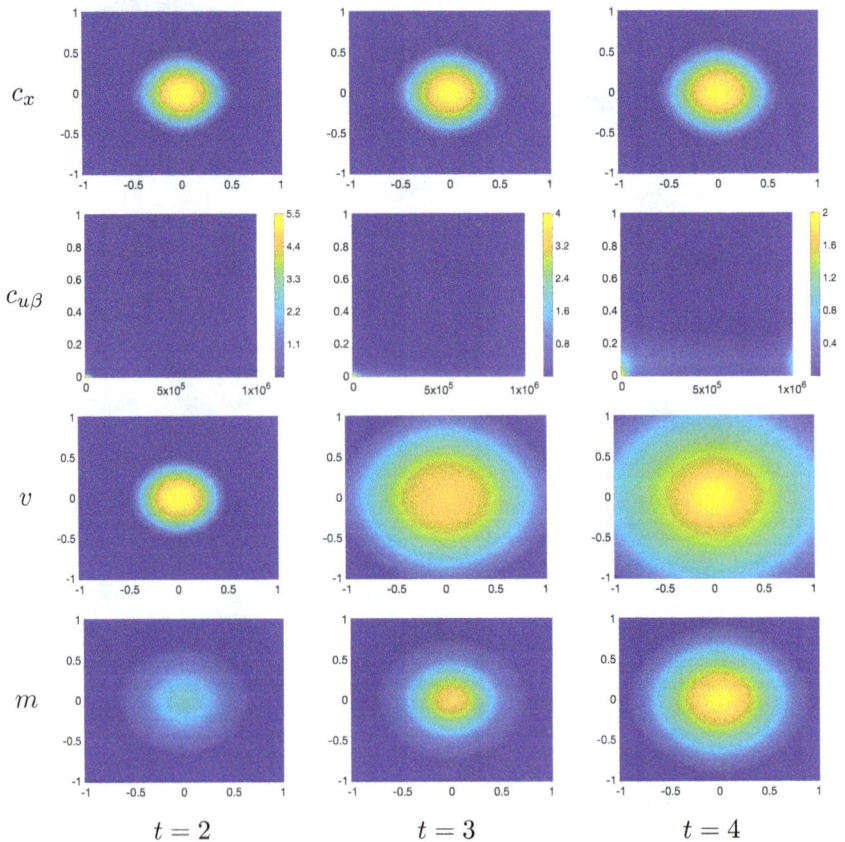

Fig. 4.   Simulated results for (19) given in space for the cancer, c, and OV, v, populations and $t \in \{2, 3, 4\}$ alongside an IIR.

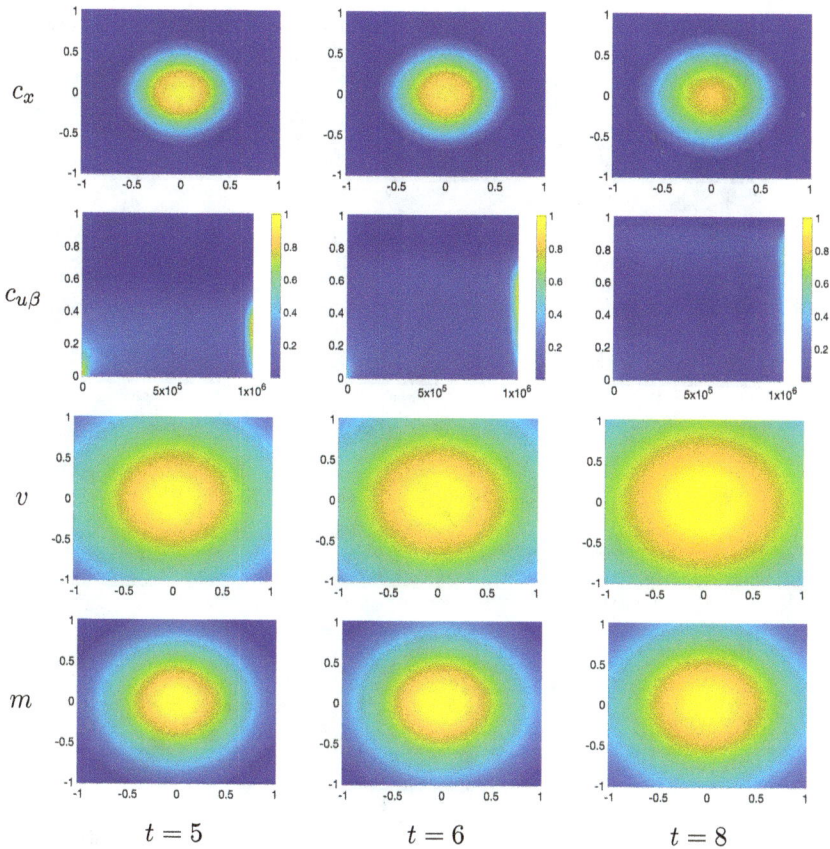

Fig. 5.   Simulated results for (19) given in space for the cancer, c, and OV, v, populations and $t \in \{5, 6, 8\}$ alongside an IIR.

cell population, $c_x := \int_{\mathcal{B}} \int_{\mathcal{V}} c \, du \, d\beta$; the structural cancer cell population, $c_{u\beta} := \iint_{\mathcal{D}} c \, dx$; the spatial OV population, v; and the (now non-zero) spatial IFN population, m. These are given for the same time points as the population distribution without an IIR (Section 3.2).

At the time of the initial OV dose, $t = 2$, the cancer cell population remains at its initial distribution in (u, β) (Fig. 4, $c_{u,\beta}$) while, beyond this time point, the OV mass increases and the cancer cell distribution evolves in u. At these early time points, the IFN population, m, may also be observed to increase its total mass and diffuse

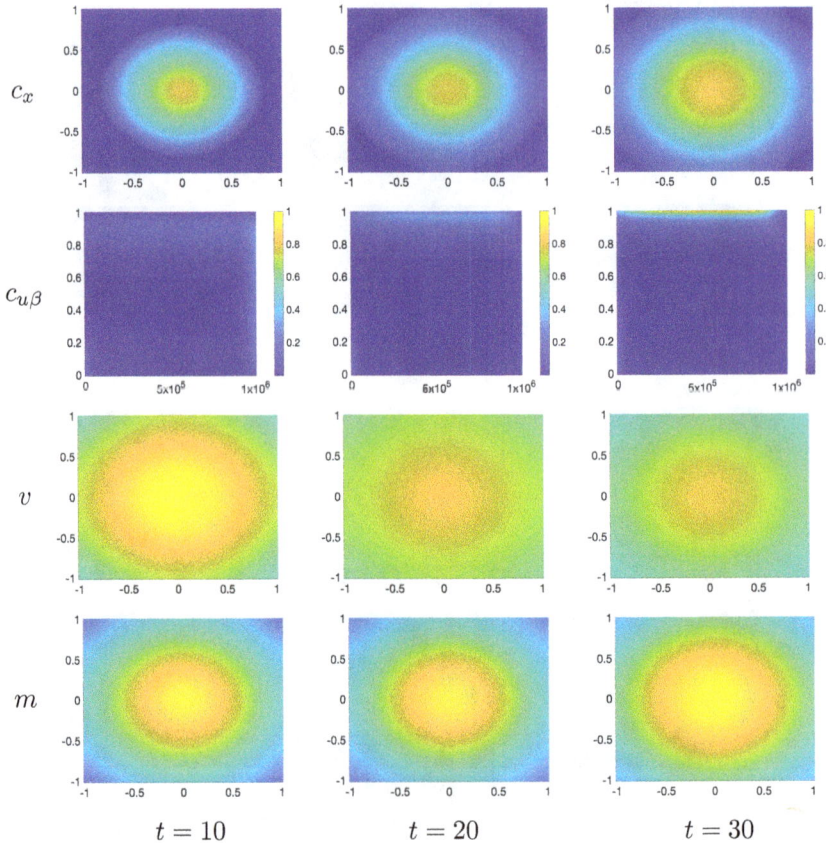

Fig. 6. Simulated results for (19) given in space for the cancer, c, and OV, v, populations and $t \in \{10, 20, 30\}$ alongside an IIR.

through the spatial domain (Fig. 4, m). At $t = 4$, one can see the concomitant increase in the position of the distribution of cancer cells, c, in the binding domain, β.

At intermediate time points (Fig. 5, $c_{u,\beta}$), the effects of the two primary drivers of cancer cell motility in u can be observed: at lower values of IFN binding, β, the major influence in the OV uptake, u, distribution is the uptake and replication of OV vectors while, at higher values of IFN binding, the major influence in the elevated distribution in OV uptake is the stochastic (overall) loss of OV vectors, eventually leading to a decrease in heterogeneity at higher time points (Fig. 6, $c_{u,\beta}$). At these higher time points, one clearly observes the effect of spatial heterogeneity on the system, where regions of low IFN concentrations yield cancer cell population at low values in the binding, β, domain and with values of OV uptake which continue to increase towards $u = 1$. That is, although the population increases overall, the protective effect of IFN binding, β, is spatially local and, in the absence of IFN, cancer cells continue to die.

4. Conclusions

We have focussed on the increasingly current fields of OV therapies and their essential counterpart in innate immunity (i.e., the IFN response), as well as the accompanying mathematical approaches to modelling these complicated biochemical systems. Although each virus is unique, there are general principles in virology which allow for the construction of mathematical models capable of capturing the generalised dynamics of these systems, while modelling of entry, replication, and lysis for specific viral vectors is ultimately desirable. The IIR, which acts rapidly and locally to protect cells from the entry and replication of viruses, has been extensively studied and the experiments and combined knowledge across centuries of research into innate immunity have culminated in a sophisticated knowledge of how these systems operate and interact with their hosts. In cancer, such protective biological systems serve to protect the cancer for lysis by OVs as opposed to protecting the host.

To accurately account for both the sophistication and correlation of these biological processes, similarly sophisticated mathematical modelling frameworks, such as spatio-temporal-structural PDEs, are becoming increasingly necessary. To demonstrate the potential for such frameworks, we have presented a novel higher-dimensional, spatio-temporal-structural model with diffusive spatial dynamics, which elucidates the interaction between OVs and cancer cell populations, as influenced by the IIR, capable of capturing spatio-structural heterogeneity across time in such biological systems.

Overall, as the biological knowledge of the scientific community increases and the mechanistic processes, which allow pharmaceutical treatments to prevail, are further elucidated, the potential for mathematical models to integrate such data becomes not only a possibility but also an imperative. Mathematical models are increasingly accurate at predicting and explaining outcomes of *in vitro* and *in vivo* experimentation, but cutting-edge techniques must be more readily embraced if the full richness of the available biological data is to be incorporated into the body of applied mathematics. We have presented one such example of a modelling technique, which allows the mathematician to capture simultaneous spatial and biochemical heterogeneity within the temporal dynamics of cell populations, though extensive work is still needed to establish rigorous functional analytic techniques for such systems. Moreover, the numerical simulation of solutions to such elaborate higher-dimensional systems of PDEs places a practical limit on the number of biochemical elements which may be explored, in such cases, and further techniques to surpass this limit will be necessary if this framework is to continue to expand and envelop the available biological data.

References

[1] P. Domschke, D. Trucu, A. Gerisch, and M. A. J. Chaplain, Structured models of cell migration incorporating molecular binding processes, *Journal of Mathematical Biology.* **75**(6–7), 1517–1561 (2017).

[2] A. Hodgkinson, O. Radulescu, G. Uzé, and D. Trucu, Signal propagation in sensing and reciprocating cellular systems with spatial and structural heterogeneity, *Bulletin of Mathematical Biology.* **80**, 1900–1936 (2018). doi: https://doi.org/10.1007/s11538-018-0439-x.

[3] A. Hodgkinson, M. A. J. Chaplain, P. Domschke, and D. Trucu, Computational approaches and analysis for a spatio-structural-temporal invasive carcinoma model, *Bulletin of Mathematical Biology.* **80**(4), 701–737 (2018).

[4] S. Ariotti, M. A. Hogenbirk, F. E. Dijkgraaf, L. L. Visser, M. E. Hoekstra, J.-Y. Song, *et al.*, Skin-resident memory CD8+ T cells trigger a state of tissue-wide pathogen alert, *Science.* **346**(6205), 101–105 (2014).

[5] C. R. Mackay, Chemokine receptors and T cell chemotaxis, *Journal of Experimental Medicine.* **184**(3), 799–802 (1996).

[6] A. Oyler-Yaniv, J. Oyler-Yaniv, B. M. Whitlock, Z. Liu, R. N. Germain, M. Huse, *et al.*, A tunable diffusion-consumption mechanism of cytokine propagation enables plasticity in cell-to-cell communication in the immune system, *Immunity.* **46**(4), 609–620 (2017).

[7] W.-L. Ng and B. L. Bassler, Bacterial quorum-sensing network architectures, *Annual Review of Genetics.* **43**(1), 197–222 (2009).

[8] D. Henrique, E. Hirsinger, J. Adam, I. Le Roux, O. Pourquié, D. Ish-Horowicz, *et al.*, Maintenance of neuroepithelial progenitor cells by delta–notch signalling in the embryonic chick retina, *Current Biology.* **7**(9), 661–670 (1997).

[9] E. Hoyos, K. Kim, J. Milloz, M. Barkoulas, J.-B. Pénigault, E. Munro, *et al.*, Quantitative variation in autocrine signaling and pathway crosstalk in the Caenorhabditis vulval network, *Current Biology.* **21**(7), 527–538 (2011).

[10] T. Maire and H. Youk, Molecular-level tuning of cellular autonomy controls the collective behaviors of cell populations article molecular-level tuning of cellular autonomy controls the collective behaviors of cell populations, *Cell Systems.* **1**, 349–360 (2015).

[11] E. P. Olimpio and H. Youk, Out-of-equilibrium statistical dynamics of spatial pattern generating cellular automata, *bioRxiv* (2017). doi: 10.1101/151050.

[12] Y. Hart, S. Reich-Zeliger, Y. E. Antebi, I. Zaretsky, A. E. Mayo, U. Alon, *et al.*, Paradoxical signaling by a secreted molecule leads to homeostasis of cell levels, *Cell.* **158**(5), 1022–1032 (2014).

[13] M. Gavutis, S. Lata, P. Lamken, P. Müller, and J. Piehler, Lateral ligand-receptor interactions on membranes probed by simultaneous fluorescence-interference detection, *Biophysical Journal.* **88**(6), 4289–4302 (2005).

[14] M. Gavutis, E. Jaks, P. Lamken, and J. Piehler, Determination of the two-dimensional interaction rate constants of a cytokine receptor complex, *Biophysical Journal.* **90**(9), 3345–3355 (2006).

[15] G. R. Stark, I. M. Kerr, B. R. Williams, R. H. Silverman, and R. D. Schreiber, How cells respond to interferons, *Annual Review of Biochemistry.* **67**, 227–264 (1998).

[16] C. E. Samuel, Antiviral actions of interferons, *Clinical Microbiology Reviews.* **14**(4), 778–809 (2001).

[17] R. Lin, C. Heylbroeck, P. M. Pitha, and J. Hiscott, Virus-dependent phosphorylation of the IRF-3 transcription factor regulates nuclear translocation, transactivation potential, and proteasome-mediated degradation, *Molecular and Cellular Biology.* **18**(5), 2986–2996 (1998).

[18] O. Haller, G. Kochs, and F. Weber, The interferon response circuit: Induction and suppression by pathogenic viruses, *Virology.* **344**, 119–130 (2006).

[19] V. François-Newton, G. M. de Freitas Almeida, B. Payelle-Brogard, D. Monneron, L. Pichard-Garcia, J. Piehler, S. Pellegrini, *et al.*,

USP18-based negative feedback control is induced by type i and type iii interferons and specifically inactivates interferon α response, *PLoS One.* **6**(7), e22200 (2011).

[20] G. Randall, L. Limin Chen, M. Panis, A. K. Fischer, B. D. Lindenbach, J. Sun, *et al.*, Silencing of usp18 potentiates the antiviral activity of interferon against hepatitis c virus infection, *Gastroenterology.* **131**, 1584–1591 (2006).

[21] S. Wilmes, O. Beutel, Z. Li, V. Francois-Newton, C. P. Richter, D. Janning, *et al.*, Receptor dimerization dynamics as a regulatory valve for plasticity of type I interferon signaling, *Journal of Cell Biology.* **209**(4), 579–593 (2015).

[22] K.-i. Arimoto, S. Löchte, S. A. Stoner, C. Burkart, Y. Zhang, S. Miyauchi, *et al.*, Stat2 is an essential adaptor in usp18-mediated suppression of type I interferon signaling, *Natural Structural Molecular Biology.* **24**(3), 279–289 (2017).

[23] D. J. Lenschow, C. Lai, N. Frias-Staheli, N. Giannakopoulos, A. Andrew Lutz, T. Wolff, *et al.*, IFN-stimulated gene 15 functions as a critical antiviral molecule against influenza, herpes, and sindbis viruses, *Proceedings of the National Academy of Sciences.* **104**(4), 1371–1376 (2007).

[24] D. J. Hui, C. R. Bhasker, W. C. Merrick, and G. C. Sen, Viral stress-inducible protein p56 inhibits translation by blocking the interaction of eIF3 with the ternary complex eIF2-GTP-Met-tRNA$_i$, *The Journal of Biological Chemistry.* **278**(41), 39477–39482 (2003).

[25] Z. Tallóczy, W. Jiang, H. W. Virgin IV, D. A. Leib, D. Scheuner, R. J. Kaufman, *et al.*, Regulation of starvation- and virus-induced autophagy by the eIF2α kinase signaling pathway, *Proceedings of the National Academy of Sciences.* **99**(1), 190–195 (2002).

[26] R. E. Randall and S. Goodbourn, Interferons and viruses: An interplay between induction, signalling, antiviral responses and virus countermeasures, *Journal of General Virology.* **89**, 1–47 (2008).

[27] M. J. V. Vähä-Koskela, J. E. Heikkilä, and A. E. Hinkkanen, Oncolytic viruses in cancer therapy, *Cancer Letters.* **254**, 178–216 (2007).

[28] M. Zheng, J. Huang, A. Tong, and H. Yang, Oncolytic viruses for cancer therapy: Barriers and recent advances, *Molecular Therapy: Oncolytics.* **15**, 2019 (2019).

[29] D. M. Rommelfanger, M. C. Grau, R. M. Diaz, E. Ilett, L. Alvarez-Vallina, J. M. Thompson, *et al.*, The efficacy versus toxicity profile of combination virotherapy and TLR immunotherapy highlights the danger of administering TLR agonists to oncolytic virus-treated mice, *Molecular Therapy.* **21**(2), 348–357 (2013).

[30] S. Z. Shalhout, D. M. Miller, K. S. Emerick, and H. L. Kaufman, Therapy with oncolytic viruses: progress and challenges, *Nature Reviews Clinical Oncology.* **20**(3), 160–177 (2023).

[31] O. Hemminki, J. M. dos Santos, and A. Hemminki, Oncolytic viruses for cancer immunotherapy, *Journal of Hematology & Oncology.* **13**, 84 (2020).

[32] V. Beljanski and J. Hiscott, The use of oncolytic viruses to overcome lung cancer drug resistance, *Current Opinion in Virology.* **2**, 629–635 (2012).

[33] K. Tamura, H. Wakimoto, A. S. Agarwal, S. D. Rabkin, D. Bhere, R. L. Martuza, *et al.*, Multimechanistic tumor targeted oncolytic virus overcomes resistance in brain tumors, *Molecular Therapy.* **21** (1), 68–77 (2013).

[34] Y. Liu, J. Cai, W. Liu, Y. Lin, L. Guo, X. Liu, *et al.*, Intravenous injection of the oncolytic virus M1 awakens antitumor T cells and overcomes resistance to checkpoint blockade, *Cell Death & Disease.* **11**, 1062 (2020).

[35] T. P. Cripe, P.-Y. Wang, P. Marcato, Y. Y. Mahller, and P. W. K. Lee, Targeting cancer-initiating cells with oncolytic viruses, *Molecular Therapy.* **17**(10), 1677–1682 (2009).

[36] C. E. Stewart, R. E. Randall, and C. S. Adamson, Inhibitors of the interferon response enhance virus replication in vitro, *PLoS ONE.* **9** (11), e112014 (2014).

[37] C. Groeneveldt, T. van Hall, S. H. van der Burg, P. ten Dijke, and N. van Montfoort, Immunotherapeutic potential of TGF-β inhibition and oncolytic viruses, *Trends in Immunology.* **41**(5), 406–420 (2020).

[38] J.-S. Diallo, F. Le Boeuf, F. Lai, J. Cox, M. Vaha-Koskela, H. Abdelbary, *et al.*, A high-throughput pharmacoviral approach identifies novel oncolytic virus sensitizers, *Molecular Therapy.* **18**(6), 1123–1129 (2010).

[39] R. Arulanandam, C. Batenchuk, F. A. Angarita, K. Ottolino-Perry, S. Cousineau, A. Mottashed, *et al.*, VEGF-mediated induction of PRD1-BF1/Blimp1 expression sensitizes tumor vasculature to oncolytic virus infection, *Cancer Cell.* **28**, 210–224 (2015).

[40] C. Dold, C. Rodriguez Urbiola, G. Wollmann, L. Egerer, A. Muik, L. Bellmann, *et al.*, Application of interferon modulators to overcome partial resistance of human ovarian cancers to vsv-gp oncolytic viral therapy, *Molecular Therapy: Oncolytics.* **3**, 16021 (2016).

[41] M. Cronin, F. Le Boeuf, C. Murphy, D. G. Roy, T. Falls, J. C. Bell, *et al.*, Bacterial-mediated knockdown of tumor resistance to an oncolytic virus enhances therapy, *Molecular Therapy.* **22**(6), 1188–1197 (2014).

[42] B.-H. Park, T. Hwang, T.-C. Liu, D. Y. Sze, J.-S. Kim, H.-C. Kwon, *et al.*, Use of a targeted oncolytic poxvirus, JX-594, in patients with refractory primary or metastatic liver cancer: A phase I trial, *Lancet Oncology.* **9**(6), 533–542 (2008).

[43] R. Bhat, S. Dempe, C. Dinsart, and J. Rommelaere, Enhancement of NK cell antitumor responses using an oncolytic parvovirus, *International Journal of Cancer.* **128**, 908–919 (2011).

[44] H. Ogbomo, F. J. Zemp, X. Lun, J. Zhang, D. Stack, M. M. Rahman, *et al.*, Myxoma virus infection promotes NK lysis of malignant gliomas in vitro and in vivo, *PLoS ONE.* **8**(6), e66825 (2013).

[45] S. Guedan and R. Alemany, CAR-T cells and oncolytic viruses: Joining forces to overcome the solid tumor challenge, *Frontiers in Immunology.* **9**, 2460 (2018).

[46] N. C. Turner and J. S. Reis-Filho, Genetic heterogeneity and cancer drug resistance, *Lancet Oncology.* **13**, e178–185 (2012).

[47] S. C. Baca, D. Prandi, M. S. Lawrence, J. M. Mosquera, A. Romanel, Y. Drier, *et al.*, Punctuated evolution of prostate cancer genomes, *Cell.* **153**, 666–677 (2013).

[48] N. McGranahan and C. Swanton, Biological and therapeutic impact of intratumor heterogeneity in cancer evolution, *Cancer Cell.* **12**, 15–26 (2015).

[49] N. Almuallem and R. Eftimie, A mathematical model for the role of macrophages in the persistence and elimination of oncolytic viruses, *Mathematics in Applied Sciences and Engineering.* **1**(2), 126–149 (2020).

[50] N. Almuallem, D. Trucu, and R. Eftimie, Oncolytic viral therapies and the delicate balance between virus-macrophage-tumour interactions, *Mathematical Biosciences and Engineering.* **18**(1), 764–799 (2021).

[51] G. P. Karev, A. S. Novozhilov, and E. V. Koonin, Mathematical modeling of tumor therapy with oncolytic viruses: Effects of parametric heterogeneity on cell dynamics, *Biology Direct.* **1**, 30 (2006).

[52] D. N. Santiago, J. P. W. Heidbuechel, W. M. Kandell, R. Walker, J. Djeu, C. E. Engeland, *et al.*, Fighting cancer with mathematics and viruses, *Viruses.* **9**(239), v9090239 (2017).

[53] D. Wodarz and N. Komarova, Towards predictive computational models of oncolytic virus therapy: Basis for experimental validation and model selection, *PLoS ONE.* **4**(1), e4271 (2009).

[54] A. Ardaševa, A. R. A. Anderson, R. A. Gatenby, H. M. Byrne, P. K. Maini, and T. Lorenzi, Comparative study between discrete and continuum models for the evolution of competing phenotype-structured cell populations in dynamical environments, *PRE.* **102**(4), 042404 (2020).

[55] D. Wodarz, A. Hofacre, J. W. Lau, Z. Sun, H. Fan, and N. L. Komarova, Complex spatial dynamics of oncolytic viruses in vitro: Mathematical and experimental approaches, *PLoS Computational Biology.* **8**(6), e1002547 (2012).

[56] J. Humplik, A. L. Hill, and M. A. Nowak, Evolutionary dynamics of infectious diseases in finite populations, *Journal of Theoretical Biology.* **360**, 149–162 (2014).

[57] W. Ghang and M. A. Nowak, Stochastic evolution of staying together, *Journal of Theoretical Biology.* **360**, 129–136 (2014).

[58] I. Bozic and M. A. Nowak, Timing and heterogeneity of mutations associated with drug resistance in metastatic cancers, *Proceedings of the National Academy of Sciences of the United States of America.* **111**(45), 15964–8 (2014).

[59] A. Kleinman, The mathematics of random mutation and natural selection for multiple simultaneous selection pressures and the evolution of antimicrobial drug resistance, *Statistics in Medicine.* **35**(29), 5391–5400 (2016).

[60] K.-A. Norton, C. Gong, S. Jamalian, and A. S. Popel, Multiscale agent-based and hybrid modeling of the tumor immune microenvironment, *Processes.* **7**, 37 (2019).

[61] B. Waclaw, I. Bozic, M. E. Pittman, R. H. Hruban, B. Vogelstein, and M. A. Nowak, A spatial model predicts that dispersal and cell turnover limit intratumour heterogeneity, *Nature.* **525**, 261–264 (2015).

[62] B. Waclaw, Evolution of drug resistance in bacteria, *Advances and Medicine and Biology.* **915**, 49–67 (2016).

[63] A. Lorz, T. Lorenzi, M. E. Hochberg, J. Clairambault, and B. Perthame, Populational adaptive evolution, chemotherapeutic resistance and multiple anti-cancer therapy, *ESAIM: Mathematical Modelling and Numerical Analysis.* **47**, 377–399 (2012).

[64] A. Lorz, T. Lorenzi, J. Clairambault, A. Escarguel, and B. Perthame, Modeling the effects of space structure and combination therapies on phenotypic heterogeneity and drug resistance in solid tumors, *Bulletin of Mathematical Biology.* **77**(1), 1–22 (2015).

[65] M. A. Boemo and H. M. Byrne, Mathematical modelling of a hypoxia-regulated oncolytic virus delivered by tumour-associated macrophages, *Journal of Theoretical Biology.* **461**, 102–116 (2019).

[66] A. Larrieux and R. Sanjuán, Cellular resistance to an oncolytic virus is driven by chronic activation of innate immunity, *iScience.* **26**, 105749 (2023).

[67] I. Liikanen, V. Monsurrò, L. Ahtiainen, M. Raki, T. Hakkarainen, I. Diaconu, *et al.*, Induction of interferon pathways mediates in vivo

resistance to oncolytic adenovirus, *Molecular Therapy.* **19**(10), 1858–1866 (2011).

[68] A. L. Huff, P. Wongthida, T. Kottke, J. M. Thompson, C. B. Driscoll, M. Schuelke, *et al.*, APOBEC3 mediates resistance to oncolytic viral therapy, *Molecular Therapy: Oncolytics.* **11** (2018).

[69] Q. Li and M. A. Tainsky, Epigenetic silencing of IRF7 and/or IRF5 in lung cancer cells leads to increased sensitivity to oncolytic viruses, *PLoS ONE.* **6**(12), e28683 (2011).

[70] A. Hodgkinson, L. Le Cam, D. Trucu, and O. Radulescu, Spatio-genetic and phenotypic modelling elucidates resistance and re-sensitisation to treatment in heterogeneous melanoma, *Journal of Theoretical Biology.* **466**, 84–105 (2019).

[71] A. Hodgkinson, L. Le Cam, M. Lacroix, D. Trucu, and O. Radulescu, Computational model of heterogeneity in melanoma: Designing therapies and predicting outcomes, *Frontiers in Oncology: Cancer Metabolism.* **12**, 857572 (2022).

[72] F. Rambow, A. Rogiers, O. Marin-Bejar, S. Aibar, J. Femel, M. Dewaele, *et al.*, Toward minimal residual disease-directed therapy in melanoma, *Cell.* **174**(4), 843–855 (2018).

Chapter 8

Malignant Transformation of Low-Grade Astrocytomas through a Mechano-Biological Triggering Hypothesis: Imaging-Informed Modelling

Meryem Abbad Andaloussi[*,†], Stéphane Urcun[*],
Andreas Husch[†], Isabel Fernandes Arroteia[‡], Giuseppe Sciumè[§],
Stéphane Bordas[*,‖], and Frank Hertel[*,‡,¶]

[*]Department of Engineering Sciences, Faculté des Sciences,
de la Technologie et de Médecine, Université du Luxembourg,
Campus Belval, Luxembourg
[†]Luxembourg Centre for Systems Biomedicine,
Université du Luxembourg,
Campus Belval, Luxembourg
[‡]Service National de Neurochirurgie,
Centre Hospitalier de Luxembourg, Luxembourg
[§]Université de Bordeaux, France
[‖]Clyde Visiting Fellow, Department of Mechanical Engineering,
The University of Utah, Salt Lake City, Utah, USA
[¶]frank.hertel@ext.uni.lu

Grade 3 and 4 astrocytomas are high-grade gliomas (HGG) that usually result from initially less aggressive low-grade gliomas (LGG) through malignant transformation (MT). This process has various definitions in the literature, clinical, and histopathological, depending on the scale of the study and researchers' interest. We introduce an overview of different aspects of MT: molecular, clinical, and the role of the microenvironment in acquiring the malignant phenotype. On the other hand, light is shed on the medical modalities that characterise LGG and the methods available to segment the tumour. These methods consist of the first step into data-driven growth models. In that scope, a novel mathematical model is introduced to assess MT of grade 2 to grade 3 astrocytoma based on a mechano-biological triggering hypothesis. The model is initialised and calibrated using data from the same patient at two different time-points and is capable of predicting the region that is more likely to be malignantly transformed 540 days later. Finally, we discuss the main limitations and perspectives for future work that aims at bringing the mathematical model closer to clinical application.

1. Introduction

Gliomas were first defined by Virchow in 1865 as 'Tumors in the central nervous system whose neoplastic cells microscopically resemble nontumourous glial cells' [1]. Since then, the World Health Organisation (WHO) classification system has evolved along with the main research breakthrough discoveries, namely the 1p/19q chromosome co-deletion and the Isocitrate DeHydrogenase (IDH) mutation status [2, 3]. The classification therefore relied not only on histopathology alone but also on additional molecular diagnosis [4]. More specifically, the WHO grading system includes grade 2 (Low-Grade Gliomas (LGG)) and 3 and 4 (High-Grade Gliomas (HGG)) [5]. The former includes two sub-types: oligodendrogliomas (IDH-mutant and 1p/19q chromosome co-deletion) and astrocytomas (IDH-mutant), while the latter separated the Astrocytoma grade 4 from the glioblastoma IDH-wild-type [6] (Fig. 1).

The IDH mutation status is the first biomarker of LGG. This enzyme intervenes in the citric cycle and catalyses the conversion of the isocitrate into α-ketoglutarate (α-KG), which has a role in the regulation of DNA methylation. When mutated, the IDH enzyme has a normal and mutated dimer as illustrated in Fig. 2. Although the normal copy still generates α-KG, the mutated one uses the α-KG to produce the oncometabolite 2-Hydroxyglutarate (2-HG). Consequently, the cell witnesses an accumulation of 2-HG levels

(a)

(b)

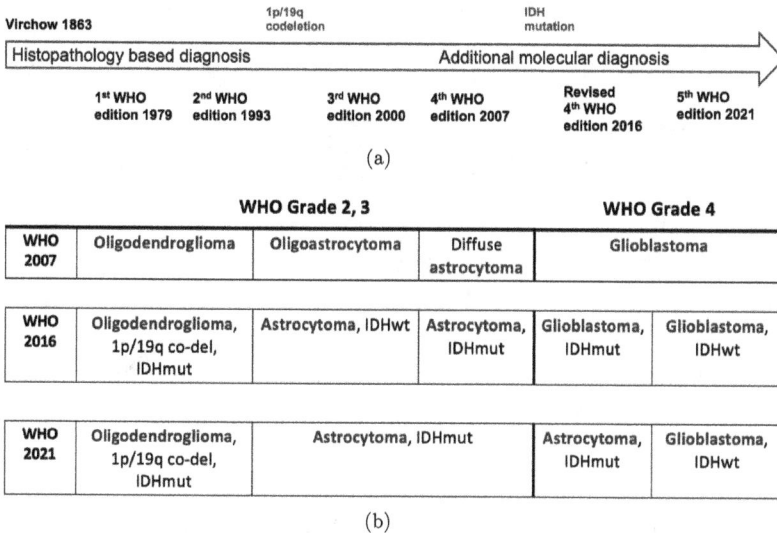

Fig. 1. General WHO evolution, classification, and grading system. (a) Evolution of the WHO Classification of Tumours of the Central Nervous System along with the main breakthrough discoveries in glioma tumours. In the recent editions, the diagnosis relies not only on histopathology but also on molecular characterisation. (b) Evolution of LGG and HGG classification according to the last 3 WHO classification editions.

leading to DNA methylation up-regulation which in turn results in some gene over-expression specifically in the case of astrocytoma tumours [7]. The general research interest has mainly been directed towards GBM growth and treatment response to the extent that, in 2011, DeAngelis *et al.* wrote in their article 'Virchow 2011 or How to ID(H) Human Glioblastoma' that 'Now we are beginning to understand exactly how multiforme glioblastoma truly is' [1]. Nevertheless, clinicians have lately shown a growing interest in malignant transformation of LGG to HGG. In fact, while the vast majority of HGG is *de novo*, the secondary type always results from an LGG that has recurred as a higher grade after resection. This phenomenon is called malignant transformation (MT). In the literature, MT can be termed 'anaplastic transformation', 'anaplastic progression', or 'malignant progression'. However, even within the LGG, the prognosis differs from 75 months in astrocytomas to 116 months in the case of oligodendrogliomas [8]. This difference may be linked to the earlier MT of astrocytoma grade 2 to astrocytoma grade 3. Consequently, in this study, the light is shed on the MT of astrocytomas grade 2–3.

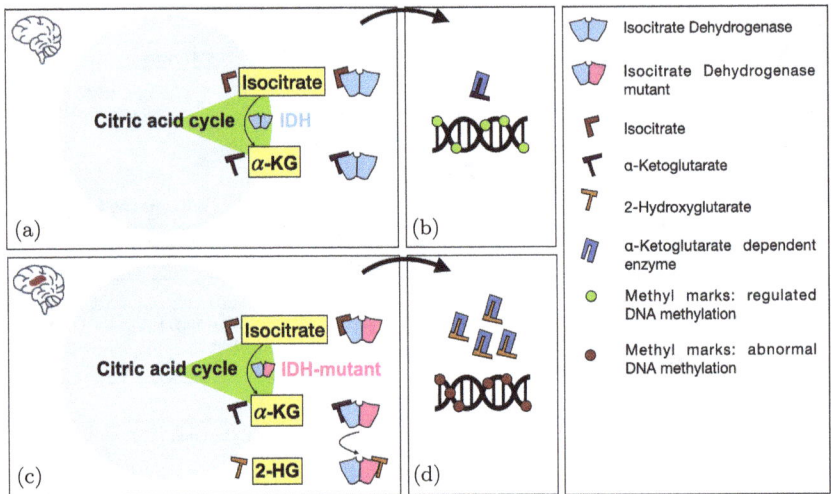

Fig. 2. (a) In a healthy cell, IDH contributes to the citric acid cycle by catalysing the conversion of Isocitrate into α-KG. The latter binds with the α-KG enzyme. (b) In the nucleus, these enzymes help regulate DNA methylation patterns. (c) In IDH-mutant tumours, IDH enzymes acquire a new mutant dimer. The normal IDH dimer copy generates α-KG which the mutated copy converts into 2-HG. (d) As a result, the 2-HG accumulates within the cell. Thanks to the chemical similarity between 2-HG and α-KG, the 2-HG binds to the α-KG-dependent enzyme inhibiting its role in DNA demethylation.

2. Malignant Transformation

There is no consensus on the definition of MT. Some researchers even describe the natural development of LGG in four stages based on imaging along with the continuously slow-growing characteristic of LGG. First, the biological birth corresponds to the occult stage, when there is neither symptom nor correlation with medical imaging. Second, the LGG reaches the detection limit of MRI. The symptoms however are still absent. The symptomatic stage 3 ensues leading to the fourth and final stage which is identified as the switch in the tumour behaviour from mild to more aggressive, therefore defining MT [9].

More generally, even though the exact causes of this transformation are unclear, two main definitions can be found in the literature: the radiological and the histological one [8,10]. The former is related to the observation of new progressive contrast enhancement, neovascularisation, and necrosis during follow-up of the patient, while the latter is based on the properties of the tissue microstructure. Nakasu *et al.* performed a meta-analysis on 41 different studies (including 7122 patients) which were divided into histologically (28 studies, 4261 patients) and radiologically defined MT (18 studies, 3714 patients). Regression lines of both approaches were plotted against the mean follow-up time and appeared to be almost parallel. The MT rate of LGG was therefore illustrated as somewhere within the area between both the radiological and the histological curves. Approximately 40% of MT was shown to occur at ten years of mean follow-up time [8]. To our knowledge, this is the only study that attempted to merge both approaches to quantify the true MT rate.

Characterisation of MT according to contrast enhancement in MRI shows some disadvantages. Contrast enhancement is not specific to HGG. In fact, nearly one-third of HGG tumours do not show enhancement in MRI, while in contrast approximately 50 % of low-grade oligodendrogliomas (LGOs) enhance [11]. The latter case makes histopathological characterisation the only relevant measure to spot malignant progression within oligodendrogliomas. Second, contrast enhancement may appear late, sometimes when MT is already observed by histopathology and not yet observed the imaging threshold.

2.1. *Molecular characterisation of malignant transformation*

Studies attempted to identify genetic alterations linked to MT. In 1995, a polymerase chain reaction (PCR)-based technique helped identify a low expression level of the human β2-chimaerin gene in high-grade astrocytomas as compared to normal brain and low-grade astrocytoma (LGA) [12]. Furthermore, TP53 and ATRX mutations were identified as hallmarks of 1p/19q intact gliomas. However, a study on a wide public dataset identified these two mutations in a small fraction of 1p1/9q co-deleted tumours of high grade, therefore indicating the possibility of these mutations to contribute to the MT of oligodendrogliomas [13]. Furthermore, other genes showed differences in incidence of mutation among grades in both 1p/19q intact and co-deleted glioma within the same study (U2AF2, U2AF65, TCF12, and ARID1A). Another study identified tumour suppressor CDKN2A deletion and MYC amplification as markers of MT [7]. Additionally, Lee *et al.* investigated the impact of CX3CL1-CX3CR1 on MT of gliomas [14]. It appeared that co-expression of CX3CL1-CX3CR1 signalling enhances vascular proliferation in immunocompetent mice models leading to promotion of malignant phenotype. These results on mice were contradictory with patients results, where CX3CL1 signalling was positively correlated with high overall survival.

Since it is unclear how molecular signalling pathways involved in MT differ from one patient to the other, a longitudinal study following five patients through MT of diffuse LGAs showed evidence of poly-T-nucleotide insertion correlated with MT of grade 2 astrocytomas [15]. On oligodendroglioma, another longitudinal study on one case showed over expressed genes in the high-grade stage: OLIG1, OLIG2, VGF, SOX4, SOX8, MYT1, and PDGFRA. Moreover, some down-regulated genes during differentiation of oligodendroglial precursor were reactivated during MT [13].

Even though these studies attempt to identify some molecular properties of MT of LGGs, one still needs to compare these findings to a non-MT control group. Furthermore, tumour heterogeneity may represent a confounder in estimating the genetic divergences even within the same patient when different regions of the tumour are sampled at different stages of tumour progression. In fact, Johnson *et al.* investigated intra-tumoural differences. Analysis on six samples of the initial tumour detected the BRAF V600E mutation in three samples but did not in all seven samples of the recurrent tumour within the same patient showing the importance of considering multiple glioma regions in such studies [16].

Despite many animal or human studies, longitudinal or not, taking or not into account the intra-tumoural heterogeneity, the genetic characteristics of MT remain an open debate.

2.2. *Clinical observations*

LGG follows white matter fiber tracts: LGGs usually occur in rich glial cell environment and then invade following white matter fibres in an anisotropic manner. This pattern makes surgical resection more challenging and more subject to uncertainties due to the absence of delineated borders [17].

In fact, multiple studies have investigated the difference in material properties between white matter and grey matter in order to attempt to explain the glioma trend to follow white matter fibre tracts. In this scope, experimental tests performed by Jamal *et al.* on brain tissue demonstrated that hydraulic permeability is significantly lower for a flow perpendicular to white matter fibres [18].

Even though the brain is structurally anisotropic, the fibre tracts are considered as functional entities, which makes the organ mechanically isotropic. Nevertheless, it has been showed that mean stresses are higher along fibres as compared to the perpendicular direction [19].

Post-surgical malignant recurrence: Surgical resection is currently the adopted approach for LGG and HGG tumour management. Previously, the "wait and see" method was preferred exclusively for LGG since resection surgery was believed to be a factor of malignant recurrence [20]. In fact, Jakola *et al.* performed a study on 46 patients to observe the spatial distribution of malignant recurrence [21]. The preoperative tumour, pre-transformation tumour and the one after transformation were overlapped. The main observation was that the post-surgical malignant recurrence correlates positively with the spatial distribution of the pre-operative tumour volume in 90% of the cases. More specifically, malignant recurrence is believed to occur at the borders of resection [22]. This observation needs to be further investigated since a study on 46 patients cannot be conclusive. In fact, another study from the same research group compared both approaches (watchful waiting and early resection) in two different Norwegian university hospitals (66 patients from hospital A and 87 patients from hospital B) [23]. The results show that, unlike the 'wait and see' approach, early surgical resection increases the overall survival and may even delay MT.

Treatment-induced malignant transformation: The same study of Jakola *et al.* shows that in 86% of the 46 cases who underwent radiotherapy after resection, a distant malignant recurrence has been observed. This leads to questions regarding the relationship between MT and treatment. It is indeed one of the reasons why the wait and see approach was preferred before the current procedure was gradually introduced.

The most optimal LGG patient management is yet unknown. In fact, some studies have linked radiotherapy with the possible activation of some mutations in glioma cells [17]. Consequently, to have a better overview of the physiological interplay, the microenvironmental role in MT of LGG needs to be acknowledged given the high heterogeneity of the central nervous system (CNS) cells' environment.

2.3. *Microenvironment role*

The extra-cellular matrix (ECM) can be considered as a structural scaffold for neurons, oligodendrocytes, and astrocytes. It is mainly made of hyaluronic acid chains bound with each other through a lectican–tenascin R complex (Fig. 3).

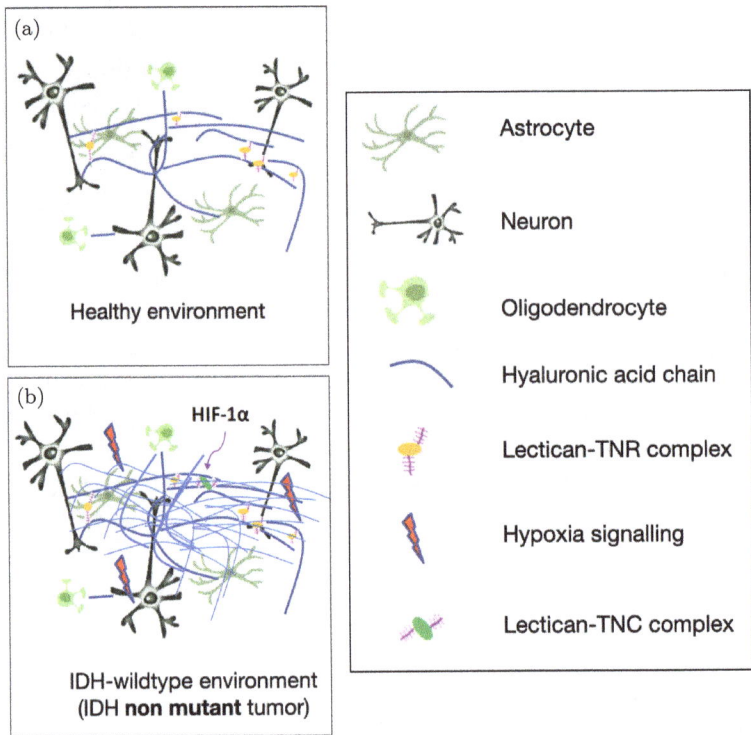

Fig. 3. Illustration of a healthy central nervous system microenvironment (a) and an IDH-wild-type tumour microenvironment (b). Focus on the hypoxia sensing cascade. Adjusted from Barnes *et al.* [24]

In the case of glioblastoma (GBM), necrotic cores and abnormal vasculature may reflect oxygen tension through the hypoxia-induced transcription factor HIF-1α. Some studies claim that this signalling will ultimately lead to a malignant phenotype [24].

On the one hand, the stiffening of the ECM triggers the IDH-wild-type tumour ability to sense hypoxia. On the other hand, when the tumour cells are inside a hypoxic environment, the hypoxia-induced transcription factor HIF-1α is produced leading to over-expression of Tenascin C (TNC) which in turn stiffens the ECM. Experimental work confirms the role of a stiff mechanical environment — and equivalently active chemical signalling — on altering the phenotype of cultured IDH-wild-type glioma cells [25].

IDH-mutant tumours, however, do not have the ability to sense hypoxia. This begs the question as to how LGG still goes through MT. In this scope, Miroshnikova *et al.* [26] investigated the role of stiffened ECM and TNC expression in the invasion of grade 4 astrocytoma IDH-mutant cells. Two main outcomes emerged. First, grade 4 astrocytoma cells are more invasive in a stiff substrate (*in vitro* experiment see Fig. 4). Second, recurrent astrocytoma shows an ECM as stiff as GBM with an over-expression of TNC (*in vivo* observation).

Following these observations, this study aims at predicting MT of LGAs. More specifically, the following hypothesis will be investigated: is MT of LGA encouraged in high mechanical stress environments? What would be the preferred path followed by the recurrent malignantly transformed LGA?

3. LGG: Imaging Techniques and Segmentation

LGGs are usually diagnosed using imaging techniques. The clinician visually examines the images to detect the right tumour location and estimate the malignancy. In practice, the clinician segregates the tumour region from the healthy brain manually or using a software-based algorithm. This process is called segmentation. In this section, the conventional imaging techniques are introduced followed by the state of the art segmentation methods.

3.1. *Imaging techniques*

Medical imaging and more specifically Magnetic Resonance Imaging (MRI) is the most commonly used method for patient diagnosis

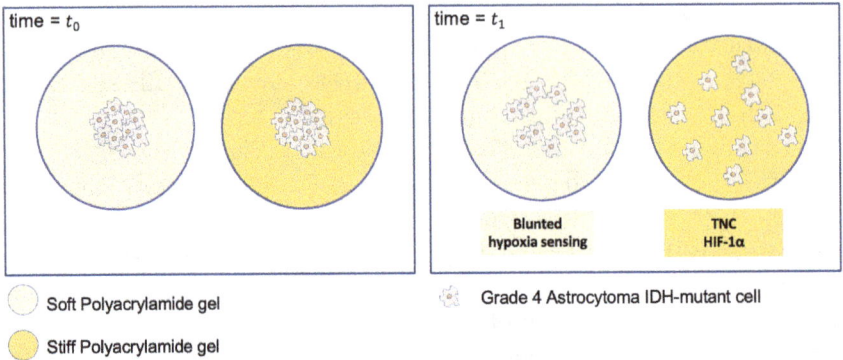

Fig. 4. Illustration of an experiment performed by Miroshnikova *et al.* [26] aiming at increasing aggression of grade 4 astrocytoma IDH-mutant cells by enhancing mechano-signalling. At time t_0, the cells are plated on 2D soft (140 Pa, representative of the normal brain and similar to soft ECM measured *in vitro*) and stiff (6000 Pa, upper range of HGG stiffness) polyacrylamide gel substrates. At time t_1, they are noticed to spread better on the stiff substrate. When plated on a soft substrate, the grade 4 astrocytoma IDH-mutant cells showed a blunted hypoxia signalling, meanwhile, an over-expression of TNC and HIF-1 α is noticed in the stiff substrate. Similarly, an important up-regulation of TNC and HIF-1 α is observed when the cells are in a hypoxic environment: the ECM stiffness may override the blunted hypoxia sensing.

and treatment to identify and track brain tumour progression. The patient is placed in a strong uniform magnetic field, aligning positively charged hydrogen ions (H^+, referred to as *hydrons* or *protons*) in the patient's tissue in a known direction. By applying magnetic pulses (excitation), the tissue property-dependent response of the previously aligned protons can be measured by a detector, without any exposure to ionising radiation. This non-invasive mapping method is controlled by different parameters, such as the time from excitation to detection (TE) and the time between pulses (TR). By varying these parameters, different image contrasts can be obtained since different tissue types show different pulse responses. Additionally, contrast agents that temporarily change the magnetic response properties of certain tissue types, such as blood vessels, could be applied. Conventional MRI sequences commonly used for diagnosis and follow-up of gliomas include the following:

- **T1-weighted MRI (T1 MRI)**: Grey matter appears darker than white matter. Cerebro-spinal fluid (CSF) is dark.

- **T1-weighted Contrast Enhanced MRI (T1-CE MRI)**: Contrast enhancement informs on vascular changes and disruption of the blood–brain barrier (BBB).
- **T2-weighted MRI (T2 MRI)**: Grey matter appears lighter than white matter.
- **T2-weighted Fluid-Attenuated Inversion Recovery (FLAIR)**: Grey matter appears lighter than white matter while CSF is dark.

In general, LGGs are hypointense on T1 MRI and hyperintense on T2 MRI, including FLAIR. On the other hand, T1-CE MRI helps detect areas where the BBB is compromised and may be representative of aggressive lesions, such as HGG. However, even though it is used as an indicator of HGGs in longitudinal studies of MT, contrast enhancement can be representative of LGOs in approximately 50% of the cases [11]. In some cases, some HGGs may not show contrast enhancement in T1-CE MRI, as in the case of molecular glioblastoma, for instance [27].

These sequences are available in 95% of the hospitals in Europe [28]. Moreover, some advanced techniques may provide more pathophysiological properties of tumours and consequently bring more insight into tumour aggressiveness and biology. Diffusion-Weighted Imaging (DWI MRI), for instance, helps estimate brain fibre structures using water molecules' diffusion properties: restricted diffusion areas are bright on DWI, while dark areas represent free water motion. As fibre structures restrict diffusion perpendicular to the fibre, information about the fibre arrangement could be obtained by multiple DWI scans each acquiring information about a certain direction. From such raw DWI data, diffusion tensors describing the potential orientation of the local fibre structure can be obtained. However, the actual (absolute) water diffusion coefficient cannot be measured directly by MRI. While true diffusion is related to the concentration gradient according to Fick's first law [29], this interplay cannot be distinguished from pressure gradients, thermal gradients, or ionic interactions in MRI. Consequently, molecular motion detected by diffusion imaging can only be calculated with the apparent diffusion coefficient (ADC) which is obtained from orthogonal diffusion-weighted MRI in all three planes [30, 31].

Perfusion-Weighted MRI (PWI MRI) is another advanced imaging method that informs about the altered microvascular environment and therefore characterises the hypoxic state of the tumour. The most relevant parameters for our study are the cerebral blood volume (CBV) and the relative cerebral blood volume (rCBV) which is the CBV calculated relatively to a control value. These are routinely calculated using commercial radiology softwares in hospitals, where suggested methods in the literature are mainly based on calculating the area under the curve of the PWI MRI voxel signal versus time [32–34].

3.2. *Low-grade glioma segmentation*

Localising the tumour, defining its size, components, and the eloquent neighbouring regions, is a main interest of the neurosurgeon and radiologist from the first diagnosis step to the treatment follow-up after surgery. However, interobserver and intraobserver variability may affect the precision of tumour segmentation [35]. Moreover, the time-consuming manual procedure limits widespread adoption in clinical routine. Machine learning algorithms for automatic segmentation are promising to serve the doctors and help gain time, precision, and reproducibility during the segmentation process. In that scope, the multi-modal Brain Tumour image Segmentation benchmark (BraTS) challenge provides reference segmentations [36].

According to a recent literature review on automatic brain tumour segmentation performed by Van Kempen *et al.* [37], among the 42 studies on brain tumour segmentation, only 2 study LGG exclusively. Three studies exclusively deal with HGG, and 37 studies deal with both tumour types. Furthermore, the BraTS challenge segmentation (before 2017) ground truth is the reference segmentation for all models.

This meta-analysis does not include the model of Van der Voort *et al.* published in 2020 that uses multi-task deep learning to automatically segment and classifies LGG and HGG according to the WHO 2016 [38]. The training dataset includes four private datasets and five public ones from the TCIA *(REMBRANDT* [39], *Ivy GAP* [40]*, CPTAC-GBM, and Brain-Tumour-Progression* [41]*)* and BraTS challenge 2020. The model was then tested with sub-datasets from the publically available TCGA-LGG and TCGA-GBM datasets.

The subsets for both training and testing were used to contain pre-operative pre- and post-contrast T1w, T2w, and T2w FLAIR.

15% of the training dataset was used to validate the model which performed an AUC for validation of 88%, 76%, and 75% for the IDH mutation, 1p/19q and grade, respectively, and a DICE score of 81% for segmentation.

The model performed even better on the test dataset with an AUC of 90%, 85%, and 81% for IDH mutation, 1p/19q and grade respectively and a DICE score of 84% for segmentation.

Finally, the model gathers both LGG and HGG in its segmentation. However, these two types of tumour are segmented differently in the clinics and the tumour 'boundaries' are not defined in the same way. Post-contrast T1 imaging provides a clear boundary of GBM, which is not representative of the entire tumour region. This post-contrast offers possible differentiation between the necrotic core, enhancing and non-enhancing tumour (the latter being visible in T2w FLAIR sequences). Conversely, LGG boundaries are less clear in post-contrast T1 imaging and are closer to a density map. This may raise the question of whether it is better to train a model segmenting LGGs alone. Moreover, the model seems to perform better on HGG than LGG. More specifically, it had difficulty differentiating IDH mutated, 1p/19q co-deleted LGG from other LGG and exhibited a low sensitivity for predicting grade 3 glioma. To address this issue, the authors propose further improving their model by adding PWI and DWI images [38].

4. Modelling Malignant Transformation of LGGs: State of the Art

4.1. *Statistical models*

Multiple statistical analyses attempted to define factors of MT. While Jung *et al.* [42] and Aoki *et al.* [43] focussed on progression-free survival (PFS), overall survival (OS), and MT, Bobek-Billewicz *et al.* [44] focussed on MRI parameters of MT. Non-eloquent location, gross total removal, and oligodendroglial diagnosis were found to correlate positively with PFS and OS in the univariate analysis of the first study which included 86 patients with LGG. Overall, oligodendroglioma (IDH-mutant, with 1p/19q co-deletion) diagnosis correlates with longer OS, PFS, and later MT, while the adjuvant therapies did not show significant influence [43]. Furthermore, Bobek-Billewicz et al. investigated the influence of new parameters on MT. The study, on 46 supratentorial glioma patients, showed that the mean and maximum normalised rCBV were higher within the MT group. ADC values also showed significant differences between different groups in the follow-up and final MRIs.

Nakasu et al., more generally, performed a meta-analysis covering 41 previous studies, including those introduced previously in this section. The study included overall 7122 patients and distinguished between radiologically and histologically defined MT. The hazard ratio was calculated and finally the crucial factors of MT were identified as histological and molecular diagnoses, pre- and post-operative volume, extent of removal, and contrast enhancement on MRI. Furthermore, the univariate analysis of studies showed significance of age, gender, and the Karnofsky performance scale (KPS). However, these parameters only reproduced this significance in few multivariate analyses [8].

4.2. Physical-based models

Numerous mathematical models in the literature attempted to describe the growth mechanisms of LGG and HGG, with different levels of complexity. However, only a few study MT.

The proliferation-invasion model constitutes the basis of tumour cell concentration evolution studies. Swanson et al. and Bogdanska et al. built on this equation to track the malignant progression of LGG [10, 45]. Both continuous models rely on the hypothesis that angiogenesis differentiates between the LGG and HGG states. However, while the first models MT as a cascade of events involving interactions between normoxic, hypoxic, and necrotic cells, the second model introduces a rather more simplified interplay between LGG and HGG cells. As a matter of fact, the latter relies on the assumption that the first step of the MT is the increase in tumour density above a critical threshold after which angiogenesis and hypoxia, representative of HGG, occur. A switch function identifies the irreversible evolution of LGG cells into HGG depending on the total cell density and the rate $1/\tau$, with τ the time it takes the cells to acquire a more aggressive high-grade behaviour after the onset of MT. More specifically, as long as the total tumour cell density is lower than $L_{crit} - \Delta_{crit}$, there is no MT. Δ_{crit} is the sensitivity of the MT switch function and is described as a variation in density L_{crit} (the L_{crit} value comes from the mathematical modelling of Pérez-García *et al.* [46]).

Choosing parameters in such models usually relies on the literature, previous experiments, or calibration. More specifically, a wide heterogeneity has been observed within the proliferation and invasion rates, even within the same glioma grade [47]. Consequently, bounds for both diffusion and proliferation where introduced by Swanson *et al.* while the other parameters were extracted from the literature. Furthermore, MT is assumed to vary spatially within the same tumour. For the predicted grading to be consistent with the WHO classification, virtual biopsies were performed randomly at different locations within the tumour region. Depending on the level of hyper-cellularity, mitoses, neovasculature, and necrosis observed, the lesion is classified as either a LGG or a HGG. In contrast, Bogdanska *et al.* did not take into account the grading variability within the same tumour. Furthermore, the number of parameters is only half the one considered by Swanson *et al.* Both models only share one parameter, the carrying capacity, with the same value of 10^8.

Since the proliferation ρ and invasion D rates vary within a range previously observed from different HGG by both research groups, Swanson *et al.* introduce 225 (ρ, D) combinations representing 225 virtual patients to explore the changes in prognosis. The survival time was calculated from T2-MRI images from the moment the tumour radius is approximately 1 cm to the fatal tumour burden 4 cm (from a clinical point of view, this fatal burden is more likely estimated at 7–8 cm). The main observation was that short survival is related to high ρ and D. Furthermore, simulations showed that for small tumours to achieve the histologic features of a HGG, there must be both low D and high ρ; however, for larger tumours, there is a wider range of D and ρ that will generate the features of HGG. Following these results, the authors claim that growth kinetics alone can drive MT and that genetic alterations may not be necessary for the phenotypic change of MT.

Bogdanska *et al.* also considered a fatal tumour burden of (4 cm) in radius, although it may change depending on the tumour location. In this study, however, the influence of both the proliferation rate of the LGG and HGG states on patient survival was studied. The effect of the former was found to be the largest. This result seems to be consistent with the observation that LGGs invade more slowly than HGGs, giving the tumour more time to grow to a larger size. Once the density reaches a critical level, the change in phenotypic rate τ does not seem to affect the virtual patient survival. Finally, the main objective of this chapter was to produce an analytical formula that can be used in the hospital. Following multiple approximations, expressions of tumour size and time to MT were provided.

None of these models distinguishes growth patterns of LGAs from LGOs nor take into account the porous nature of the brain and tumour media. Regarding HGGs, to our knowledge, only two studies develop a poromechanical description [48, 49]. In the following sections, a novel mathematical model that aims at predicting MT of a grade 2 astrocytoma is introduced.

5. A Grade 2 Astrocytoma Growth Model

5.1. *Patient information*

The data of one patient with histologically confirmed grade 2 astrocytoma are used in this study. In this study, two MRI datasets with an interval of 69 days were used. The first one was taken at the initial diagnosis, while the second was performed right after the resection surgery. Because the tumour was located in an eloquent region, only sub-total resection could be achieved. We therefore used this timepoint to calibrate the model parameters. The MRIs were acquired from a 'GE Medical Systems, Signa HDxt' scanner. Both timepoints show a grade 2 astrocytoma and no surgical intervention was performed between both images. The first contrast uptake was observed 540 days after the second MRI, leading to confirmation of the histopathological report of the MT 59 days later. T1 and T1-CE MRIs of the patient are compared in Fig. 5 to identify contrast linked to MT. Available patient information is shown in Table 1.

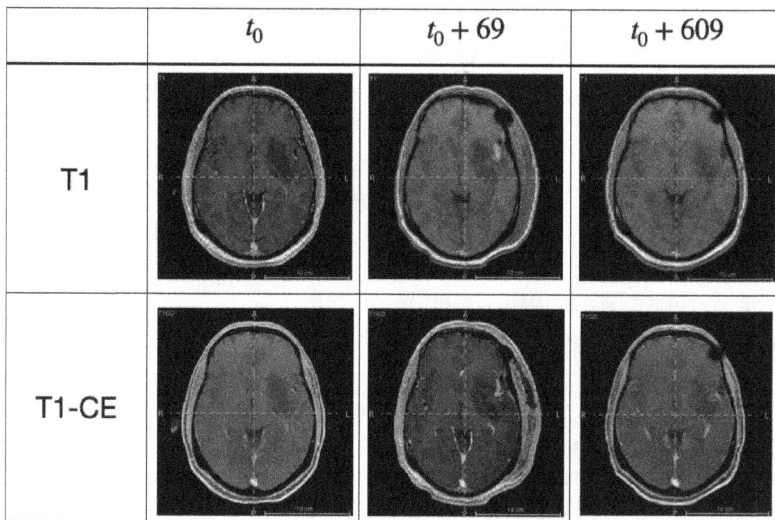

(a)

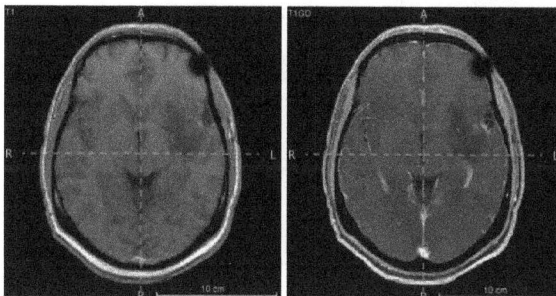

(b)

Fig. 5. Patient longitudinal MRI sequences from first diagnosis to MT. (a) T1 and T1-CE MRI sequences of the patient at $t_0, t_0 + 69$ days, and $t_0 + 609$ days. The T1 sequences are shown to distinguish the contrast noticed in the T1-CE sequences between contrast due to blood vessels and one due to the malignantly transformed tumour. (b) T1 MRI (left) and T1-CE MRI (right) at $t_0 + 609$ days. A newly gained contrast is noticed.

Table 1. Available patient information.

Age	Sex	Tumour type at first and second MR	Tumour location	Interval between two MR visits
40	Male	Grade 2 astrocytoma	Insular	69 days

5.2. *MRI data*

At the first MRI visit, six MRI sequences were acquired: (1) a pre-contrast T1-weighted image (T1), (2) a post-contrast T1-weighted image (T1-CE), (3) T2-weighted image (T2), (4) T2-FLAIR image (FLAIR), (5) Diffusion Tensor image (DTI), and (6) Perfusion-Weighted image (PWI), while only the five first sequences were taken at the second timepoint. The T1, T1-CE, T2, and FLAIR images were used to segment the tumour using the convolutional neural network PrognosAIs at both timepoints [50].

The ADC calculated from the DTI was used to inform on tumour cellularity.

The rCBV was calculated from perfusion imaging and used to estimate the nutrient intake by the tumour.

Figure 6 illustrates the modelling workflow along with the clinical follow-up of the patient.

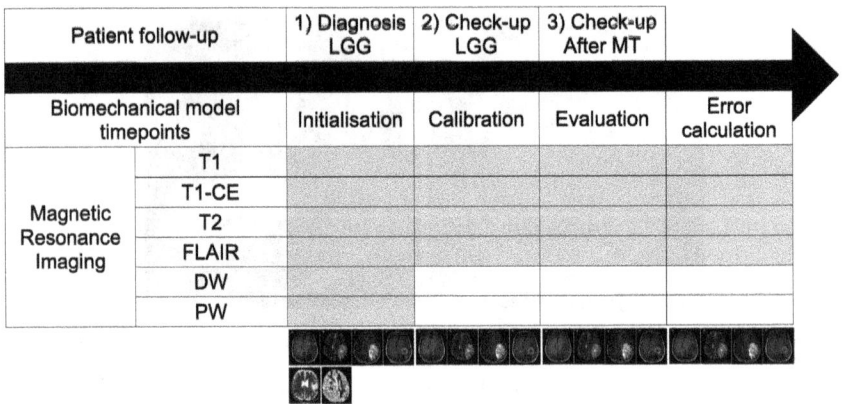

Patient follow-up		1) Diagnosis LGG	2) Check-up LGG	3) Check-up After MT	
Biomechanical model timepoints		Initialisation	Calibration	Evaluation	Error calculation
Magnetic Resonance Imaging	T1				
	T1-CE				
	T2				
	FLAIR				
	DW				
	PW				

Fig. 6. Mathematical model workflow. (1) First, a LGG is diagnosed. T1 MRI, T1-CE MRI, T2 MRI, FLAIR-MRI, DW-MRI, and PW-MRI sequences at this timepoint are necessary for model initialisation: the first four are needed for tumour segmentation by PrognosAIs, while the diffusion-weighted MRI informs on the tumour cellularity and the perfusion on the nutrient level. (2) Model calibration is performed at the second timepoint which clinically corresponds to a routinely performed check-up, while the glioma is still low grade. (3) Usually, MT appears as new contrast enhancement on T1CE MRI during a routine check-up. The model results at this date are evaluated against MRIs acquired at this step. Tumour segmentation is still needed at steps 2 and 3 to inform on the tumours as well as for error calculation.

6. Mathematical Model

The brain parenchyma may be considered a porous medium, according to several studies [48, 51–54]. Budday *et al.* [19] made a comprehensive review of brain tissue mechanics and devoted one of its sections to poromechanics. The mechanical properties of the healthy tissue are deduced from several experimental sources [55, 56] and adapted to the poromechanical framework [57]. In the mathematical model, the brain parenchyma is considered as a porous medium; in other words, a continuum where two main components can be distinguished at every point: a solid scaffold and a porosity. Let ε^s be the volume fraction occupied by the solid scaffold and ε, the volume fraction occupied by the fluid phases:

$$\varepsilon + \varepsilon^s = 1. \tag{1}$$

The porosity is saturated by three fluid phases (t, tumour, h, healthy, and l, liquid). The liquid phase corresponds to the interstitial fluid (IF). Defining their own saturation degree as $S^\beta = \varepsilon^\beta / \varepsilon$ (with $\beta = t, h, l$ the index associated to extra-vascular fluids), we obtain

$$S^l + S^t + S^h = 1. \tag{2}$$

Their respective volume fractions are defined by $\varepsilon^\beta = \varepsilon S^\beta$. Within this porous medium, the nutrient source ω^{bs}, informed by the rCBV, is considered as a fraction of the solid scaffold. Its volume fraction is defined as $\varepsilon^s \omega^{bs}$.

Governing equations: The solid scaffold being deformable, we use the chain rule to define the material derivative:

$$\frac{D^\alpha f^\pi}{Dt} = \frac{\partial f^\pi}{\partial t} + \nabla f^\pi \cdot \mathbf{v}^\alpha. \tag{3}$$

We define the mass conservation of phases and express derivatives with respect of the solid phase ε^s. Introducing porosity ε and the saturation degrees of its phases t, h, and l, the mass balance equations of s, t, h, and l phases read, respectively,

$$\frac{D^s}{Dt}(\rho^s \varepsilon^s) + \rho^s \varepsilon^s \nabla \cdot \mathbf{v}^{\bar{s}} = 0, \tag{4}$$

$$\frac{D^s}{Dt}\left(\rho^t \varepsilon S^t\right) + \nabla \cdot \left(\rho^t \varepsilon S^t \mathbf{v}^{\overline{ts}}\right) + \rho^t \varepsilon S^t \nabla \cdot \mathbf{v}^{\overline{s}} = \overset{l\to t}{M}, \tag{5}$$

$$\frac{D^s}{Dt}\left(\rho^h \varepsilon S^h\right) + \nabla \cdot \left(\rho^h \varepsilon S^h \mathbf{v}^{\overline{hs}}\right) + \rho^h \varepsilon S^h \nabla \cdot \mathbf{v}^{\overline{s}} = 0, \tag{6}$$

$$\frac{D^s}{Dt}\left(\rho^l \varepsilon S^l\right) + \nabla \cdot \left(\rho^l \varepsilon S^l \mathbf{v}^{\overline{ls}}\right) + \rho^l \varepsilon S^l \nabla \cdot \mathbf{v}^{\overline{s}} = -\overset{l\to t}{M}. \tag{7}$$

This system may be read as follows: when the tumourous phase grows, it takes its mass from the interstitial fluid phase, the exchange being represented by $\overset{l\to t}{M}$. As the porous medium is deformable, we follow the same procedure as Sciumé et al. [58]. However, we keep the saturation of the phases unknown, as previously described by the same authors [59], instead of defining the capillary pressure as unknown. Therefore, the four unknowns of this system are the solid displacement $\mathbf{u}^s$ and the saturation of the three fluid phases S^t, S^h, and S^l. The mass equations are complemented by the momentum conservation of all phases:

$$\nabla \cdot \mathbf{t}^{\overline{\overline{T}}} = 0, \tag{8}$$

where $\mathbf{t}^{\overline{\overline{T}}}$ is the total Cauchy stress tensor.

Constitutive relationships: We define the momentum equation through Biot's effective stress principle [60]. We assume that all phases are incompressible, that is, their densities ρ^α (with $\alpha = s, t, l$) are constant and the Biot's coefficient $\beta = 1$. In the absence of external force, the total Cauchy stress tensor equation (8) is expressed as follows:

$$\mathbf{t}^{\overline{\overline{T}}} = \mathbf{t}^{\overline{\overline{E}}} - \beta p^s \overline{\overline{\mathbb{1}}}, \tag{9}$$

with $\mathbb{1}$ the identity tensor, and $p^s = S^t p^t + S^h p^h + S^l p^l$, which is denoted the solid pressure in poroelasticity. In this model, we identify the solid pressure as the intracranial pressure, as each component of the multi-phase system contributes to the pressure on the solid scaffold. Regarding the latter, the solid scaffold is considered as linear elastic:

$$\mathbf{t}^{\overline{\overline{E}}} = \lambda tr(\overline{\overline{\epsilon}})\overline{\overline{\mathbb{1}}} + 2\mu \overline{\overline{\epsilon}}, \tag{10}$$

with $\bar{\bar{\epsilon}}(\mathbf{u}^s) = \frac{1}{2}(\nabla\mathbf{u}^s + (\nabla\mathbf{u}^s)^T)$ the linearised strain tensor, and the Lamé constants $\lambda = \frac{E\nu}{(1+\nu)(1-2\nu)}$ and $\mu = \frac{E}{2(1+\nu)}$.

The relationships between saturation and pressure are designed to take into account the specificity of intracranial pressure. The tumour phase is considered as the wetting phase, i.e., the phase that preferentially adheres to the solid scaffold (here, the ECM), and first contributes to the intracranial pressure. The other, non-wetting, phases h, l add their pressures to the pressure of the wetting phase. Therefore, the saturations of the non-wetting phases define a pressure jump between the phases:

$$p_t = \Gamma_t \left(S^t\right)^{b_t} \quad p_{ht} = \Gamma_h \left(S^h\right)^{b_h} \quad p_{lh} = \Gamma_l \left(S^l\right)^{b_l}, \qquad (11)$$

where $p_{ht} = p^h - p^t$ and $p_{lh} = p^l - p^h$ are the pressure jumps between the respective phases. Γ_α $\alpha = t, h, l$ represents the intensity of the interfacial tension between the fluid and its surrounding medium and where b_α $\alpha = t, h, l$ governs the evolution of the saturation-pressure relationship. Each pair of parameters is first estimated by clinical findings (see the following paragraph *Initial conditions and parameters settings*).

The interaction between fluid phases and the solid scaffold is modelled by a generalised Darcy's law [57, 58], deduced from the linear momentum conservation of fluid phases:

$$-\frac{(S^\alpha)^2 k_{\text{int}}^s}{\mu^\alpha}\nabla p_\alpha = \varepsilon S^\alpha(\mathbf{v}^{\alpha s}) \quad \alpha = t, h, l, \qquad (12)$$

where $\mathbf{v}^{\alpha s} = \mathbf{v}^s - \mathbf{v}^\alpha$ is the relative velocity, k_{int}^s is the intrinsic permeability of the solid scaffold, and μ^α and p_α are respectively the dynamic viscosity and the pressure of each fluid phase $\alpha = t, h, l$.

The tumour growth term $\overset{l \to t}{M}$ is directly dependent on the nutrient supply, here quantified by ω^{bs}, the tumour volume fraction itself ε^t, and a parameter specific to the cell line, the growth rate $\overset{l \to t}{\gamma}$ to calibrate. Finally, the tumour growth can be limited by the tumour density itself through the function $\mathcal{H}(S^t)$ and can be inhibited by the mechanical pressure (a phenomenon shared by a wide category of cancer types [61]), represented by the function $\mathcal{H}_p(p^s)$. Therefore, the growth term $\overset{l \to t}{M}$ takes the following form:

$$\overset{l \to t}{M} = \overset{l \to t}{\gamma} \varepsilon^t [1 - \mathcal{H}(S^t)][1 - \mathcal{H}(p^s)] \frac{\omega^{bs}}{\omega^{bs}_{\max}}, \tag{13}$$

where $\omega^{bs}_{\max}$ is defined by the maximum value of the rCBV in the patient dataset and $\mathcal{H}$ is a regularised step function, already used in several studies [62–64]. If $\mathcal{H}(S^t)$ has a classic form because $S^t \in [0,1]$, $\mathcal{H}(p^s)$ is defined by two parameters, p_{start} and p_{crit}. These two values represent the beginning mechanical stimulation p_{start} and the critical value where the growth is totally stopped by mechanical pressure p_{crit}. $\mathcal{H}(p^s)$ takes the following form:

$$\mathcal{H}(p^s, p_{\text{start}}, p_{\text{crit}})$$
$$= \begin{cases} 0 & \text{if } p^s \leq p_{\text{start}}, \\ \dfrac{1}{2} - \dfrac{1}{2} \cos\left(\pi \dfrac{p^s - p_{\text{start}}}{p_{\text{crit}} - p_{\text{start}}} \right) & \text{if } p_{\text{start}} \leq p^s \leq p_{\text{crit}}, \\ 1 & \text{if } p^s \geq p_{\text{crit}}. \end{cases} \tag{14}$$

6.1. *Initial conditions and parameter settings*

All the initial settings described in this subsection are summarised in Table 2 for the parameters fixed or bounded by the experimental literature and Table 3 for the parameters left to be calibrated.

Segmentations: Let Ω be the computational domain. The PrognosAIs output provides the tumour sub-domain Ω_{TC} which defines $S^t > 0 \in \Omega_{\text{TC}}$ and $S^t = 0$ else. The FAST segmentation [65] provides the anatomical sub-domains of CSF Ω_{CSF}, grey Ω_{G}, and white matter Ω_{W}, where $\Omega_{\text{CSF}} \cup \Omega_{\text{G}} \cup \Omega_{\text{W}} = \Omega$. Young's moduli of brain tissues are attributed following this partition, their values based on the results of Budday *et al.* [56] adapted to the poromechanical framework in Urcun *et al.* [57]. The boundary of Ω is constituted by the dura matter, to prevent any significant deformation, the Young's modulus of this surface is set to $E = 600\,\text{kPa} \in \partial\Omega$.

Tumor saturation estimation: The initial distribution of the fluid phases S^h and S^l is bounded by physiological findings [66,67]. As the contrast of the ADC method is inversely correlated with the cellularity [68], the higher contrast corresponds to the lower value of S^h and the higher value of S^l. Between these two bonds, the values are linearly interpolated as follows:

$$S_0^l(x,y,z) = \frac{S_{\max}^l - S_{\min}^l}{\mathrm{ADC}_{\max} - \mathrm{ADC}_{\min}} (\mathrm{ADC}(x,y,z) - \mathrm{ADC}_{\min}) + S_{\min}^l.$$

(15)

In the cancerous sub-domain Ω_{TC} defined by the segmentation, the quantity corresponding to S^t is subtracted from S^h. The range provided in Table 2 corresponds to the histological measurements in

Table 2. Parameters estimation deduced from *ex vivo* mechanical testing [57] and from clinical literature.

Symb.	Range	Unit	Meaning	Source
S^l	0.148 ± 0.083	[1]	IF saturation	[66]
S^h	0.881 ± 0.053	[1]	HC saturation	[66, 67]
S^t	0.12 ± 0.07	[1]	TC saturation	[76]*
ε	0.55 ± 0.05	[1]	Porosity	[24, 66, 67, 70]
ν	0.48 ± 0.01	[1]	Poisson's ratio	[72, 73]
E_{Cortex}	3.23 ± 2.8	kPa	Young's Modulus of Cortex tissue	[56, 57]
k_{Cortex}	$1.5 \pm 1.4 \cdot 10^{-12}$	m^2	Permeability of Cortex tissue	[18, 57]
μ_l	$5.5 \pm 2.5 \cdot 10^{-3}$	Pa·s	Dynamic viscosity of IF	[57, 71]
μ_h	32.5 ± 2.5	Pa·s	Dynamic viscosity of HC	[57]
†Γ_l	26500	[1]	Interfacial tension between IF and the surrounding medium	[74, 75]
†Γ_h	1000	[1]	Interfacial tension between HC and the surrounding medium	[74, 75]
†b_l	1	[1]	Exponent of IF saturation–pressure relationship	[74, 75]
†b_h	1	[1]	Exponent of HC saturation–pressure relationship	[74, 75]

Notes: *from HGG cases. †These parameters are dependent on equations (16a) and (16b).

HGG cases, which are denser than LGG. We choose to set the maximum LGG cell saturation S^t to the lower bound $S^t = 0.07$, which corresponds to a volume fraction of cancerous cells ε^t around 3.5%. The minimum volume fraction of LGG cells is set to $\varepsilon^t = 0.1\%$. Similar to S^l and S^h, S^t is linearly interpolated with the ADC contrast using equation (15). Regarding brain tissue permeability k^s_{int}, we keep the base values of [57] and follow the results of Jamal et al. [18] by prescribing a value 15 times higher in the white matter sub-domain Ω_W.

Nutrient fraction estimation: The growth term $\overset{l \to t}{M}$ is informed by the PW-MRI. We attempted to provide an estimate that can serve to calculate ω^{bs}. The reflexivity–time curve, a parameter related to the contrast solution in a voxel, was obtained using the formula: $\Delta2((t)) = -\ln(S(t)/S_{\text{base}})/TE$. S is the dynamic signal intensity, S_{base} is the baseline, and TE is the echo time [69]. From this formula, the timepoint corresponding to the maximum $\Delta2((t))$ was detected and ω^{bs} calculated. The maximum contrast of the selected timepoint is termed ω^{bs}_{max}. We interpret it as the maximum value of the nutrient fraction. To inform $\overset{l \to t}{M}$, the ratio $\frac{\omega^{bs}(x,y,z)}{\omega^{bs}_{\text{max}}}$ is provided at all nodes of the computational domain.

Experimental data and literature: Using several experimental sources [24, 66, 67, 70], we define the bounds of the porosity (i.e., the volume fraction occupied by the fluid phases: interstitial, glial, and glioma phases) as $\varepsilon = 0.55 \pm 0.05$. The dynamic viscosity of the liquid phase μ_l comes from the estimation of Sowinski et al. [71] and was adapted to the poromechanical model in [57]. Regarding the dynamic viscosities of the other two phases, the lack of experimental data forced us to keep the generic values of the modelling literature [58]. Regarding Poisson's ratio ν, the global consensus in the literature considers brain tissue to be nearly incompressible [72,73]. For further details on the experimental data and literature, the interested reader is referred to Urcun et al. [57].

Saturation–pressure relationships: We bound these relationships by the physiological measurements of intracranial pressure [74,75], p^s, and the liquid phase saturation in the brain [66], S^l. In the case of a healthy brain, if we adopt the very simplifying hypothesis that only the liquid phase saturation S^l is responsible for the increase of intracranial pressure p^s, we obtain the following relationships:

$$0.07\,\Gamma^l(0.07)^{b^l} + 0.93\,\Gamma^h(0.93)^{b^h} = 1000\,\text{Pa} \ (\approx 7.5\,\text{mmHg}), \quad (16\text{a})$$

$$0.23\,\Gamma^l(0.23)^{b^l} + 0.77\,\Gamma^h(0.77)^{b^h} = 2000\,\text{Pa} \ (\approx 15\,\text{mmHg}). \quad (16\text{b})$$

For the case of $b^l = b^h = 1$, we obtain an interfacial tension Γ^l 26.5-fold higher than Γ^h. These values are kept as initial guesses. Regarding the interfacial tension of the astrocytoma cells, we choose as initial guess to set Γ^t 10-fold higher than Γ^h; unrelated to the intrinsic properties of astrocytoma cells but because of inflammatory activities which accompany these cells.

6.2. *Computational framework*

Finite element framework: We implemented the above model with Dolfin, the C++ libraries of the FEniCS framework [77], with staggered resolution methods commonly adopted (see [58]). An updated Lagrangian approach has been adopted and the incremental resolution allows us to update primary variables as follows:

$$\mathbf{X}_{n+1} = \mathbf{X}_n + \delta\mathbf{X}, \quad (17)$$

with $\delta\mathbf{X}$ the vector of unknowns

$$\delta\mathbf{X} = \begin{pmatrix} \delta u^s_x \\ \delta u^s_y \\ \delta u^s_z \\ \delta S^t \\ \delta S^h \\ \delta S^l \end{pmatrix}.$$

After each time step, $\mathcal{X}^s \in \mathbb{R}^3$, the geometrical space occupied by the porous medium is updated as follows:

$$\mathcal{X}^s_{n+1} = \mathcal{X}^s_n + \delta\mathbf{u}^s. \quad (18)$$

The finite element code is run on 180 Xeon cores (18 nodes, 10 cores per node) and provides the results at $t_0 + 69$ days in 12 hours. Therefore, each iteration of the calibration process takes 12 hours.

Boundary conditions: Homogeneous Dirichlet conditions are prescribed on the domain boundary for all unknowns. This is a consequence of the incremental formulation. For each unknown α, we prescribed $\delta X_\alpha = 0$ on $\partial\Omega$, the domain boundary. In other words, the initial settings of the unknowns remain unchanged at the domain boundary during the simulation. To ensure that these boundary conditions do not influence the simulation, the boundaries of the computational domain were chosen far from the segmented tumour $(2.35 \pm 0.35\,\text{cm}$, see Fig. 7).

Quantities evaluated: The relevant quantities for the model calibration and evaluation are the volume fraction ε^α, with α one of the system phase. Indeed, the saturation of tumour cells S^t could be meaningless without indicating the porosity ε. For instance, if we want to delineate a tumour area, the significance of a high S^t could be diminished by a small ε. Hence, we adopt the following measure

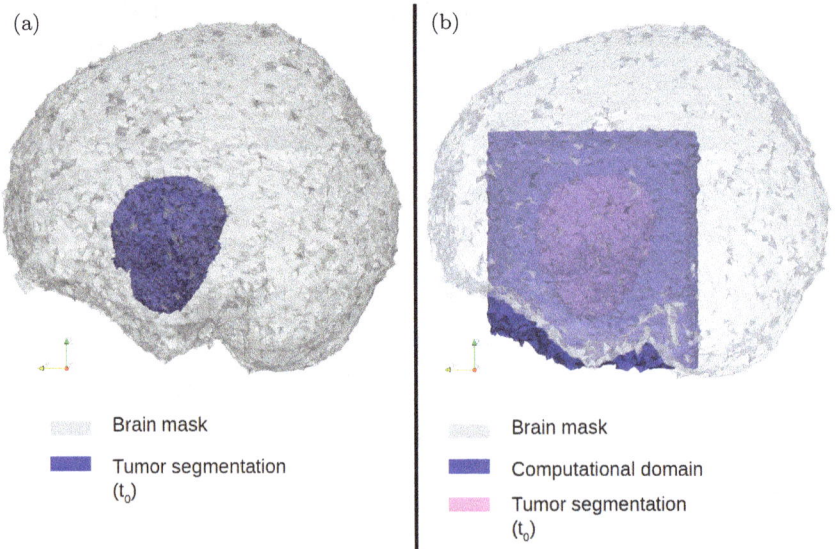

(a)

(b)

Brain mask

Tumor segmentation (t_0)

Brain mask

Computational domain

Tumor segmentation (t_0)

Fig. 7. Definition of the computational domain. (a) Brain mask (grey transparent); Tumour segmentation (blue). (b) Brain mask (grey transparent); Computational domain (blue); Tumour segmentation (pink). The computational domain was designed to ensure its boundaries do not influence the simulation. The boundaries are defined with a distance to the segmented tumour of $2.35 \pm 0.35\,\text{cm}$.

for the interpretation of the results:

$$\text{Vol}_{\text{TC}} = \varepsilon S^t. \tag{19}$$

Calibration and evaluation criterion: At $t_0 + 69\,\text{days}$, the numerical outputs are calibrated against patient data through the cost function J_{over}, which quantifies the error between the numerical results and the patient segmentation, by measuring the spatial overlap:

$$J_{\text{over}} = \frac{\sum_j |\,(\mathbb{K}_{\text{exp}}(j) - \mathbb{K}_{\text{num}}(\text{Vol}_{TC\,j}))\,|\Delta_j}{\sum_j \Delta_j} \quad j \in \Omega, \tag{20}$$

with

$$\mathbb{K}_{\text{num}}(\text{Vol}_{\text{TC}}) = \begin{cases} 0 & \text{if } \text{Vol}_{\text{TC}} \le 0.001, \\ 1 & \text{else,} \end{cases} \tag{21}$$

$$\mathbb{K}_{\text{exp}}(j) = \begin{cases} 0 & \text{if } j \notin \Omega_{TC}, \\ 1 & \text{else,} \end{cases} \tag{22}$$

where Δ_i is the volume of the ith tetrahedron, where $\mathbb{K}_{\text{exp}}(j)$ is the characteristic function of the patient segmentation at $t_0 + 69\,\text{days}$, and $\mathbb{K}_{\text{num}}(\text{Vol}_{\text{TC}})$ the characteristic function of the numerical results at the same timepoint.

The hypotheses of this study regarding MT, sustained mechanical stimulation coupled with oxygen deprivation, are evaluated with a patient dataset at $t_0 + 18\,\text{months}$ where MT was observed through a contrast uptake in the MRI. The zone in the numerical results $t_0 + 69\,\text{days}$ considered at risk are subjected to three conditions:

- belong to the tumour area $\text{Vol}_{\text{TC}} \le 0.001$,
- subjected to mechanical stimulation $p^s \ge p_{\text{start}}$,
- being hypoxic $\omega^{bs} \le 0.25\omega^{bs}_{\text{max}}$.

The hypoxic threshold is defined by the following measures: the maximum value of rCBV corresponds to the artery where the oxygen partial pressure is evaluated to 90 mmHg [78] and the hypoxic level is reached at 20 mmHg [79]. Therefore, $0.25\omega^{bs}_{\text{max}}$ is a reasonable assumption for the hypoxic threshold.

7. Results

Calibration: Starting with the parameters presented in Table 3 (overlapping error 52.3%), the Newton–Raphson algorithm stabilised at an overlapping error of 30.0% after 8 iterations. The seven previous iterations provided the following overlapping errors: 35.7% 34.6% 32.5% 31.4% 30.3% 30.1%, and 30.0%. At $T_0 + 69$ days, we obtain a tumour of $136.1 \, \text{cm}^3$, the segmented tumour of the patient at the same time being of $155.1 \, \text{cm}^3$. The calibration result gives a tumour with a volume error of 12.7%, which overlaps 70.0% of the patient tumour. The values of the parameters obtained at the 8th iteration are shown in Table 4. The exponent b_t of the saturation–pressure relationship in equation (11) was not calibrated. This parameter being an integer, we found that other values than 1 provided meaningless results from the physiological point of view (below or above the physiological range of intracranial pressure for the law density of tumour cells). The results against patient data are shown in Fig. 8.

Evaluation: After calibration, we extract the numerical results which correspond to our mechano-biological hypothesis on malignant transformation (see Fig. 9(a)): the isoline of tumour domain $\text{Vol}_{\text{TC}} = 0.001$ and the isoline of the calibrated parameter p_{start}. From our initial conditions, we extract the lower quarter of the nutrient function ω^{bs} which corresponds to the zone of nutrient deprivation. The intersection of these three conditions corresponds to zones considered as risky, respectively, to our hypothesis. These zones occupy a small volume of the numerical tumour. An MT was observed in

Table 3. Parameters left to be calibrated.

Symb.	Value	Unit	Meaning
p_{start}	1000	Pa	Mechanical stimulation start
p_{crit}	2000	Pa	Mechanical inhibition of growth
Γ_t	26500	[1]	Interfacial tension between TC and the surrounding medium
b_t	1	[1]	Exponent of TC saturation–pressure relationship
μ_t	35	Pa·s	Dynamic viscosity of TC
$\overset{l \to t}{\gamma}$	$2 \cdot 10^{-3}$	kg/(m³·s)	TC growth term

Table 4. Parameters calibrated.

Symb.	Value	Unit
p_{start}	1030	Pa
p_{crit}	1620	Pa
Γ_t	43725	[1]
μ_t	44.5	Pa · s
$\gamma^{l \to t}$	$1.6 \cdot 10^{-3}$	kg/(m³·s)

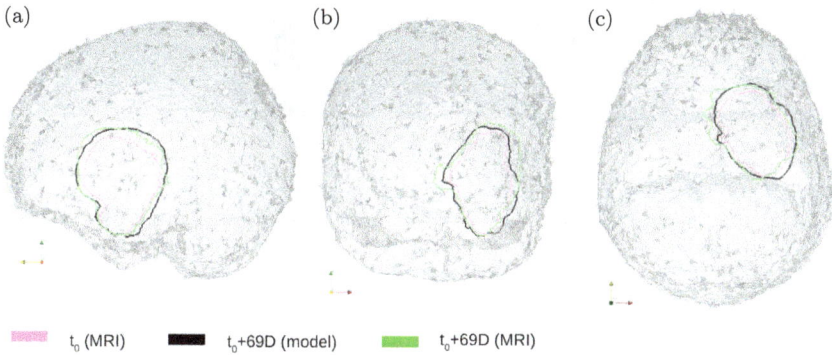

Fig. 8. Calibration results. (a) Sagittal view. (b) Coronal view. (c) Axial view. Brain mask (grey transparent); patient data at T_0 (pink); numerical data at $T_0 + 69$ days (black); patient data at $T_0 + 69$ days (green). Calibration results give a tumour with a volume error of 12.7%, which overlaps 70.0% of the patient tumour.

the patient data by a contrast uptake at $t_0 + 609$ days and confirmed by histopathology at $t_0 + 666$ days. The overlap of the zones marked as risky and the contrast uptake in the patient are shown in Fig. 9(b).

8. Discussion

In this chapter, an overview of MT of LGG is introduced. Radiological, histological and molecular characterisation attempts are introduced along with clinical observations related to MT. Moreover, the study of the microenvironmental role in acquiring the malignant phenotype led to questioning the mechano-biological role in MT of LGA. More specifically, in this study, we introduced a model that aimed at

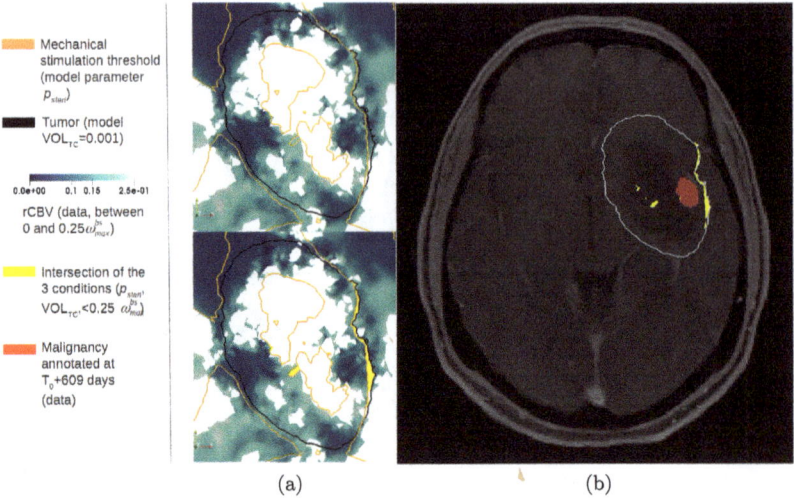

Fig. 9. Model evaluation. Isoline of mechanical stimulation threshold p_{start} 1030 Pa $\approx$ 8 mmHg (orange); isoline of tumour cell volume fraction $\text{Vol}_{\text{TC}} = 0.001$ (black); lower quarter of rCBV values, between 0 and $0.25\omega_{\max}^{bs}$ (linear blue); intersection of the three previous conditions $\geq p_{\text{start}}$, $\text{Vol}_{\text{TC}} \geq 0.001$, and $\omega^{bs} \leq 0.25\omega_{\max}^{bs}$ (yellow); malignant zone annotated at $t_0 + 609$ days (red). (a) The intersection of the three conditions of the mechano-biological hypothesis (yellow) occupies a small volume of the numerical results. (b) T1-CE MRI of the patient. The white contour represents the tumour segmentation provided by the model. The annotation of a malignant zone in the patient data is in the centre of the zone considered at risk in the numerical model.

predicting the MT of LGA. The criteria for MT were established in regions with low nutrient uptake $\omega^{bs} \leq 0.25\omega_{\max}^{bs}$ [78, 79] and an intracranial pressure above the calibrated mechanical stimulation threshold $p^s \geq p_{\text{start}}$.

The patient's T1-CE MRI taken 540 days after the second checkup indicates a new contrast in the red zone in Fig. 9(b). The newly observed contrast uptake zone lied within the region at risk predicted by the model. In other words, since this was the first clinical evidence of malignant transformation available, the model informed on the region that was more likely to be malignantly transformed first, 540 days earlier. The histopathological report confirming MT was issued 57 days after the contrast was first noticed in T1-CE MRI.

This study was only a first proof of concept for MT prediction through a mechano-biological hypothesis and shows various limitations. The tumour contours provided by the model were evaluated against the segmentations performed by PrognosAIs. These segmentations were validated by an expert. However, variability between and within observers is usually observed with respect to tumour segmentation [35].

In this study, the model was only applied to one patient. Of course, more patients that ideally underwent the 'wait and see' approach until MT would be preferred to assess the model performance.

Numerical results overlap only 70.0% of the patient's tumour. Furthermore, the second MRIs were taken right after the partial resection surgery. This may be due to the brain shift which was not taken into account as well as the reduction in the tumour volume. This may also explain the error in the overlap results.

Disregarding the uncertainties coming from segmentation and imaging methods, the model can be improved in several ways: in-depth evaluation of the parameters pre-calibrated by *ex vivo* mechanical testing [57], assessment of anisotropic permeability of the brain [18] using the DTI method, as already proposed in GBM modelling [80]. In this study, the solid scaffold, as the sum of the ECM, neurons, and wall vessels, was described as an heterogeneous elastic solid. A detailed study of brain tissue deformation would lead to a more complex and relevant constitutive relationship [19, 81].

Last but not least, the mechanical stimulation threshold $p_{\text{start}} \approx$ 8 mmHg has a physiological value but seems low comparing to intracranial pressure measured in case of edema or glioma [82]. Further improvements are to be added to this work. The model will be tested on new patients for whom PW-MRI sequences are included at each timepoint. This would inform us on the evolution of nutrient uptake, allowing us to test the robustness of the hypothesis.

Acknowledgements

MAA was supported by the Institute of Advanced Studies (IAS) of the University of Luxembourg, project U-AGR-6046-00-B. SU thanks the Agence National de la Recherche (ANR) (France) and the Fond National de la Recherche (FNR) (Luxembourg) joint grant number ANR-21-CE45-0025-01. The results presented in this chapter were carried out using the HPC facilities of the University of Luxembourg [83] (see https://hpc.uni.lu).

References

[1] L. M. DeAngelis and I. K. Mellinghoff, Virchow 2011 or how to id (h) human glioblastoma, *Journal of Clinical Oncology.* **29**(34), 4473–4474 (2011).

[2] J. Reifenberger, G. Reifenberger, L. Liu, C. D. James, W. Wechsler, and V. P. Collins, Molecular genetic analysis of oligodendroglial tumors shows preferential allelic deletions on 19q and 1p, *The American Journal of Pathology.* **145**(5), 1175 (1994).

[3] D. W. Parsons, S. Jones, X. Zhang, J. C.-H. Lin, R. J. Leary, P. Angenendt, *et al.*, An integrated genomic analysis of human glioblastoma multiforme, *Science.* **321**(5897), 1807–1812 (2008).

[4] F. P. Barthel, K. C. Johnson, P. Wesseling, and R. G. Verhaak, Evolving insights into the molecular neuropathology of diffuse gliomas in adults, *Neurologic Clinics.* **36**(3), 421–437 (2018).

[5] M. J. van den Bent and S. M. Chang, Grade ii and iii oligodendroglioma and astrocytoma, *Neurologic Clinics.* **36**(3), 467–484 (2018).

[6] D. N. Louis, A. Perry, P. Wesseling, D. J. Brat, I. A. Cree, D. Figarella-Branger, *et al.*, The 2021 who classification of tumors of the central nervous system: A summary, *Neuro-Oncology.* **23**(8), 1231–1251 (2021).

[7] D. Bready and D. G. Placantonakis, Molecular pathogenesis of low-grade glioma, *Neurosurgery Clinics.* **30**(1), 17–25 (2019).

[8] S. Nakasu and Y. Nakasu, Malignant progression of diffuse low-grade gliomas: A systematic review and meta-analysis on incidence and related factors, *Neurologia Medico-Chirurgica* (2022). 10.2176/jns-nmc.2021-0313.

[9] G. L. D. O. Lima, M. Zanello, E. Mandonnet, L. Taillandier, J. Pallud, and H. Duffau, Incidental diffuse low-grade gliomas: From early detection to preventive neuro-oncological surgery, *Neurosurgical Review.* **39**(3), 377–384 (2016).

[10] M. U. Bogdańska, M. Bodnar, M. J. Piotrowska, M. Murek, P. Schucht, J. Beck, *et al.*, A mathematical model describes the malignant transformation of low grade gliomas: Prognostic implications, *PLoS One.* **12**(8), e0179999 (2017).

[11] W.B. Pope and G. Brandal, Conventional and advanced magnetic resonance imaging in patients with high-grade glioma, *The Quarterly*

Journal of Nuclear Medicine and Molecular Imaging, **62**(3), 239–253 (2018).

[12] S. Yuan, D. W. Miller, G. H. Barnett, J. F. Hahn, and B. R. Williams, Identification and characterization of human β2-chimaerin: Association with malignant transformation in astrocytoma, *Cancer Research.* **55**(15), 3456–3461 (1995).

[13] C.-K. Park, I. Park, S. Lee, C.-H. Sun, Y. Koh, S.-H. Park, *et al.*, Genomic dynamics associated with malignant transformation in idh1 mutated gliomas, *Oncotarget.* **6**(41), 43653 (2015).

[14] S. Lee, K. Latha, G. Manyam, Y. Yang, A. Rao, and G. Rao, Role of cx3cr1 signaling in malignant transformation of gliomas, *Neuro-Oncology.* **22**(10), 1463–1473 (2020).

[15] T. Tunthanathip, S. Sangkhathat, and K. Kanjanapradit, Molecular landscape for malignant transformation in diffuse astrocytoma, *Global Medical Genetics.* **8**(03), 116–122 (2021).

[16] B. E. Johnson, T. Mazor, C. Hong, M. Barnes, K. Aihara, C. Y. McLean, *et al.*, Mutational analysis reveals the origin and therapy-driven evolution of recurrent glioma, *Science.* **343**(6167), 189–193 (2014).

[17] J. Wang, L. Yi, Q.-M. Kang, J. Zhou, T.-Q. Chen, J.-P. Hugnot, *et al.*, Glioma invasion along white matter tracts: A dilemma for neurosurgeons, *Cancer Letters.* **526**, 103–111 (2022).

[18] A. Jamal, M. T. Mongelli, M. Vidotto, M. Madekurozwa, A. Bernardini, D. R. Overby, *et al.*, Infusion mechanisms in brain white matter and their dependence on microstructure: An experimental study of hydraulic permeability, *IEEE Transactions on Biomedical Engineering.* **68**(4), 1229–1237 (2020).

[19] S. Budday, T. C. Ovaert, G. A. Holzapfel, P. Steinmann, and E. Kuhl, Fifty shades of brain: A review on the mechanical testing and modeling of brain tissue, *Archives of Computational Methods in Engineering.* **27**(4), 1187–1230 (2020).

[20] A. S. Jakola and I. Reinertsen, Radiological evaluation of low-grade glioma: Time to embrace quantitative data? *Acta Neurochirurgica.* **161**(3), 577–578 (2019).

[21] A. S. Jakola, D. Bouget, I. Reinertsen, A. J. Skjulsvik, L. M. Sagberg, H. K. Bø, *et al.*, Spatial distribution of malignant transformation in patients with low-grade glioma, *Journal of Neuro-Oncology.* **146**(2), 373–380 (2020).

[22] F.-X. Ferracci, K. Michaud, and H. Duffau, The landscape of postsurgical recurrence patterns in diffuse low-grade gliomas, *Critical Reviews in Oncology/Hematology.* **138**, 148–155 (2019).

[23] A. S. Jakola, A. J. Skjulsvik, K. Myrmel, K. Sjåvik, G. Unsgård, S. H. Torp, *et al.*, Surgical resection versus watchful waiting in low-grade gliomas, *Annals of Oncology.* **28**(8), 1942–1948 (2017).

[24] J. M. Barnes, L. Przybyla, and V. M. Weaver, Tissue mechanics regulate brain development, homeostasis and disease, *Journal of Cell Science.* **130**(1), 71–82 (2017).

[25] K. Pogoda, R. Bucki, F. J. Byfield, K. Cruz, T. Lee, C. Marcinkiewicz, *et al.*, Soft substrates containing hyaluronan mimic the effects of increased stiffness on morphology, motility, and proliferation of glioma cells, *Biomacromolecules.* **18**(10), 3040–3051 (2017).

[26] Y. A. Miroshnikova, J. K. Mouw, J. M. Barnes, M. W. Pickup, J. N. Lakins, Y. Kim, *et al.*, Tissue mechanics promote idh1-dependent hif1α–tenascin c feedback to regulate glioblastoma aggression, *Nature Cell Biology.* **18**(12), 1336–1345 (2016).

[27] N. Upadhyay and A. Waldman, Conventional mri evaluation of gliomas, *The British Journal of Radiology.* **84**(special_issue_2), S107–S111 (2011).

[28] S. Thust, S. Heiland, A. Falini, H. R. Jäger, A. Waldman, P. Sundgren, *et al.*, Glioma imaging in Europe: A survey of 220 centres and recommendations for best clinical practice, *European Radiology.* **28**(8), 3306–3317 (2018).

[29] A. Fick, Poggendorff's flannel, *Physik.* **94**(59), 297 (1855).

[30] P. W. Schaefer, P. E. Grant, and R. G. Gonzalez, Diffusion-weighted MR imaging of the brain, *Radiology.* **217**(2), 331–345 (2000).

[31] D. A. Hamstra, A. Rehemtulla, and B. D. Ross, Diffusion magnetic resonance imaging: A biomarker for treatment response in oncology, *Journal of Clinical Oncology.* **25**(26), 4104–4109 (2007).

[32] G. Zaharchuk, Theoretical basis of hemodynamic MR imaging techniques to measure cerebral blood volume, cerebral blood flow, and permeability, *American Journal of Neuroradiology.* **28**(10), 1850–1858 (2007).

[33] G.-H. Jahng, K.-L. Li, L. Ostergaard, and F. Calamante, Perfusion magnetic resonance imaging: A comprehensive update on principles and techniques, *Korean Journal of Radiology.* **15**(5), 554–577 (2014).

[34] M. Villien. Méthodologie et application de l'imagerie de la perfusion cérébrale et de la vasoréactivité par IRM. PhD thesis, Université de Grenoble (2012).

[35] H. K. Bø, O. Solheim, A. S. Jakola, K.-A. Kvistad, I. Reinertsen, and E. M. Berntsen, Intra-rater variability in low-grade glioma segmentation, *Journal of Neuro-Oncology.* **131**(2), 393–402 (2017).

[36] U. Baid, S. Ghodasara, S. Mohan, M. Bilello, E. Calabrese, E. Colak, *et al.*, The rsna-asnr-miccai brats 2021 benchmark on brain tumor segmentation and radiogenomic classification (2021). *arXiv preprint* arXiv:2107.02314.

[37] E. J. van Kempen, M. Post, M. Mannil, R. L. Witkam, M. Ter Laan, A. Patel, *et al.*, Performance of machine learning algorithms for glioma segmentation of brain MRI: A systematic literature review and meta-analysis, *European Radiology.* **31**(12), 9638–9653 (2021).

[38] S. R. van der Voort, F. Incekara, M. M. Wijnenga, G. Kapsas, R. Gahrmann, J. W. Schouten, *et al.*, The erasmus glioma database (egd): Structural MRI scans, who 2016 subtypes, and segmentations of 774 patients with glioma, *Data in Brief.* **37**, 107191 (2021).

[39] L. Scarpace, A. E. Flanders, R. Jain, T. Mikkelsen, and D. W. Andrews, Data from REMBRANDT. *The Cancer Imaging Archive.* (2015).

[40] N. Shah, X. Feng, M. Lankerovich, R. B. Puchalski, and B. Keogh, Data from ivy gap, *The Cancer Imaging Archive.* **10**, K9 (2016).

[41] K. Schmainda and M. Prah, Data from brain-tumor-progression, *The Cancer Imaging Archive* (2018).

[42] T.-Y. Jung, S. Jung, J.-H. Moon, I.-Y. Kim, K.-S. Moon, and W.-Y. Jang, Early prognostic factors related to progression and malignant transformation of low-grade gliomas, *Clinical Neurology and Neurosurgery.* **113**(9), 752–757 (2011).

[43] K. Aoki, H. Suzuki, T. Yamamoto, K. N. Yamamoto, S. Maeda, Y. Okuno, *et al.*, Mathematical modeling and mutational analysis reveal optimal therapy to prevent malignant transformation in grade ii idh-mutant gliomas, *Cancer Research* (2021).

[44] B. Bobek-Billewicz, G. Stasik-Pres, A. Hebda, K. Majchrzak, W. Kaspera, and M. Jurkowski, Anaplastic transformation of low-grade gliomas (WHO ii) on magnetic resonance imaging, *Folia Neuropathologica.* **52**(2), 128–140 (2014).

[45] K. R. Swanson, R. C. Rockne, J. Claridge, M. A. Chaplain, E. C. Alvord, and A. R. Anderson, Quantifying the role of angiogenesis in malignant progression of gliomas: In silico modeling integrates imaging and histology, *Cancer Research.* **71**(24), 7366–7375 (2011).

[46] V. M. Pérez-García and L. A. Pérez-Romasanta, Extreme protraction for low-grade gliomas: Theoretical proof of concept of a novel therapeutical strategy, *Mathematical Medicine and Biology: A Journal of the IMA.* **33**(3), 253–271 (2016).

[47] H. L. Harpold, E. C. Alvord Jr., and K. R. Swanson, The evolution of mathematical modeling of glioma proliferation and invasion, *Journal of Neuropathology & Experimental Neurology.* **66**(1), 1–9 (2007).

[48] W. Ehlers and A. Wagner, Multi-component modelling of human brain tissue: A contribution to the constitutive and computational description of deformation, flow and diffusion processes with application to the invasive drug-delivery problem, *Computer Methods in*

Biomechanics and Biomedical Engineering. **18**(8), 861–879 (2015). doi: 10.1080/10255842.2013.853754. PMID: 24261340.

[49] S. Urcun, D. Baroli, P.-Y. Rohan, W. Skalli, V. Lubrano, S. P. Bordas, *et al.*, Non-operable glioblastoma: Proposition of patient-specific forecasting by image-informed poromechanical model, *Brain Multiphysics.* 100067 (2023). doi: https://doi.org/10.1016/j.brain.2023.100067.

[50] S. R. van der Voort, F. Incekara, M. M. Wijnenga, G. Kapsas, R. Gahrmann, J. W. Schouten, *et al.*, Who 2016 subtyping and automated segmentation of glioma using multi-task deep learning (2020).

[51] J. A. Lefever, J. Jaime García, and J. H. Smith, A patient-specific, finite element model for noncommunicating hydrocephalus capable of large deformation, *Journal of Biomechanics.* **46**(8), 1447–1453 (2013). doi: https://doi.org/10.1016/j.jbiomech.2013.03.008.

[52] G. E. Lang, P. S. Stewart, D. Vella, S. L. Waters, and A. Goriely, Is the donnan effect sufficient to explain swelling in brain tissue slices? *Journal of The Royal Society Interface.* **11**(96), 20140123 (2014). doi: 10.1098/rsif.2014.0123.

[53] T. L. Fletcher, A. G. Kolias, P. J. A. Hutchinson, and M. P. F. Sutcliffe, Development of a finite element model of decompressive craniectomy, *PLOS One.* **9**(7), 1–9 (2014). doi: 10.1371/journal.pone.0102131.

[54] T. Dutta-Roy, A. Wittek, and K. Miller, Biomechanical modelling of normal pressure hydrocephalus, *Journal of Biomechanics.* **41**(10), 2263–2271 (2008). doi: https://doi.org/10.1016/j.jbiomech.2008.04.014.

[55] G. Franceschini, D. Bigoni, P. Regitnig, and G. Holzapfel, Brain tissue deforms similarly to filled elastomers and follows consolidation theory, *Journal of the Mechanics and Physics of Solids.* **54**(12), 2592–2620 (2006). doi: https://doi.org/10.1016/j.jmps.2006.05.004.

[56] S. Budday, R. Nay, R. de Rooij, P. Steinmann, T. Wyrobek, T. C. Ovaert, *et al.*, Mechanical properties of gray and white matter brain tissue by indentation, *Journal of the Mechanical Behavior of Biomedical Materials.* **46**, 318–330 (2015). doi: 10.1016/j.jmbbm.2015.02.024.

[57] S. Urcun, P.-Y. Rohan, G. Sciumè, and S. P. Bordas, Cortex tissue relaxation and slow to medium load rates dependency can be captured by a two-phase flow poroelastic model, *Journal of the Mechanical Behavior of Biomedical Materials.* **126**, 104952 (2022). doi: https://doi.org/10.1016/j.jmbbm.2021.104952.

[58] G. Sciumè, R. Santagiuliana, M. Ferrari, P. Decuzzi, and B. A. Schrefler, A tumor growth model with deformable ECM, *Physical Biology.* **11**(6) (2014).

[59] G. Sciumè, W. G. Gray, F. Hussain, M. Ferrari, P. Decuzzi, and B. A. Schrefler, Three phase flow dynamics in tumor growth, *Computational Mechanics.* **53**(3), 465–484 (2014).

[60] M. A. Biot, General theory of three-dimensional consolidation, *Journal of Applied Physics.* **12**(2), 155–164 (1941). 10.1063/1.1712886. https://doi.org/10.1063/1.1712886.

[61] S. Urcun, G. Lorenzo, D. Baroli, P.-Y. Rohan, G. Sciumè, W. Skalli, et al., Oncology and mechanics: Landmark studies and promising clinical applications. In *Advances in Applied Mechanics* (Elsevier, 2022). doi: https://doi.org/10.1016/bs.aams.2022.05.003.

[62] R. Santagiuliana, M. Milosevic, B. Milicevic, G. Sciumè, V. Simic, A. Ziemys, et al., Coupling tumor growth and bio distribution models, *Biomedical Microdevices.* **21** (2019).

[63] V. Le Maout, K. Alessandri, B. Gurchenkov, H. Bertin, P. Nassoy, and G. Sciumè, Role of mechanical cues and hypoxia on the growth of tumor cells in strong and weak confinement: A dual in vitro–in silico approach, *Science Advances.* **6** (2020).

[64] S. Urcun, P.-Y. Rohan, W. Skalli, P. Nassoy, S. P. A. Bordas, and G. Sciumè, Digital twinning of cellular capsule technology: Emerging outcomes from the perspective of porous media mechanics, *PLOS One.* **16**(7), 1–30 (2021). doi: 10.1371/journal.pone.0254512. https://doi.org/10.1371/journal.pone.0254512.

[65] Y. Zhang, M. Brady, and S. Smith, Segmentation of brain MR images through a hidden Markov random field model and the expectation-maximization algorithm, *IEEE Transactions on Medical Imaging.* **20**(1), 45–57 (2001). doi: 10.1109/42.906424.

[66] B. Bender and U. Klose, Cerebrospinal fluid and interstitial fluid volume measurements in the human brain at 3t with epi, *Magnetic Resonance in Medicine.* **61**(4), 834–841 (2009). doi: https://doi.org/10.1002/mrm.21915.

[67] F. A. Azevedo, L. R. Carvalho, L. T. Grinberg, J. M. Farfel, R. E. Ferretti, R. E. Leite, et al., Equal numbers of neuronal and nonneuronal cells make the human brain an isometrically scaled-up primate brain, *Journal of Comparative Neurology.* **513**(5), 532–541 (2009). doi: https://doi.org/10.1002/cne.21974.

[68] T. E. Yankeelov, N. Atuegwu, D. Hormuth, J. A. Weis, S. L. Barnes, M. I. Miga, et al., Clinically relevant modeling of tumor growth and treatment response, *Science Translational Medicine.* **5**(187) (2013). doi: 10.1126/scitranslmed.3005686.

[69] P. Korfiatis, T. L. Kline, Z. S. Kelm, R. E. Carter, L. S. Hu, and B. J. Erickson, Dynamic susceptibility contrast-mri quantification software tool: Development and evaluation, *Tomography.* **2**(4), 448–456 (2016).

[70] Y. Lei, H. Han, F. Yuan, A. Javeed, and Y. Zhao, The brain interstitial system: Anatomy, modeling, in vivo measurement, and applications, *Progress in Neurobiology.* **157** (New Perspectives on Healthy Aging), 230–246 (2017). doi: https://doi.org/10.1016/j.pneurobio.2015.12.007.

[71] D. R. Sowinski, M. D. J. McGarry, E. E. W. Van Houten, S. Gordon-Wylie, J. B. Weaver, and K. D. Paulsen, Poroelasticity as a model of soft tissue structure: Hydraulic permeability reconstruction for magnetic resonance elastography in silico, *Frontiers in Physics.* **8**, 637 (2021). doi: 10.3389/fphy.2020.617582. https://www.frontiersin.org/article/10.3389/fphy.2020.617582.

[72] A. D. C. Smith, W. R. Crum, D. L. G. Hill, N. A. Thacker, and P. A. Bromiley. Biomechanical simulation of atrophy in MR images. In M. Sonka and J. M. Fitzpatrick (eds.), *Medical Imaging 2003: Image Processing*, Vol. 5032 (SPIE, 2003), pp. 481–490. doi: 10.1117/12.480412. https://doi.org/10.1117/12.480412.

[73] P. Schiavone, F. Chassat, T. Boudou, E. Promayon, F. Valdivia, and Y. Payan, In vivo measurement of human brain elasticity using a light aspiration device, *Medical Image Analysis.* **13**(4), 673–678 (2009). doi: https://doi.org/10.1016/j.media.2009.04.001.

[74] N. Canac, J. K. Jalaleddini, S. G. Thorpe, C. M. Thibeault, and R. B. Hamilton, Review: Pathophysiology of intracranial hypertension and noninvasive intracranial pressure monitoring, *Fluids and Barriers of the CNS.* **17**(1), 40 (2020). doi: 10.1186/s12987-020-00201-8.

[75] V. Singh and R. Cheng. Chapter 5 - Neurovascular physiology and neurocritical care. In S. W. Hetts and D. L. Cooke (eds.), *Interventional Neuroradiology. Handbook of Clinical Neurology*, Vol. 176 (Elsevier, 2021), pp. 71–80. doi: https://doi.org/10.1016/B978-0-444-64034-5.00014-6.

[76] F. Zaccagna, F. Riemer, A. N. Priest, M. A. McLean, K. Allinson, J. T. Grist, *et al.*, Non-invasive assessment of glioma microstructure using verdict MRI: Correlation with histology, *European Radiology.* **29**, 5559–5566 (2019). doi: https://doi.org/10.1007/s00330-019-6011-8.

[77] M. Alnæs, J. Blechta, J. Hake, A. Johansson, B. Kehlet, A. Logg, *et al.*, The fenics project version 1.5, *Archive of Numerical Software.* **3**(100) (2015). http://journals.ub.uni-heidelberg.de/index.php/ans/article/view/20553.

[78] E. Ortiz-Prado, J. F. Dunn, J. Vasconez, D. Castillo, G. Viscor, F. Warner, *et al.*, Partial pressure of oxygen in the human body: A general review, *American Journal of Blood Research.* **9**(1), 1–14 (2019).

[79] N. Khan, B. B. Williams, H. Hou, H. Li, and H. M. Swartz, Repetitive tissue po2 measurements by electron paramagnetic resonance oximetry: Current status and future potential for experimental and clinical studies, *Antioxidants & Redox Signaling.* **9**(8), 1169–1182 (2007). doi: 10.1089/ars.2007.1635. https://doi.org/10.1089/ars.2007.1635. PMID: 17536960.

[80] S. Angeli, K. E. Emblem, P. Due-Tonnessen, and T. Stylianopoulos, Towards patient-specific modeling of brain tumor growth and formation of secondary nodes guided by DTI-MRI, *NeuroImage: Clinical.* **20**, 664–673 (2018).

[81] N. Reiter, B. Roy, F. Paulsen, and S. Budday, Insights into the microstructural origin of brain viscoelasticity, *Journal of Elasticity* (2021). doi: 10.1007/s10659-021-09814-y.

[82] J. Lipková, B. Menze, B. Wiestler, P. Koumoutsakos, and J. S. Lowengrub, Modelling glioma progression, mass effect and intracranial pressure in patient anatomy, *Journal of the Royal Society Interface.* **19**(188), 20210922 (2022). doi: 10.1098/rsif.2021.0922.

[83] S. Varrette, P. Bouvry, H. Cartiaux, and F. Georgatos. Management of an academic HPC cluster: The UL experience. In *Proceedings of the 2014 International Conference on High Performance Computing & Simulation (HPCS 2014)*, July, Bologna, Italy (IEEE, 2014), pp. 959–967.

Chapter 9

Brain Tumour Evolution Backwards in Time via Reaction–Diffusion Models and Sobolev Regularisation

**George Baravdish*, B. Tomas Johansson[†],
Lukáš Malý[‡], and Olof Svensson[§]**

*Department of Science and Technology,
Linköping University,
Norrköping, Sweden*
*george.baravdish@liu.se
[†]tomas.johansson@liu.se
[‡]lukas.maly@liu.se
[§]olof.svensson@liu.se

Evolution of brain tumours backwards in time is studied using well-established brain tumour growth models being semilinear parabolic equations of reaction–diffusion type. To run the models backwards, the tumour cell density data at a fixed (final) time is used, rendering an inverse ill-posed problem. This problem is recast as the minimisation of a cost functional matching the data against the solution at a final time of a forward parabolic model having the initial cell density as a control function. Regularisation is incorporated via penalising terms involving Sobolev norms. Mathematical properties of the semilinear parabolic equations are shown in Sobolev–Bochner spaces including uniqueness of a solution to the inverse problem. Differentiability of the control-to-state map is established rendering a sensitivity problem. The derivative

of the cost functional is calculated and the adjoint state is derived via
the Lagrange formalism. A nonlinear conjugate gradient (NCG) method
is presented for the minimisation. Numerical realisation of the minimisation on the BraTS'20 dataset is included using a standard finite difference discretisation of the space and time derivatives, showing that
tumour evolution backwards in time can be accomplished and that the
initial tumour cell density can be reconstructed. Comparison is done
with a nonlinear Landweber method.

1. Introduction

Tumour growth models, based on a reaction–diffusion partial differential equations formalism, have been studied for decades since
their introduction by Murray and co-workers in the early 1990s [1],
in particular for aiding medical imaging techniques and improving
treatment planning of gliomas. Models of this type can be formulated as a semilinear parabolic partial differential equation with a
Neumann boundary condition and a given initial condition:

$$
\begin{cases}
\partial_t u(x,t) - \operatorname{div}(D(x,t)\nabla u(x,t)) = f(x,t,u(x,t)) & \text{in } \Omega \times (0,T), \\
D(x,t)\nabla u(x,t) \cdot n(x) = 0 & \text{on } \partial\Omega \times (0,T), \\
u(x,0) = \varphi(x) & \text{in } \Omega,
\end{cases}
\tag{1}
$$

where $u(x,t)$ is the (normalised) spatio-temporal evolution of the
density of the cells of the tumour at the spatial position x of the brain
region Ω (the skull) for a time $t > 0$, $\operatorname{div}(D\nabla u)$ is the diffusion term
with a positive definite matarix D, the diffusion matrix of the cells
in the brain tissue, and it models the passive diffusion (random cell
movement also known as a Brownian or Fickian process) of tumour
cells as a diffusive flux proportional to the cell density gradient. Cell
migration (active motion of cells) and cell invasion (destruction of
the extra-cellular matrix) processes are not modelled. The function
$f(x,t,u)$ is known as the reaction term, which is a function that models the reproduction of cells in the brain; it describes the tumour cell
population growth which can be exponential, $f(u) = \rho u$ with a constant proliferation rate ρ, stating that cellular division obeys a cycle
with doubling time $(\ln(2)/\rho)$, or logistic $f(u) = \rho u^a (1 - u^b)^c$, where
a, b, and c are positive real numbers, with decreasing proliferation

parameter ρ in areas of high cellular density. Moreover, the Neumann boundary condition in (1) ensures that tumour cells do not diffuse outside the brain region. In the model, n denotes the outward unit normal to the boundary of Ω, and the parameter φ is the initial density of tumour cells given at time $t = 0$. For the diffusion, a different parameter is used for white matter and grey matter:

$$D(x,t) = \begin{cases} d_w\, I & \text{if } x \in \text{white matter,} \\ d_g\, I & \text{if } x \in \text{grey matter,} \end{cases} \tag{2}$$

where $d_w \gg d_g > 0$ are the respective diffusion coefficients in the white and grey matter and I is a 3-by-3 identity matrix.

These reaction–diffusion growth models have been continuously improved to successively integrate, for example, a variable tumour cell diffusion rate in white versus grey matter, an anisotropic diffusion tensor field accounting for the preferred migration of tumour cells along white matter tracts, as well as multi-scale modelling. Moreover, tumour-induced effects of, for example, surgery, chemotherapy, and radiotheraphy have also been included into the models as well as necrosis and hypoxia. The research into reaction–diffusion growth models is too prolific to be adequately listed here; for some guidance, we refer the reader to [2–21] and references therein, and the survey [22].

A key issue and limitation is the collection and acquisition of information of the initial tumour cell density. We shall not go into this issue here but mention that there are ideas for its estimation, most recently via deep learning, for an overview see the introduction in [23]. Cell density maps computed from histological slides of a non-operated brain with glioblastoma are presented in [24] and also combined with deep learning for estimates of the cell density.

Rather than direct modelling, our focus is on mathematical properties of running the governing equation in (1) backwards in time. We thus consider the inverse problem consisting of (1), where the initial cell density $u(x,0) = \varphi(x)$ is not known but instead additional data

$$u(x,T) = \psi(x), \quad x \in \Omega \tag{3}$$

is provided with the aim of estimating $\varphi(x)$. This is a parabolic equation backwards in time and known to be severely ill-posed. Research on backward problems has been prolific in particular for the case of a linear governing equation; for a general overview and references, see [25, Chapter 3.1].

Being able to run the governing reaction–diffusion model backwards in time can give further insights into the tumour growth and its origin. Moreover, it can help generating additional synthetic data to be fed into deep learning models of tumour detection and classification [26]. Also, the mathematical machinery developed to backward evolution is general and can be applied for parameter identification in (1), for example, in identifying a response parameter [27]. For more on inverse problem approaches in cancer modelling, see [28, 29]. Equations in the form (1) can model other phenomena than tumours; for an overview see [30], and for a recent application in the control of the spread of Dengue fever, see [31].

In [32], a numerical procedure is outlined based on the Landweber method [33] for the nonlinear inverse ill-posed problem of reconstructing the initial location of a brain tumour. In this chapter, we consider a similar problem but apply instead the framework developed in [34–37] in combination with results on optimal control of partial differential equations [38] to derive a nonlinear conjugate gradient (NCG) method for the backward evolution. The inverse problem consisting of (1) and (3) is reformulated as the minimisation of a cost functional matching the given data (3) against the solution of (1) at $t = T$, having the initial cell density φ as a control function. Regularisation is incorporated via penalising terms involving Sobolev norms. Moreover, for the numerical implementation, we use a standard finite difference scheme.

We mention that a general mathematical analysis of backward reaction–diffusion models is presented in [39, 40] and a numerical algorithm for the identification of φ is presented in [17]. Furthermore, a backward problem for a system of nonlinear parabolic equations is investigated in [41]. Both the results and methods in those references are different from this study. We use a cost functional with Sobolev regularisation and employ a control theoretic framework with accompanying mathematical analysis in Sobolev–Bochner spaces not present in those works.

For the outline of this chapter, in the remaining part of this section, we introduce some notation and spaces and discuss existence and uniqueness of a solution to (1) and of the backward problem (1) and (3) for various reaction terms f. In Section 2, sensitivity of the solution to (1) with respect to the initial data is investigated, see Theorem 1. As a corollary, the Fréchet derivative of the control-to-state map taking the initial condition to the value of the solution (1) at $t = T$ is calculated leading to a solution of a so-called sensitivity problem, see Corollary 3. In Section 3, we reformulate the backward problem as the minimisation of a cost functional. Existence of a minimiser is shown in Section 3.1. The derivative of the cost functional is calculated via the Lagrange formalism, see Section 3.2. In Section 3.3, a NCG method is given for the stable minimisation of the introduced cost functional. As an alternative, a nonlinear Landweber method for the minimisation is briefly presented in Section 4. In Section 5, we present numerical results on the BraTS'20 dataset. For comparison, we also give results obtained with the nonlinear Landweber method.

Spaces and notation: The standard linear space of square integrable functions in Ω is denoted by $L^2(\Omega)$. The space $W^{k,2}(\Omega)$, $k > 0$, denotes the standard Sobolev space of functions with weak and square integrable derivatives up to order k. We write $u \in W_0^{1,2}(\Omega)$ if the Sobolev function $u \in W^{1,2}(\Omega)$ has zero trace on $\partial\Omega$. Let I be the time interval $(0, T)$ with $T > 0$. For a Banach space X, we use the Bochner spaces

$$L^2(I; X) = \left\{ u : I \to X : \|u\|_{L^2(I;X)} = \left(\int_0^T \|u(t)\|_X^2 \, dt \right)^{1/2} < \infty \right\},$$

$$L^\infty(I; X) = \left\{ u : I \to X : \|u\|_{L^\infty(I;X)} = \operatorname*{ess\,sup}_{t \in I} \|u(t)\|_X < \infty \right\},$$

and

$$\mathcal{C}(I; X) = \left\{ u : I \to X \text{ is continuous} : \|u\|_{\mathcal{C}(I;X)} \right.$$

$$\left. = \sup_{t \in I} \|u(t)\|_X < \infty \right\}.$$

Moreover, for two Banach spaces X_1 and X_2, we have the Sobolev–Bochner space (sometimes denoted a Lions space)

$$W^{1,p}(I; X_1, X_2) = \{ u \in L^p(I; X_1) : u_t' \in L^p(I; X_2) \},$$

with norm

$$\|u\|_{W^{1,p}(I;X_1,X_2)} = \|u\|_{L^p(I;X_1)} + \|u'_t\|_{L^p(I;X_2)}.$$

Here, the derivative with respect to time t, u'_t, is in the weak (distributional) sense. We use either $p = 2$ or $p = \infty$. We typically take $W^{1,2}(\Omega)$ and its dual as X_1 and X_2, respectively, and then shorten the notation of $W^{1,p}(I; X_1, X_2)$ into $W^{1,p}(I; W^{1,2}(\Omega))$. The above spaces can also be defined, with obvious modifications, for the closed interval $\bar{I} = [0, T]$.

We assume that Ω is a bounded domain with a Lipschitz boundary so that we can apply arguments based on continuous and compact embeddings of Sobolev spaces $W^{1,2}(\Omega)$, cf. [42, Chapter 12].

Forward existence and uniqueness: The parabolic equation (1) with initial value data $\varphi \in W^{1,2}(\Omega)$ has a unique strong (and also weak) solution by [43, Theorems 8.30–34] provided that the differential operator $Au = \mathrm{div}(D(x,t)\nabla u(x,t)) - f(x,t,u(x,t))$ is pseudomonotone and semicoercive, uniformly in t. Pseudomonotonicity follows from [43, Lemmata 8.8 and 8.29], and semicoercivity can be easily proven whenever $D(x,t)$ is a positive definite matrix for all $(x,t) \in \Omega \times \bar{I}$, and $f(x,t,u)$ is Lipschitz continuous with respect to the variable u.

It is important with appropriate conditions on f. Otherwise the solution to (1) can blow up in finite time. An example of this phenomena with $f(x,t,u) = u^2$ is given in [44, p. 6]. For more on blow-up of solutions to nonlinear evolution equations with history and references, see the overview [45] as well as [46].

Backward existence and uniqueness: We briefly discuss uniqueness for the inverse problem considered, i.e., for the semilinear parabolic equation (1) backwards in time given the additional data (3). Uniqueness is important in terms of tumour modelling, since having multiple or spurious solutions can hinder correct medical decisions.

We start with a logistic growth, where $f(x,t,u) = \rho(x,t)u(1-u)$. Assume that there exist two solutions u and u_1 both satisfying the first two equations in (1) together with (3). Define $w = u - u_1$. Then, as can be directly verified,

$$\begin{cases} \partial_t w(x,t) - \text{div}(D(x,t)\nabla w(x,t)) = \beta(x,t)w & \text{in } \Omega \times (0,T), \\ \qquad\qquad D(x,t)\nabla w(x,t) \cdot n(x) = 0 & \text{on } \partial\Omega \times (0,T), \\ \qquad\qquad\qquad w(x,T) = 0 & \text{in } \Omega, \qquad (4) \end{cases}$$

with $\beta(x,t) = \rho(x,t)(1 - u - u_1)$. Since the solutions we are considering will be uniformly bounded, the element β is in particular bounded and we can appeal to classical backward uniqueness results for linear parabolic equations, for example, [47, Theorem 6 in Chapter 6, Section 7], alternatively see [48,49], to conclude that w in (4) is identically zero implying $u = u_1$. An overview of results for backward parabolic equations is given in [25, Chapter 3, Section 1].

In the general case, there are criteria on $f(t,u)$ that generates uniqueness, such as a Lipschitz-type condition,

$$\|f(t,v) - f(t,w)\| \leq L\|v - w\|,$$

with L independent of t, v, and w, see [50–52]; for a local Lipschitz condition generating uniqueness, see [53, 54]. A general condition guaranteeing uniqueness is presented in [55]. Conditional stability for backward problems for degenerate semilinear parabolic equations is derived in [56].

Note that there are criteria guaranteeing that there exists a solution to the backward problem for a dense set of data (3), see [57].

2. Perturbation of the Initial Data: The Sensitivity Problem

In this section, we investigate the effects of initial data perturbations, provided that we have a solution $u(x,t)$ to (1) with initial data replaced by $u(x,0) = u_0(x)$, $x \in \Omega$.

Theorem 1. *Let $\varepsilon > 0$, u_0, $v_0 \in W^{1,2}(\Omega)$. Assume that $f = f(x,t,u)$ is twice continuously differentiable with respect to u with both derivatives being uniformly bounded. Assume also that there are numbers $m < M$ such that $f(\cdot,\cdot,m) = f(\cdot,\cdot,M) = 0$ and both u_0 and*

$u_0 + \varepsilon v_0$ *attain values only within the interval* $[m, M]$. *Let* $u_\varepsilon(x, t)$ *be a solution to* (1) *with initial data replaced by* $u_\varepsilon(x, 0) = u_0(x) + \varepsilon v_0(x)$. *Then, the difference quotient*

$$q_\varepsilon(x, t) := \frac{u_\varepsilon(x, t) - u(x, t)}{\varepsilon}, \quad (x, t) \in \Omega \times \bar{I},$$

converges to a function $v(x, t)$ *weakly in* $W^{1,2}([0, T]; W^{1,2}(\Omega))$ *and in norm in* $C([0, T]; L^2(\Omega))$ *as* $\varepsilon \to 0$, *where* v *is the solution to the sensitivity problem*

$$\begin{cases} \partial_t v(x, t) - \operatorname{div}(D(x, t)\nabla v(x, t)) \\ \quad = \partial_u f(x, t, u(x, t))v(x, t) & \text{in } \Omega \times I, \\ D(x, t)\nabla v(x, t) \cdot n(x) = 0 & \text{on } \partial\Omega \times I, \\ v(x, 0) = v_0(x) & \text{in } \Omega. \end{cases} \quad (5)$$

Moreover, $u_\varepsilon(\cdot, t) = u(\cdot, t) + \varepsilon v(\cdot, t) + o(\varepsilon)$ *with equality in* $L^2(\Omega)$, *uniformly for all* $t \in [0, T]$.

Remark 2. The requirement of boundedness of $\partial^2_{uu} f$ is in fact not very restrictive since we may premultiply $f(x, t, u)$ by a smooth compactly supported cut-off function that equals 1 whenever $u \in [m, M]$.

Sketch of proof. From the proof of Lipschitz dependence on initial data [43, Theorem 8.35 (ii)], we obtain a uniform bound

$$\|u_\varepsilon(\cdot, t) - u(\cdot, t)\|_{W^{1,2}(\Omega)} \leq C\|\varepsilon v_0\|_{W^{1,2}(\Omega)}, \quad t \in \bar{I}. \quad (6)$$

In other words, the set of functions $\{q_\varepsilon : \varepsilon > 0\}$ is bounded in the Bochner space $C(\bar{I}; W^{1,2}(\Omega)) \subset L^2(I; W^{1,2}(\Omega))$. We aim however to show boundedness in the Sobolev–Bochner space $W^{1,2}(I; W^{1,2}(\Omega))$.

Since u and u_ε are solutions to (1) with modified initial data, we obtain that q_ε is a solution to

$$\begin{cases} \partial_t q_\varepsilon(x, t) - \operatorname{div}(D(x, t)\nabla q_\varepsilon(x, t)) \\ \quad = \dfrac{f(x, t, u_\varepsilon) - f(x, t, u)}{\varepsilon} & \text{in } \Omega \times I, \\ D(x, t)\nabla q_\varepsilon(x, t) \cdot n(x) = 0 & \text{on } \partial\Omega \times I, \\ q_\varepsilon(x, 0) = v_0(x) & \text{in } \Omega. \end{cases} \quad (7)$$

It follows from [58] that $\max\{|u(x,t)|, |u_\epsilon(x,t)|\} \le M < \infty$ uniformly for all $(x,t) \in \Omega \times \bar{I}$. Taylor's expansion of f of second order in the third variable, together with this bound, yields that

$$\frac{f(x,t,u_\varepsilon(x,t)) - f(x,t,u(x,t))}{\varepsilon}$$
$$= \partial_u f(x,t,u(x,t))q_\varepsilon(x,t) + \varepsilon B(x,t,q_\varepsilon(x,t)),$$

for some uniformly bounded function B.

Let $\eta \in (W^{1,2}(\Omega))^{**} \cong W^{1,2}(\Omega)$ be an arbitrary test function in the unit ball of $W^{1,2}(\Omega)$. In particular, $\|\eta\|_{L^2(\Omega)} \le 1$ and $\|\nabla\eta\|_{L^2(\Omega)} \le 1$ holds true. For every $t \in \bar{I}$, we then have that

$$|\langle \eta(\cdot), \partial_t q_\varepsilon(\cdot,t)\rangle|$$
$$= \left| \int_\Omega (D(x,t)\nabla q_\varepsilon(x,t)) \cdot \nabla\eta(x) \right.$$
$$\left. + (\partial_u f(x,t,u(x,t))q_\varepsilon(x,t) + \varepsilon B(x,t,q_\varepsilon(x,t)))\eta(x)\, dx \right|$$
$$\le \left\| \|D(x,t)\|_{\mathbb{R}^3 \to \mathbb{R}^3} \right\|_{L^\infty(\Omega)} \|\nabla q_\varepsilon(\cdot,t)\|_{L^2(\Omega)} \|\nabla\eta\|_{L^2(\Omega)}$$
$$+ (\|\partial_u f\|_{L^\infty(\Omega \times I \times \mathbb{R})} \|q_\varepsilon(\cdot,t)\|_{L^2(\Omega)} + \varepsilon\|B\|_{L^\infty(\Omega \times I \times \mathbb{R})} \|\eta\|_{L^2(\Omega)})$$
$$\le C\left(\|q_\varepsilon(\cdot,t)\|_{W^{1,2}(\Omega)} + \varepsilon\right) \le C\left(\|v_0\|_{W^{1,2}(\Omega)} + \varepsilon\right).$$

We have thus shown a uniform bound for $\|\partial_t q_\varepsilon(\cdot,t)\|_{W^{1,2}(\Omega)^*}$ with $t \in \bar{I}$. Therefore, the set of functions $\{q_\varepsilon : 0 < \varepsilon < 1\}$ is bounded in the Sobolev–Bochner space $W^{1,2}(I; W^{1,2}(\Omega))$. By reflexivity of $W^{1,2}(I; W^{1,2}(\Omega))$, there is a sequence $\{\varepsilon_n\}_{n=1}^\infty$ with $\varepsilon_n \to 0$ and a function $v \in W^{1,2}(I; W^{1,2}(\Omega))$ such that $q_{\varepsilon_n} \rightharpoonup v$.

Note that $v \in \mathcal{C}(I; W^{1,2}(\Omega))$ due to the continuous embedding $W^{1,2}(I; W^{1,2}(\Omega)) \subset \mathcal{C}(I; W^{1,2}(\Omega))$, see [43, Section 7.2]. A generalised Aubin–Lions lemma as in [59, Theorem 5.1], see also [43, Lemma 7.10], yields a compact embedding $W^{1,2}(\bar{I}, W^{1,2}(\Omega)) \Subset \mathcal{C}(\bar{I}, L^2(\Omega))$. Hence, $u_{\varepsilon_n}(\cdot,t) \to v(\cdot,t)$ in $L^2(\Omega)$ for every $t \in \bar{I}$.

Let $\zeta \in W^{1,\infty}(I; W^{1,2}(\Omega))$ be an arbitrary test function. Since q_ε is a weak solution to (7) in the sense of [43, Definition 8.2], it satisfies the integral equation

$$\int_0^T \int_\Omega -q_\varepsilon(x,t)\partial_t\zeta(x,t) + (D(x,t)\nabla q_\varepsilon(x,t)) \cdot \nabla\zeta(x,t)$$

$$- \left(\partial_u f(x,t,u(x,t))q_\varepsilon(x,t) + \varepsilon B(x,t,q_\varepsilon(x,t))\right)\zeta(x,t)\,dx\,dt$$

$$= \int_\Omega v_0(x)\zeta(x,0) - q_\varepsilon(x,T)\zeta(x,T)\,dx.$$

Since both $q_{\varepsilon_n} \rightharpoonup v \in L^2(I;W^{1,2}(\Omega))$ and $q_{\varepsilon_n} \to v \in \mathcal{C}(I;L^2(\Omega))$ as $n \to \infty$, we may pass to the limit with $\varepsilon = \varepsilon_n \to 0$ in the integral equation above to obtain that

$$\int_0^T \int_\Omega - v(x,t)\partial_t\zeta(x,t) + \left(D(x,t)\nabla v(x,t)\right) \cdot \nabla\zeta(x,t)$$

$$- (\partial_u f(x,t,u(x,t))v(x,t))\zeta(x,t)\,dx\,dt$$

$$= \int_\Omega v_0(x)\zeta(x,0) - v(x,T)\zeta(x,T)\,dx.$$

In particular, the limit function v is a weak solution to (5). By [43, Lemma 8.4], it is a strong solution as well. Since $\partial_u f$ is uniformly Lipschitz, one can verify the assumptions of [43, Theorem 8.34], which guarantees the existence of a unique strong solution of (5). Due to the uniqueness of a weak limit v, there is no need to extract a convergent subsequence q_{ε_n}, but $q_\varepsilon \rightharpoonup v$ in $W^{1,2}(I;W^{1,2}(\Omega))$ and hence $q_\varepsilon \to v$ in $\mathcal{C}(I;L^2(\Omega))$ as $\varepsilon \to 0$.

Observe that the norm convergence $q_\varepsilon \to v$ in $\mathcal{C}(I;L^2(\Omega))$ implies immediately that

$$u_\varepsilon(\cdot,t) = u(\cdot,t) + \varepsilon v(\cdot,t) + o(\varepsilon)$$

as $L^2(\Omega)$-functions uniformly in $t \in \bar{I}$.   □

Corollary 3. *The mapping $u_0 \mapsto u(\cdot,T)$ from $W^{1,2}(\Omega)$ to $L^2(\Omega)$, where u solves (1), is Lipschitz continuous. Furthermore, this mapping is Fréchet differentiable, that is, there exists a bounded linear operator $\mathcal{A}$ (depending on u_0) from $W^{1,2}(\Omega)$ to $L^2(\Omega)$ such that for any $v_0 \in W^{1,2}(\Omega)$,*

$$\lim_{\varepsilon \to 0} \frac{\|u_\varepsilon(\cdot,T) - u(\cdot,T) - \varepsilon\mathcal{A}v_0\|_{L^2(\Omega)}}{\|\varepsilon v_0\|_{W^{1,2}(\Omega)}} = 0, \tag{8}$$

where $u_\varepsilon(x,t)$ *is a solution to* (1) *with initial data replaced by* $u_\varepsilon(x,0) = u_0(x) + \varepsilon v_0(x)$. *The element* $\mathcal{A}v_0$ *equals* $v(\cdot, T)$, *where* v *is a solution to the sensitivity problem* (5).

3. Nonlinear Conjugate Gradient Method

Given regularisation parameters $m_1, m_2, \mu_1, \mu_2 \geq 0$ and an arbitrary cut-off function $\chi \in W_0^{2,2}(\Omega)$ that satisfies $0 \leq \chi \leq 1$ pointwise in Ω, e.g.,

$$\chi(x) = \tilde{\chi}\big(\min\{1, \operatorname{dist}(x, \partial\Omega)\}\big), \quad x \in \Omega, \quad \text{where}$$
$$\tilde{\chi}(t) = 3t^2 - 2t^3, \qquad\qquad t \in [0, 1],$$

we aim to reconstruct the unknown parameter φ in the inverse problem consisting of (1) and (3) by minimising the functional

$$E(u_0) = \frac{m_1}{2}\|u(\cdot, T) - \psi(\cdot)\|_{L^2(\Omega)}^2$$
$$+ \frac{m_2}{2}\left\|\nabla\Big((u(\cdot, T) - \psi(\cdot))\chi(\cdot)\Big)\right\|_{L^2(\Omega)}^2$$
$$+ \frac{\mu_1}{2}\|u_0\|_{L^2(\Omega)}^2 + \frac{\mu_2}{2}\|\nabla u_0\|_{L^2(\Omega)}^2, \tag{9}$$

subject to $u(x,t)$ being a (weak) solution of (1) with the initial condition $u(x,0) = u_0(x)$. The cut-off function χ is really only important in the case $m_2 \neq 0$. Without such a cut-off function that vanishes on $\partial\Omega$, when using a Green's formula in deriving the adjoint problem (11), we will obtain a boundary integral in (10) that cannot be controlled by a suitable choice of the final value condition in (11). A solution to (1) with a modified initial condition does indeed exist as outlined earlier and can be proven by discretising (1) in time, approximating the time-derivative with a backward difference quotient, and thereby generating a sequence of elliptic problems. Solving these yields a rather direct proof of existence and uniqueness of a solution of the direct problem (1), see [60, Section 4] for details. Note that [60] considered only f independent of x and t, nevertheless the argument there still applies even in our setting. A complete, though abstract, proof of existence and uniqueness is given in [43, Chapter 8].

If $\mu_1 = \mu_2 = 0$, then $E(\varphi) = 0$. In other words, the sought unknown parameter φ is the minimiser of E. However, in order to handle the ill-posedness of the backward problem and to improve numerical stability, Tikhonov regularisation terms are included in the functional by letting μ_1 and/or μ_2 be non-zero. Then, the minimiser of E is an approximate reconstruction of φ but need not of course be equal to φ. Typically, in practise, there will be measurement errors in the data (3) and there is then an interplay between the parameters in the functional and the error level in order to obtain a stable approximation converging to the sought φ as the error level tends to zero. For Tikhonov regularisation of nonlinear ill-posed problems in Banach spaces and criteria for convergence, see [61, Chapter 4].

3.1. *Existence of a minimiser*

First, we show that there exists a minimiser to the functional in (9) under the assumption that $\mu_1, \mu_2 > 0$ and start with the case when $m_2 = 0$. Let $\{u_0^n\} \subset W^{1,2}(\Omega)$ be a minimising sequence such that

$$\lim_{n \to \infty} E(u_0^n) = \inf_{u_0 \in W^{1,2}(\Omega)} E(u_0).$$

Thus, due to the structure of the functional E, it follows that the sequence $\{u_0^n\}$ is uniformly bounded in $W^{1,2}(\Omega)$. This implies that there exists a subsequence of $\{u_0^n\}$, denoted for simplicity by the same index, and an element $u_0^* \in W^{1,2}(\Omega)$ such that u_0^n converges weakly to u_0^* in $W^{1,2}(\Omega)$. We show that u_0^* is a minimiser of E.

Let u^n and u^* solve (1) with initial data u_0^n and u_0^*, respectively. As in the proof of Theorem 1, one can show that $u^n(\cdot, T)$ converges strongly to $u^*(\cdot, T)$ in $L^2(\Omega)$. Combining this with the weak lower semicontinuity of the norms, we obtain that

$$\frac{m_1}{2} \|u^*(\cdot, T) - \psi(\cdot)\|_{L^2(\Omega)}^2 + \frac{\mu_1}{2} \|u_0^*\|_{L^2(\Omega)}^2 + \frac{\mu_2}{2} \|\nabla u_0^*\|_{L^2(\Omega)}^2$$

$$\leq \liminf_{n \to \infty} \Big(\frac{m_1}{2} \|u^n(\cdot, T) - \psi(\cdot)\|_{L^2(\Omega)}^2 + \frac{\mu_1}{2} \|u_0^n\|_{L^2(\Omega)}^2$$

$$+ \frac{\mu_2}{2} \|\nabla u_0^n\|_{L^2(\Omega)}^2 \Big).$$

This shows that u^* is a minimiser of E in the case $m_2 = 0$.

Let us now consider the case when $m_2 > 0$. Then, the sequence of functions $\{(u^n(\cdot, T) - \psi(\cdot))\chi(\cdot)\}$ is uniformly bounded in $W^{1,2}(\Omega)$ since $\|\nabla((u^n(\cdot, T) - \psi(\cdot))\chi(\cdot))\|_{L^2(\Omega)}$ is bounded due to the structure of E and

$$(u^n(\cdot, T) - \psi(\cdot))\chi(\cdot) \to (u^*(\cdot, T) - \psi(\cdot))\chi(\cdot) \quad \text{in } L^2(\Omega)$$

as χ is pointwise bounded and $u^n(\cdot, T) \to u^*(\cdot, T)$ in $L^2(\Omega)$. By reflexivity of $W^{1,2}(\Omega)$, there is a subsequence (denoted by the same index) such that

$$(u^n(\cdot, T) - \psi(\cdot))\chi(\cdot) \rightharpoonup (u^*(\cdot, T) - \psi(\cdot))\chi(\cdot) \quad \text{in } W^{1,2}(\Omega).$$

In particular,

$$\nabla((u^n(\cdot, T) - \psi(\cdot))\chi(\cdot)) \rightharpoonup \nabla((u^*(\cdot, T) - \psi(\cdot))\chi(\cdot)) \quad \text{in } L^2(\Omega; \mathbb{R}^3).$$

The weak lower semicontinuity of the norms then implies that

$$E(u_0^*) \leq \liminf_{n \to \infty} E(u_0^n) = \inf_{u_0 \in W^{1,2}(\Omega)} E(u_0).$$

Thus, u_0^* is a minimiser of the functional E.

Remark 4. Since (1) is nonlinear, the functional E is not convex, in general. Thus, there can potentially exist several elements giving the minimal value of E, see further [62, 63].

Remark 5. The existence of a minimiser can be also shown if $\mu_1 = 0$ but $\mu_2 > 0$. This is due to the Poincaré inequality

$$\int_\Omega |u(x)|^2 \, dx \leq C_\Omega \int_\Omega |\nabla u(x)|^2 \, dx,$$

which holds true in Lipschitz domains for all functions $u \in W^{1,2}(\Omega)$ that satisfy $|\{x \in \Omega : u(x) = 0\}| \geq c|\Omega|$ for some fixed $c \in (0,1)$, which follows from [42, Theorem 13.27]. Note that the value of C_Ω depends on the constant c. In our case, u_0 describes the cell density of tumour cells in a brain of a living individual, and hence it is reasonable to assume that the cell density satisfies $u_0(x) = 0$ in at least half of the brain region.

Remark 6. In case $\mu_2 = 0$ and $\mu_1 \geq 0$, we can apply the earlier argument if we additionally impose an *a priori* bound on the Sobolev norm of the initial data. In other words, given $M > 0$, there exists $u_0^* \in W^{1,2}(\Omega)$ with $\|u_0^*\|_{W^{1,2}(\Omega)} \leq M$ such that

$$E(u_0^*) = \inf\{E(u_0) : \|u_0\|_{W^{1,2}(\Omega)} \leq M\}.$$

3.2. The steepest descent direction via the adjoint problem

We use the Lagrange multiplier method to rewrite the constrained minimisation problem in (9) as an unconstrained minimisation of the Lagrange functional

$$
\mathcal{E}(u_0) := E(u_0) + \int_0^T \int_\Omega \lambda(x,t)[f(x,t,u(x,t))
$$
$$
+ \operatorname{div}(D(x,t)\nabla u(x,t)) - \partial_t u(x,t)]\, dx\, dt,
$$

where $u(x,0) = u_0(x)$ and $\lambda \in W^{1,2}(\bar{I}, W^{1,2}(\Omega))$ is a Lagrange multiplier.

In case $m_2 \neq 0$, the set Ω is required to have a $\mathcal{C}^2$-smooth boundary so that $u(\cdot, T)$ will be of regularity $W^{2,2}(\Omega)$ by [64, Theorem 15.1], which is needed in Green's formula applied in (10) below.

Given $v_0 \in W^{1,2}(\Omega)$, we may compute the directional derivative

$$
D_{v_0}\mathcal{E}(u_0) = \lim_{\varepsilon \to 0} \frac{\mathcal{E}(u_0 + \varepsilon v_0) - \mathcal{E}(u_0)}{\varepsilon}
$$
$$
= \lim_{\varepsilon \to 0} \frac{E(u_0 + \varepsilon v_0) - E(u_0)}{\varepsilon}
$$
$$
+ \int_0^T \int_\Omega \lambda(x,t)[\partial_u f(x,t,u(x,t))v(x,t)
$$
$$
+ \operatorname{div}(D(x,t)\nabla v(x,t)) - \partial_t v(x,t)]\, dx\, dt,
$$

where $v \in W^{1,2}(\bar{I}; W^{1,2}(\Omega))$ is the solution to the sensitivity problem (5) as we applied the differentiable dependence on initial data as stated in Theorem 1.

Let us first investigate each term of E, as defined in (9), in the difference quotient above. By Theorem 1, we have that

$$
\frac{\|u_\varepsilon(\cdot,T) - \psi(\cdot)\|_{L^2(\Omega)}^2 - \|u(\cdot,T) - \psi(\cdot)\|_{L^2(\Omega)}^2}{\varepsilon}
$$
$$
= \frac{\|u(\cdot,T) + \varepsilon v(\cdot,T) + o(\varepsilon) - \psi(\cdot)\|_{L^2(\Omega)}^2 - \|u(\cdot,T) - \psi(\cdot)\|_{L^2(\Omega)}^2}{\varepsilon}
$$

$$= 2 \int_\Omega \left(v(x,T) + \frac{o(\varepsilon)}{\varepsilon} \right) (u(x,T) - \psi(x) + O(\varepsilon)) \, dx$$

$$\to 2 \int_\Omega v(x,T)(u(x,T) - \psi(x)) \, dx \quad \text{as } \varepsilon \to 0.$$

As for the second term in E, the product rule for Sobolev functions yields that

$$\nabla((u(x,T) - \psi(x))\chi(x)) = \chi(x)\nabla(u(x,T) - \psi(x))$$
$$+ (u(x,T) - \psi(x))\nabla\chi(x).$$

For the sake of brevity, let us define the functions $U(x) = u(x,T) - \psi(x)$ and $U^\varepsilon(x) = u^\varepsilon(x,T) - \psi(x)$, $x \in \Omega$. It follows from (6) that $U^\varepsilon \to U$ and $\nabla U^\varepsilon \to \nabla U$ in $L^2(\Omega)$ as $\varepsilon \to 0$. Moreover, $(\nabla U^\varepsilon - \nabla U)/\varepsilon \rightharpoonup \nabla v(\cdot, T)$ weakly in $L^2(\Omega)$ as $\varepsilon \to 0$ by Theorem 1. Then,

$$\frac{\|\chi \nabla U^\varepsilon - U^\varepsilon \nabla \chi\|^2_{L^2(\Omega)} - \|\chi \nabla U - U\nabla\chi\|^2_{L^2(\Omega)}}{\varepsilon}$$

$$= \int_\Omega \chi(x)^2 \left(\nabla U^\varepsilon(x) + \nabla U(x) \right) \cdot \frac{\nabla U^\varepsilon(x) - \nabla U(x)}{\varepsilon} \, dx$$

$$+ \int_\Omega U^\varepsilon(x)\chi(x) \frac{\nabla U^\varepsilon(x) - \nabla U(x)}{\varepsilon} \cdot \nabla\chi(x) \, dx$$

$$+ \int_\Omega \frac{U^\varepsilon(x) - U(x)}{\varepsilon}\chi(x) \nabla U(x) \cdot \nabla\chi(x) \, dx$$

$$+ \int_\Omega \frac{U^\varepsilon(x) - U(x)}{\varepsilon}(U^\varepsilon(x) + U(x))|\nabla\chi(x)|^2 \, dx$$

$$\to 2 \int_\Omega (\chi(x)\nabla v(x,T) + v(x,T)\nabla\chi(x)) \cdot (\chi(x)\nabla U(x)$$

$$+ U(x)\nabla\chi(x)) \, dx$$

$$= 2 \int_\Omega \nabla(v(x,T)\chi(x)) \cdot \nabla((u(x,T) - \psi(x))\chi(x)) \, dx$$

$$= 2 \int_\Omega v(x,T)\chi(x) \, \Delta((u(x,T) - \psi(x))\chi(x)) \, dx. \tag{10}$$

Here, we used the fact that $\int_\Omega f_n(x)g_n(x) \, dx \to \int_\Omega f(x)g(x) \, dx$ whenever $f_n \rightharpoonup f$ and $g_n \to g$ in $L^2(\Omega)$. The very last equality was obtained by Green's formula, utilising that $\chi = 0$ on $\partial\Omega$. Observe that it is in this last step where we require the higher $W^{2,2}$-regularity of $u(\cdot, T)$ and ψ.

For the Tikhonov regularisation terms, we obtain rather immediately that

$$\frac{\|u_0 + \varepsilon v_0\|^2_{L^2(\Omega)} - \|u_0\|^2_{L^2(\Omega)}}{\varepsilon} = 2 \int_\Omega u_0(x) v_0(x) \, dx + \varepsilon \|v_0\|^2_{L^2(\Omega)}$$

$$\to 2 \int_\Omega u_0(x) v_0(x) \, dx \quad \text{as } \varepsilon \to 0,$$

and similarly

$$\frac{\|\nabla(u_0 + \varepsilon v_0)\|^2_{L^2(\Omega)} - \|\nabla u_0\|^2_{L^2(\Omega)}}{\varepsilon}$$

$$\to 2 \int_\Omega \nabla u_0(x) \cdot \nabla v_0(x) \, dx \quad \text{as } \varepsilon \to 0.$$

Let us now focus on the Lagrangian terms. Integration by parts in the time variable as stated in [43, Lemma 7.3] yields that

$$\int_0^T \lambda(\cdot, t) \, \partial_t v(\cdot, t) \, dt = \lambda(\cdot, T) v(\cdot, T) - \lambda(\cdot, 0) v(\cdot, 0)$$

$$- \int_0^T v(\cdot, t) \, \partial_t \lambda(\cdot, t) \, dt.$$

Applying Green's formula (see [43, Theorem 1.31]) twice in the spatial variable implies that

$$\int_\Omega \lambda(x, t) \, \text{div}(D(x, t) \nabla v(x, t)) \, dx$$

$$= \int_\Omega v(x, t) \, \text{div}(D(x, t)^\mathsf{T} \nabla \lambda(x, t)) \, dx$$

provided that $\lambda(\cdot, t)$ satisfies the Neumann condition

$$D(x, t)^\mathsf{T} \nabla \lambda(x, t) \cdot n(x) = 0, \quad x \in \partial\Omega.$$

Combining all of the above, we obtain that the directional derivative of $\mathcal{E}(u_0)$ can be expressed by

$$D_{v_0}\mathcal{E}(u_0) = \int_\Omega \left(m_1 v(x, T) \Big(u(x, T) - \psi(x) \Big) \right)$$

$$+ m_2(v(x,T)\chi(x)\,\Delta((u(x,T) - \psi(x))\chi(x))$$
$$+ \mu_1 u_0(x)v_0(x) + \mu_2 \nabla u_0(x) \cdot \nabla v_0(x)$$
$$- \lambda(x,T)v(x,T) + \lambda(x,0)v_0(x)\Big)dx$$
$$+ \int_0^T \int_\Omega v(x,t)(\partial_u f(x,t,u(x,t))\lambda(x,t)$$
$$+ \operatorname{div}(D(x,t)^\mathsf{T}\nabla\lambda(x,t)) + \partial_t\lambda(\cdot,t))\,dx\,dt.$$

Assuming that $\lambda \in W^{1,2}(\bar{I}, W^{1,2}(\Omega))$ is a solution to the *adjoint problem*

$$\begin{cases} \partial_t\lambda(x,t) + \operatorname{div}(D(x,t)^\mathsf{T}\nabla\lambda(x,t)) = -\partial_u f(x,t,u(x,t))\lambda(x,t), \\[2mm] (D(x,t)^\mathsf{T}\nabla\lambda(x,t)) \cdot n(x) = 0, \\[2mm] \lambda(x,T) = m_1(u(x,T) - \psi(x)) \\[2mm] \qquad\qquad + m_2\chi(x)\,\Delta\Big((u(x,T) \\[2mm] \qquad\qquad\qquad - \psi(x))\chi(x)\Big), \end{cases} \tag{11}$$

we obtain that

$$D_{v_0}\mathcal{E}(u_0) = \int_\Omega (\mu_1 u_0(x) + \lambda(x,0))v_0(x) + \mu_2\nabla u_0(x)\cdot\nabla v_0(x)\,dx. \tag{12}$$

It is clear from this expression that the mapping $v_0 \mapsto D_{v_0}\mathcal{E}(u_0)$ is a bounded linear functional on $W^{1,2}(\Omega)$. By Riesz representation theorem, there is a function $w \in W^{1,2}(\Omega)$ such that

$$D_{v_0}\mathcal{E}(u_0) = \langle w, v_0\rangle_{W^{1,2}(\Omega)} = \int_\Omega w(x)v_0(x) + \nabla w(x)\cdot\nabla v_0(x)\,dx, \tag{13}$$

i.e., $w \in W^{1,2}(\Omega)$ represents the derivative $\mathcal{E}'(u_0) \in W^{1,2}(\Omega)^*$. Note that $w = \tilde{w} + \mu_2 u_0$, where $\tilde{w} \in W^{1,2}(\Omega) \cap W^{2,2}_{\text{loc}}(\Omega)$ is a solution to the Neumann problem

$$\begin{cases} -\Delta \tilde{w}(x) + \tilde{w}(x) = (\mu_1 - \mu_2)u_0(x) + \lambda(x,0) & \text{in } \Omega, \\ \nabla \tilde{w}(x) \cdot n(x) = 0 & \text{on } \partial\Omega. \end{cases}$$

See [65, Chapter 6] for proofs of existence and regularity of solutions of this linear elliptic partial differential equation.

Remark 7. If either $\mu_2 = 0$ or $u_0 \in W_0^{2,2}(\Omega)$, then the Fréchet derivative $\mathcal{E}'(u_0) \in W^{1,2}(\Omega)^* \cong W^{1,2}(\Omega) \subset L^2(\Omega) \cong L^2(\Omega)^*$ can also be expressed using L^2-dual pairing, namely

$$D_{v_0}\mathcal{E}(u_0) = \langle \mu_1 u_0 + \lambda(\cdot,0) - \mu_2 \Delta u_0, v_0 \rangle_{L^2(\Omega)}$$

$$= \int_\Omega (\mu_1 u_0(x) + \lambda(x,0) - \mu_2 \Delta u_0(x))v_0(x)\,dx, \qquad (14)$$

which can be seen by applying Green's formula in (12).

3.3. *An iterative method with conjugate gradients*

In order to find a minimiser of the cost functional E, defined in (9), one may use an iterative gradient method. Given an initial guess $u_0^{(0)}$ of the sought data $\varphi \in W^{1,2}(\Omega)$, one computes the derivative of $\mathcal{E}'(u_0^{(0)})$ to determine a direction of the steepest descent. The initial guess is then updated to $u_0^{(1)}$ following this direction. In subsequent iterations, one uses the direction of a conjugate gradient instead to produce $u_0^{(k)}$, $k = 2, 3, \ldots$, that give better estimates of φ.

Note that it is not obvious how the initial guess $u_0^{(0)}$ is supposed to be chosen. In our numerical experiments, we have seen that $u_0^{(0)} = 0$ or $u_0^{(0)} = \psi$ do, in fact, work reasonably well.

The descent direction in the $(k+1)^{\text{st}}$ iteration is given by

$$d^{(k)} = \begin{cases} -\mathcal{E}'(u_0^{(0)}) & \text{if } k = 0, \\ -\mathcal{E}'(u_0^{(k)}) + \gamma^{(k)}d^{(k-1)} & \text{if } k > 0, \end{cases} \qquad (15)$$

where $\gamma^{(k)}$ is the *Fletcher–Reeves-type conjugate gradient coefficient* given by

$$\gamma^{(k)} = \frac{\|\mathcal{E}'(u_0^{(k)})\|^2}{\|\mathcal{E}'(u_0^{(k-1)})\|^2}, \quad k > 0, \qquad (16)$$

with the function norm being either $L^2(\Omega)$ or $W^{1,2}(\Omega)$ depending on whether the Fréchet derivative $\mathcal{E}'(u_0^{(\cdot)})$ is being represented in the L^2-dual or $W^{1,2}$-dual pairing. Note that it is possible to use other types of conjugate gradient coefficients. For reference, see [66, Section 5.2].

Having determined a descent direction $d^{(k)}$, then the initial data update can be symbolically written as $u_0^{(k+1)} = u_0^{(k)} + \beta^{(k)}d^{(k)}$, where $\beta^{(k)}$ is a step size found by, for example, optimising the function $s(\beta) = E(u_0^{(k)} + \beta d^{(k)})$, $\beta > 0$. Let $v(x,t)$ be a solution to the sensitivity problem (5) with initial data $v(x,0) = d^{(k)}(x)$. We apply the linearisation $u^{(k+1)}(x,t) \approx u^{(k)}(x,t) + \beta^{(k+1)}v(x,t)$, $t \in \bar{I}$, which is a good approximation for small values of β in the norm of $L^2(\Omega)$ and weakly in $W^{1,2}(\Omega)$ by Theorem 1. The derivative

$$s'(\beta) = \lim_{\varepsilon \to 0} \frac{E(u_0^{(k)} + (\beta + \varepsilon)d^{(k)}) - E(u_0^{(k)} + \beta d^{(k)})}{\varepsilon}$$

can be computed similarly as in Subsection 3.2. Then,

$$
\begin{aligned}
s'(\beta) \approx \int_\Omega &(m_1 v(x,T)(u^{(k)}(x,T) + \beta v(x,T) - \psi(x)) \\
&+ m_2 \nabla(v(x,T)\chi(x)) \cdot \nabla((u^{(k)}(x,T) + \beta v(x,T) - \psi(x))\chi(x)) \\
&+ \mu_1(u_0^{(k)}(x) + \beta d^{(k)}(x))d^{(k)}(x) \\
&+ \mu_2 \nabla(u_0^{(k)}(x) + \beta d^{(k)}(x)) \cdot \nabla d^{(k)}(x))\, dx.
\end{aligned}
\tag{17}
$$

This is a linear expression in β making $s'(\beta) = 0$ easy to solve for $\beta^{(k)}$.

For convergence of NCG methods, see [67,68] and [69, Section 4.1].

The steps for reconstruction of the initial data φ from the final state ψ using the NCG method are summarised in Algorithm 1 on p. 273.

4. Nonlinear Landweber Iterations

In [32], a different method is considered, the so-called nonlinear Landweber method, for the reconstruction of the initial data φ from a given final state $u(x,T) = \psi(x)$. For an overview of the nonlinear Landweber method, we refer to [70, Section 11.1] in the case of Hilbert spaces and to [61, Chapter 7] in the case of Banach spaces. Even though the way to derive the nonlinear Landweber iterations differs significantly from the NCG method described in Section 3, there are striking connections in the actual iterations.

Let us consider the nonlinear operator F that maps $u_0 \in W^{1,2}(\Omega)$ to $u(\cdot, T) \in L^2(\Omega)$, where u is the solution to (1). It has been shown in Corollary 3 that F is Lipschitz continuous and has a Fréchet derivative $F'(u_0) = \mathcal{A} : W^{1,2}(\Omega) \to L^2(\Omega)^* \cong L^2(\Omega)$, which maps $v_0 \mapsto v(\cdot, T)$, where v is a solution to the sensitivity problem (5).

We aim to find a solution $\varphi \in W^{1,2}(\Omega)$ to the equation

$$F(\varphi) = \psi. \tag{18}$$

An initial guess $u_0^{(0)}$ of the solution φ is updated by *Landweber iterations*

$$u_0^{(k+1)} = u_0^{(k)} - \mathcal{A}^*(F(u_0^{(k)}) - \psi), \quad k = 0, 1, 2, \ldots, \tag{19}$$

where $\mathcal{A}^* : L^2(\Omega)^{**} \to W^{1,2}(\Omega)^*$ is the *adjoint operator* of $\mathcal{A}$, i.e., it satisfies $\langle \mathcal{A}v_0, \lambda_T \rangle_{L^2(\Omega)} = \langle v_0, \mathcal{A}^*\lambda_T \rangle_{W^{1,2}(\Omega)}$ for every $\lambda_T \in L^2(\Omega)$. Assuming that $v(\cdot, t)$ is a solution to the sensitivity problem (5) with the initial data v_0 and that $\lambda(\cdot, t)$ is a solution to the adjoint problem (11) with the final data λ_T, we obtain that

$$\langle \mathcal{A}v_0, \lambda_T \rangle_{L^2(\Omega)} = \int_\Omega v(x, T)\lambda(x, T) - v(x, 0)\lambda(x, 0)$$

$$+ v(x, 0)\lambda(x, 0)\, dx$$

$$= \int_0^T \int_\Omega \lambda(x, t)\partial_t v(x, t) + v(x, t)\partial_t \lambda(x, t)\, dx\, dt$$

$$+ \langle v_0, \lambda(\cdot, 0) \rangle_{L^2(\Omega)}$$

$$= \int_0^T \int_\Omega \lambda(x, t)(\mathrm{div}(D(x, t)\nabla v(x, t))$$

$$+ \partial_u f(x, t, u(x, t))v(x, t))$$

$$- v(x, t)(\mathrm{div}(D(x, t)^{\mathsf{T}}\nabla \lambda(x, t))$$

Algorithm 1. Nonlinear conjugate gradient method

Input: Final data $\psi \in W^{1,2}(\Omega)$ and initial guess $u_0^{(0)} \in W^{1,2}(\Omega)$.
Coefficients $m_1, m_2, \mu_1, \mu_2 \geq 0$ and a cut-off function $\chi \in W_0^{2,2}(\Omega)$ in the cost functional (9), where $\max\{m_1, m_2\} > 0$.
Maximal number of iterations K, a stopping condition threshold $\kappa > 0$.

Output: Reconstructed initial data $\varphi \in W^{1,2}(\Omega)$

1: **for** $k = 0$ **to** K **do**
2:     Solve the direct problem (1) with initial data $u_0^{(k)}$
3:     **if** $\|u^{(k)}(\cdot, T) - \psi(\cdot)\|_{L^2(\Omega)} < \kappa$ **or** $k = K$ **then**
4:         **return** $u_0^{(k)}$
5:     Solve the adjoint problem (11) with $u = u^{(k)}$
6:     Find the steepest descent direction as in (13) or (14)
7:     Compute the conjugate gradient coefficient (16)
        {only if $k > 0$}
8:     Find the descent direction $d^{(k)}$ as in (15)
9:     Solve the sensitivity problem (5) with $u = u^{(k)}$ and initial
        data $d^{(k)}$
10:    Find the step length $\beta^{(k)}$ by solving $s'(\beta) = 0$ in (17)
11:    $u_0^{(k+1)} \leftarrow u_0^{(k)} + \beta^{(k)} d^{(k)}$

$$+ \partial_u f(x, t, u(x,t)) \lambda(x,t)) \, dx \, dt + \langle v_0, \lambda(\cdot, 0)\rangle_{L^2(\Omega)}$$

$$= \int_0^T \int_\Omega 0 \, dx \, dt$$

$$+ \langle v_0, \lambda(\cdot, 0)\rangle_{L^2(\Omega)}.$$

We see that $\mathcal{A}^*$ is the operator that solves (11) backwards in time for a given final data and outputs the corresponding initial data to represent an element of $W^{1,2}(\Omega)^*$ in terms of L^2-dual pairing.

Revisiting (19), we see that the nonlinear Landweber iterations correspond to a simplification of the gradient method described in Algorithm 1. Namely, let $m_1 = 1$ and $m_2 = \mu_1 = \mu_2 = 0$, and skip steps 7, 9, and 10 by setting $\gamma^{(k)} = 0$ and $\beta^{(k)} = 1$ for all $k \geq 0$.

Remark 8. The (nonlinear) Landweber iteration method requires that the operator norm $\|\mathcal{A}\|$ lies under a certain threshold in order to guarantee convergence of the iterations. In our setting, it is not feasible to compute $\|\mathcal{A}\|$ (and available estimates are too rough) to verify whether this condition is satisfied.

Note also that possible convergence issues may be mitigated by pre-multiplying the equation (18) by a constant factor $\sqrt{\beta} > 0$, which yields $\sqrt{\beta}F(\varphi) = \sqrt{\beta}\psi$. This equation leads to Landweber iterations of the form

$$u_0^{(k+1)} = u_0^{(k)} - \beta\mathcal{A}^*(F(u_0^{(k)}) - \psi), \quad k = 0, 1, 2, \ldots.$$

In other words, it is possible to incorporate a step-length $\beta > 0$ into the iterative process.

5. Numerical Experiments

In this section, we discuss an implementation of the nonlinear conjugate gradient method (NCG, Algoritm 1) and the Landweber iterations (19) for the minimisation of the cost functional (9). In our numerical experiments, we work with magnetic resonance tomography images from the BraTS'20 dataset [71–73]. We planted a tumour seed φ in the white matter of the healthy part of the brain. This seed is then grown according to the reaction–diffusion model (1) to obtain the final state ψ. Given this state, we try to reconstruct φ by minimising (9) using the NCG and Landweber methods.

Note that the images in the BraTS'20 dataset already contain tumours, however, we work with artificially seeded ones to be able to measure the performance of the proposed algorithms.

5.1. *Data obtained from magnetic resonance imaging*

We used T1-weighted MR images and segmented them into white and grey matter using the *SPM12* software package (the interested reader is referred to [74]). As an alternative, one can use the FMRIB's Automated Segmentation Tool (FAST, [75]) from the FMRIB Software Library v6.0 (FSL, [76]).

The voxel data of a T1-weighted MR image consist of scalar values (greyscale) on a 3D-grid. In the case of BraTS'20, the MR images have dimensions $240 \times 240 \times 155$ voxels, where each voxel corresponds to a cube with the side length of 1 mm.

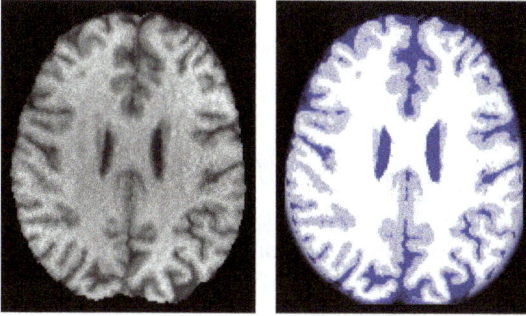

Fig. 1. An axial section of a brain (subject 79 in the BraTS'20 dataset): T1-weighted MR image to the left; its segmentation (white = WM, grey = GM, blue = CSF) done by SPM12 to the right.

The automatic segmentation gives an estimate of the proportion of grey matter (GM), white matter (WM), and cerebrospinal fluid (CSF) in a voxel, see Fig. 1. A voxel is classified as GM or WM if the respective proportion exceeds a 50 % threshold, in which case it is included in the brain region Ω. Note also that this classification determines the value of the diffusion coefficient in (2). In fact, one may also consider defining the element $D(x,t)$ as a convex combination of d_g and d_w, since each voxel has been assigned a proportion of GM and WM during the segmentation.

5.2. *Discretisation and numerical scheme*

The domain Ω and the diffusion coefficient $D(x,t)$ are both given in terms of voxels; it is thus natural to use the finite difference method to numerically solve the partial differential equations used in the earlier NCG and Landweber methods. To that end, given spacing factors $h_x, h_y, h_z > 0$ in each direction, we define a uniform three-dimensional grid as

$$\mathbb{G}^3 = \{(ih_x, jh_y, kh_z) \in \mathbb{R}^3 : (i, j, k) \in \mathbb{Z}^3\}.$$

For the sake of convenience, elements of the grid $\mathbb{G}^3$ will be referred to by their indices $(i, j, k) \in \mathbb{Z}^3$.

The spacing factors give rise to the volume element $\delta V = h_x h_y h_z$ that corresponds to the volume of a rectangular cuboid with side lengths h_x, h_y, and h_z. Given a bounded (and hence finite) set $\Omega \subset \mathbb{G}^3$, we define the discrete counterparts of Lebesgue spaces with

$p \in [1, \infty)$ by

$$\|f\|^p_{\ell^p(\Omega)} = \sum_{(i,j,k)\in\Omega} |f(i,j,k)|^p \, \delta V, \quad \text{and}$$

$$\|f\|_{\ell^\infty(\Omega)} = \max_{(i,j,k)\in\Omega} |f(i,j,k)|.$$

In order to define Sobolev-type spaces, we need to extract points in Ω that remain inside Ω when shifted by one step. Thus, we define the sets

$$\Omega^+_x = \Omega \cap \{(i,j,k) \in \mathbb{G}^3 : (i+1,j,k) \in \Omega\} \quad \text{and}$$

$$\Omega^-_x = \Omega \cap \{(i,j,k) \in \mathbb{G}^3 : (i-1,j,k) \in \Omega\},$$

and analogously Ω^+_y, Ω^-_y, Ω^+_z, and Ω^-_z when shifting along the y- or z-direction. Then, we define the forward and backward difference quotients

$$\partial^+_x f(i,j,k) = \frac{f(i+1,j,k) - f(i,j,k)}{h_x}, \quad (i,j,k) \in \Omega^+_x,$$

$$\partial^-_x f(i,j,k) = \frac{f(i,j,k) - f(i-1,j,k)}{h_x}, \quad (i,j,k) \in \Omega^-_x,$$

with analogues for the other two directions. The discrete Sobolev norm is

$$\|f\|^2_{w^{1,2}(\Omega)} = \|f\|^2_{\ell^2(\Omega)} + \|\partial^+_x f\|^2_{\ell^2(\Omega^+_x)} + \|\partial^+_y f\|^2_{\ell^2(\Omega^+_y)} + \|\partial^+_z f\|^2_{\ell^2(\Omega^+_z)}$$

$$= \|f\|^2_{\ell^2(\Omega)} + \|\partial^-_x f\|^2_{\ell^2(\Omega^-_x)} + \|\partial^-_y f\|^2_{\ell^2(\Omega^-_y)} + \|\partial^-_z f\|^2_{\ell^2(\Omega^-_z)}.$$

Since all normed linear spaces of a given finite dimension are equivalent, the sets of functions $\ell^p(\Omega)$, $p \in [1, \infty]$ and $w^{1,2}(\Omega)$ are equal and their norms are equivalent as long as $\Omega \subset \mathbb{G}^3$ is bounded. It is also worth noting that $\ell^2(\Omega)$ and hence also $w^{1,2}(\Omega)$ are endowed by an inner product

$$\langle f, g \rangle_{\ell^2(\Omega)} = \sum_{(i,j,k)\in\Omega} f(i,j,k) g(i,j,k) \, \delta V.$$

This allows us to formulate a discrete version of Green's formula.

Lemma 9. *Let $\Omega \subset \mathbb{G}^3$ be a non-empty bounded set and let $f, g \in \ell^2(\Omega)$. Then,*

$$\langle \partial_x^+ f, \partial_x^+ g \rangle_{\ell^2(\Omega_x^+)} = \left(\langle \partial_x^- f, g \rangle_{\ell^2(\partial_x^- \Omega)} - \langle \partial_x^+ f, g \rangle_{\ell^2(\partial_x^+ \Omega)} \right) \frac{1}{h_x}$$

$$- \langle \Delta_x f, g \rangle_{\ell^2(\Omega_x^\pm)}$$

$$\langle \partial_x^- f, \partial_x^- g \rangle_{\ell^2(\Omega_x^-)} = \langle \partial_x^+ f, \partial_x^+ g \rangle_{\ell^2(\Omega_x^+)},$$

where $\Delta_x f = \partial_x^+(\partial_x^- f) = \partial_x^-(\partial_x^+ f)$ and

$$\partial_x^- \Omega = \Omega_x^- \setminus \Omega_x^+, \quad \partial_x^+ \Omega = \Omega_x^+ \setminus \Omega_x^-, \quad \Omega_x^\pm = \Omega_x^+ \cap \Omega_x^-,$$

with immediate analogues for the y- and z-directions.

Proof. The identities are immediate results of reordering terms in the sums that define the respective inner products. $\qquad\square$

5.2.1. *Discretisation of the divergence term in* (1), (5), *and* (11)

Similarly as in [32, 60], we consider only a diagonal diffusion coefficient matrix D and discretise the differential operators in the reaction–diffusion model (1), the sensitivity problem (5), and the adjoint problem (11) by a finite difference method with an alternating scheme, i.e.,

$$\mathrm{div}(D\nabla u) \approx \frac{1}{2}((\partial_x^+(D_{11}\partial_x^- u) + \partial_x^-(D_{11}\partial_x^+ u))$$

$$+ (\partial_y^+(D_{22}\partial_y^- u) + \partial_y^-(D_{22}\partial_y^+ u))$$

$$+ (\partial_z^+(D_{33}\partial_z^- u) + \partial_z^-(D_{33}\partial_z^+ u))). \qquad (20)$$

This definition is however only valid in the "interior" $\Omega_x^\pm \cap \Omega_y^\pm \cap \Omega_z^\pm$, since at least one of the difference quotients is undefined outside this set. On the other hand, when we take into account the Neumann boundary condition $D\nabla u \cdot n = 0$, we may extend the definition of difference quotients by zero whenever undefined in Ω, e.g., $\partial_x^+ u(i, j, k) = 0$ in case $(i, j, k) \in \Omega \setminus \Omega_x^+$.

5.2.2. *Forward Euler scheme and discretisation of the time variable*

In order to solve the parabolic PDEs (1), (5), and (11), we adopt an explicit forward Euler scheme with discretised time variable. The time interval $[0, T]$ is divided into sub-intervals each of length $\tau \ll 1$. Then,

$$\partial_t u(x, t) \approx \frac{u(x, t + \tau) - u(x, t)}{\tau}, \quad \text{hence}$$

$$u(x, t + \tau) \approx u(x, t) + \tau \partial_t u(x, t),$$

where $\partial_t u(x, t)$ is defined by (1), having used the spatial discretisation given in (20). The sensitivity and adjoint problems (5) and (11) are solved analogously, though backwards in time for the adjoint problem, i.e., $\lambda(x, t - \tau) \approx \lambda(x, t) - \tau \partial_t \lambda(x, t)$.

5.2.3. *Discrete version of the cost functional (9)*

Due to the spatial discretisation, a cut-off function χ is no longer needed in (9) since the discrete Green formula of Lemma 9 has a boundary term whose measure is not singular but rather coincides with δV. Thus, we may use

$$E(u_0) = \frac{m_1 - m_2}{2} \|u(\cdot, T) - \psi(\cdot)\|^2_{\ell^2(\Omega)} + \frac{m_2}{2} \|u(\cdot, T) - \psi(\cdot)\|^2_{w^{1,2}(\Omega)}$$

$$+ \frac{\mu_1 - \mu_2}{2} \|u_0\|^2_{\ell^2(\Omega)} + \frac{\mu_2}{2} \|u_0\|^2_{w^{1,2}(\Omega)},$$

and modify the final value condition of the adjoint problem (11) accordingly to take into account the boundary terms that appear in the discrete counterpart of (10).

5.2.4. *Directional derivative (12) with respect to ℓ^2 and $w^{1,2}$-dual pairing*

Given $u_0, v_0 \in \ell^2(\Omega)$, we find the directional derivative of the unconstrained cost functional $D_{v_0}\mathcal{E}(u_0)$ similarly as in the continuous case and obtain

$$D_{v_0}\mathcal{E}(u_0) = \langle(\mu_1 - \mu_2)u_0 + \lambda(\cdot, 0), v_0\rangle_{\ell^2(\Omega)} + \mu_2\langle u_0, v_0\rangle_{w^{1,2}(\Omega)}. \quad (21)$$

The terms in the $w^{1,2}$-inner product can be rewritten using the Green formula stated in Lemma 9, e.g.,

$$\langle \partial_x^+ u_0, \partial_x^+ v_0\rangle_{\ell^2(\Omega_x^+)} = \left(\langle \partial_x^- u_0, v_0\rangle_{\ell^2(\partial_x^- \Omega)} - \langle \partial_x^+ u_0, v_0\rangle_{\ell^2(\partial_x^+ \Omega)}\right)\frac{1}{h_x}$$
$$- \langle \Delta_x u_0, v_0\rangle_{\ell^2(\Omega_x^\pm)},$$

with analogues in the y- and z-directions. Thereby, we can find a function $g \in \ell^2(\Omega)$ that represents the directional derivative (21) in the ℓ^2-dual pairing so that $D_{v_0}\mathcal{E}(u_0) = \langle g, v_0\rangle_{\ell^2(\Omega)}$. Thus, $\mathcal{E}'(u_0) = g$ is the Fréchet derivative in $\ell^2(\Omega)^*$.

Similarly, there is a function $G \in w^{1,2}(\Omega)$ such that

$$\langle G, v_0\rangle_{w^{1,2}(\Omega)} = \langle(\mu_1 - \mu_2)u_0 + \lambda(\cdot, 0), v_0\rangle_{\ell^2(\Omega)}.$$

It follows from Lemma 9 that G is a solution to the equation

$$G + \left(1_{\partial_x^- \Omega}\partial_x^- G - 1_{\partial_x^+ \Omega}\partial_x^+ G\right)\frac{1}{h_x} - 1_{\Omega_x^\pm}\Delta_x G$$

$$+ \left(1_{\partial_y^- \Omega}\partial_y^- G - 1_{\partial_y^+ \Omega}\partial_y^+ G\right)\frac{1}{h_y} - 1_{\Omega_y^\pm}\Delta_y G$$

$$+ \left(1_{\partial_z^- \Omega}\partial_z^- G - 1_{\partial_z^+ \Omega}\partial_z^+ G\right)\frac{1}{h_z} - 1_{\Omega_z^\pm}\Delta_z G = (\mu_1 - \mu_2)u_0 + \lambda(\cdot, 0),$$

where 1 denotes the indicator function. This equation can be rewritten in operator form as $(I + Q)G = (\mu_1 - \mu_2)u_0 + \lambda(\cdot, 0)$, where I denotes the identity operator and Q is a linear operator on $\ell^2(\Omega)$ that consists of all the difference quotients of first and second orders in the earlier equation.

It is fairly straightforward to see that the mapping Q can be expressed by a diagonally dominant matrix. In fact, $Q_{mm} = \sum_{m\neq n}|Q_{nm}| = \sum_{m\neq n}|Q_{mn}|$, where all the off-diagonal elements are non-positive. Hence, all eigenvalues of the operator Q have non-negative real part by the Geršgorin circle theorem [77]. In particular, the operator $(I + Q)$ is invertible. Moreover, $(I + Q)$ is strictly diagonally dominant and the solution to the equation

Table 1. Parameters in the reaction–diffusion model in the presented experiments.

Subject	T	d_g	d_w	ρ	$f(x,t,u)$
79	4	0.5	0.1	0.06	$\rho u(1-u^2)$
341	3	0.5	0.1	0.04	$\rho u(1-u)$

$(I+Q)G = (\mu_1 - \mu_2)u_0 + \lambda(\cdot,0)$ can be found (or at least approximated) using the Jacobi iteration method.

Finally, it holds that $D_{v_0}\mathcal{E}(u_0) = \langle G + \mu_2 u_0, v_0 \rangle_{w^{1,2}(\Omega)}$ and hence $\mathcal{E}'(u_0) = G + \mu_2 u_0$ is the Fréchet derivative in $w^{1,2}(\Omega)^*$.

We close this section pointing out that for convergence of finite difference approximations to nonlinear PDEs via discrete Sobolev spaces, see [78, Chapters 35.4–35.6].

5.3. Parameters and setup of the experiments

We have used MR images of the brains of the subjects 79 and 341 of the BraTS'20 dataset, with different time intervals $[0, T]$ and proliferation functions $f(x,t,u)$ in the reaction–diffusion model (1) to grow a synthetic tumour and then reconstruct its seed, see Table 1.

The initial state φ of the seed is defined as a pointwise maximum of two or three Gaussians with different values of standard deviation and peaks close to each other. Hence, φ lacked symmetry. The final state ψ is obtained by solving (1) using the explicit forward Euler method in time and alternating scheme for the divergence term, see Section 5.2.

In order to avoid the inverse crime when reconstructing φ from ψ, we resampled the brain image and hence also D, φ, and ψ so that voxels were no longer cubes but rather rectangular cuboids with side lengths $1.04 \leq h_x, h_y, h_z \leq 1.15$. Moreover, the time step was also chosen differently in the inverse problem.

The performance of the reconstruction of u_0 of the tumour seed φ are measured by the following quantities:

- relative distance from u_0 to φ and from $u(\cdot, T)$ to ψ, i.e.,

$$d_0 = \frac{\|u_0 - \varphi\|}{\|\varphi\|} \quad \text{and} \quad d_T = \frac{\|u(\cdot, T) - \psi\|}{\|\psi\|},$$

where the norms are either of $\ell^1(\Omega)$, $\ell^2(\Omega)$, $\ell^\infty(\Omega)$, and $w^{1,2}(\Omega)$,

- Euclidean distance between the centroids of u_0 and φ, and of $u(\cdot, T)$ and ψ, where the coordinates (E_x, E_y, E_z) of the centroid of a non-negative function $u \in \ell^2(\Omega)$ are given by

$$E_x = \frac{\sum_\Omega i\, u(i, j, k)}{\sum_\Omega u(i, j, k)} \quad \text{and analogously for } E_y \text{ and } E_z,$$

- distance between the dispersion matrices of u_0 and φ, and of $u(\cdot, T)$ and ψ, where the dispersion (covariance) matrix C of a non-negative function $u \in \ell^2(\Omega)$ is given by

$$C = \begin{pmatrix} c_{xx} & c_{xy} & c_{xz} \\ c_{yx} & c_{yy} & c_{yz} \\ c_{zx} & c_{zy} & c_{zz} \end{pmatrix},$$

$$\text{where} \quad c_{xy} = c_{yx} = \frac{\sum_\Omega (i - E_x)(j - E_y)\, u(i, j, k)}{\sum_\Omega u(i, j, k)}$$

and analogously for the other elements of C.

Note that the volume elements δV in the sums defining the centroids E_* and the dispersion matrix C have cancelled out each other.

5.4. *Results of the numerical experiments*

The graphs in Fig. 2 show that the Landweber method reconstructs the initial data in the sense of the ℓ^2-distance equally well as the NCG method with $m_1 = 1$ and $m_2 = 0$. Surprisingly enough, the best performance appears to be achieved by the NCG method with $m_2 = 1$ but $m_1 = 0$. It turns out that such a conclusion is heavily misleading since the ℓ^2 and $w^{1,2}$-distances at $t = 0$ are the only metrics, where NCG with this particular combination of coefficients appears to succeed.

When we however compare the positions of the centroids and the dispersion matrices, Figs. 3 and 4, cf. Table 2, we immediately see that the NCG with $m_1 = 0$ and $m_2 = 1$ yields an extremely poor approximation of the initial data. On the other hand, the Landweber and NCG-methods with $m_1 = 1$ perform more or less equally well.

The values of the regularising parameters μ_1 and μ_2 have only a minute effect on the performance, provided that they are small

ℓ^2-error at $t = 0$

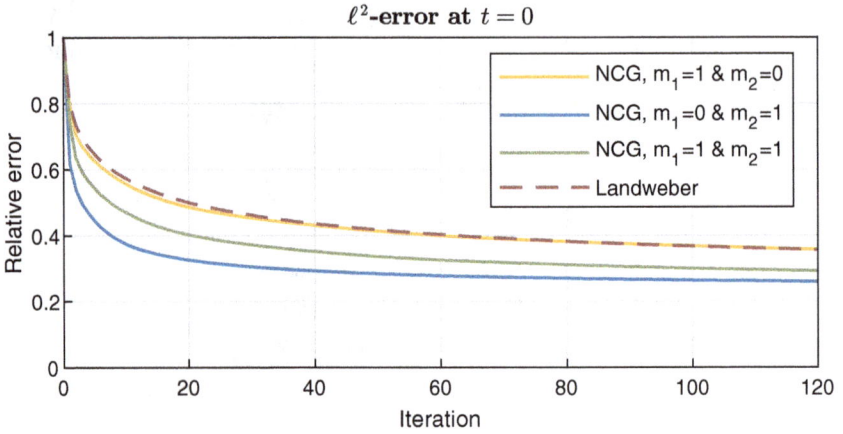

Fig. 2. Subject 79: Comparison of the relative ℓ^2-distance d_0 between φ and its reconstruction $u_0^{(k)}$, where k denotes the number of iterations completed in the respective method.

Distance between centroids of $u_0^{(k)}$ and φ

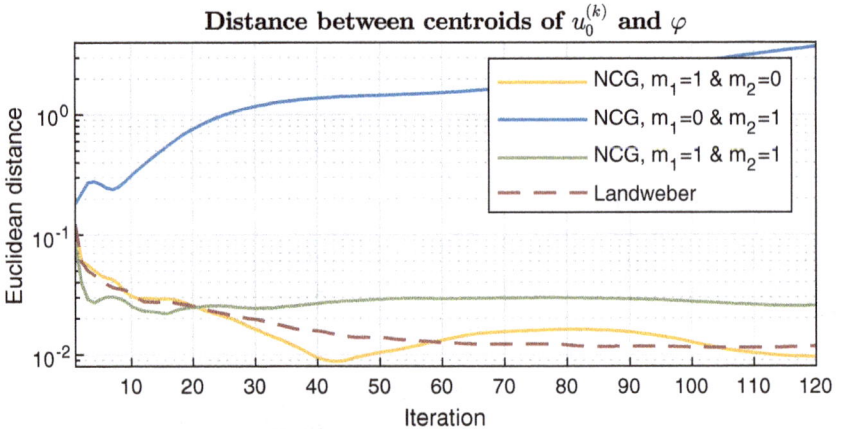

Fig. 3. Subject 79: Comparison of the Euclidean distance between the centroids of φ and $u_0^{(k)}$ for different optimisation methods.

enough. Given the data in our experiments, the reconstruction efforts fail if one chooses $\mu_1 = 1$ and/or $\mu_2 = 1$. However, values of μ_1 and μ_2 of magnitude at most 10^{-5} do not pose any obstacle for the optimisation.

The results presented in Figs. 2–4 as well as in Table 2 used the constant initial guess $u_0^{(0)} = 0$. In all our numerical experiments, we

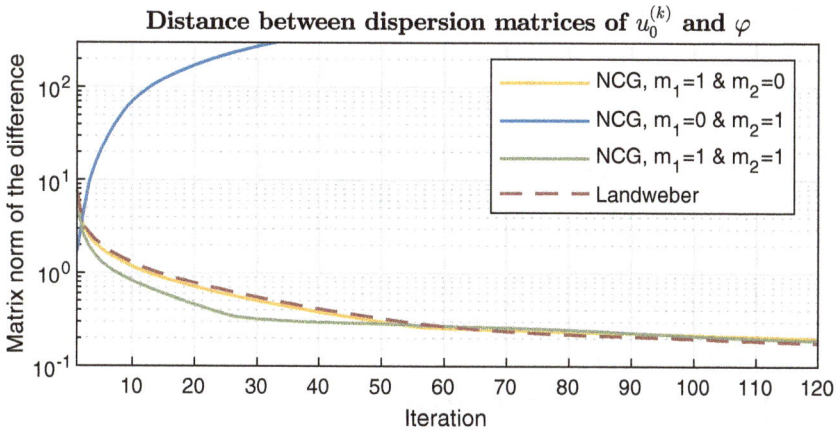

Fig. 4. Subject 79: Comparison of the norm of the difference of the dispersion matrices for φ and $u_0^{(k)}$ for different optimisation methods

Table 2. Subject 341: Results of the reconstruction of φ after 120 iterations.

Method	m_1	m_2	Rel. $w^{1,2}$-error at $t=0$	Rel. ℓ^1-error at $t=0$	Centroid distance	Dispersion difference
NCG	1	0	0.403	0.298	0.020	0.078
NCG	0	1	0.298	1.471	3.389	474.6
NCG	1	1	0.343	0.261	0.014	0.077
Landweber	–	–	0.419	0.308	0.016	0.107

have observed that the initial guess $u_0^{(0)} = \psi$ performs equally well (better in some metrics, worse in others, the differences are rather small and vary, though). The method was terminated after a fixed number of iterations (120), and well before any magnification of the resampling errors started to appear.

Generally speaking, the Landweber method is approximately 30 % faster than the nonlinear conjugate gradient (NCG) method. This is not unexpected since the sensitivity problem (5) is skipped in the Landweber iterations, while both the direct problem (1) and the adjoint problem (11) need to be solved in each iteration in both the Landweber and NCG methods.

References

[1] P. Tracqui, G. C. Cruywagen, D. E. Woodward, G. T. Bartoo, J. D. Murray, and E. C. Alvord Jr., A mathematical model of glioma growth: The effect of chemotherapy on spatio-temporal growth, *Cell Proliferation.* **28**(1), 17–31 (1995).

[2] D. E. Woodward, J. Cook, P. Tracqui, G. C. Cruywagen, J. D. Murray, and E. C. Alvord Jr., A mathematical model of glioma growth: The effect of extent of surgical resection, *Cell Proliferation.* **29**(6), 269–288 (1996).

[3] K. R. Swanson, E. C. Alvord Jr., and J. D. Murray, A quantitative model for differential motility of gliomas in grey and white matter, *Cell Proliferation.* **33**(5), 317–329 (2000).

[4] K. R. Swanson, E. C. Alvord Jr., and J. D. Murray, Quantifying efficacy of chemotherapy of brain tumors with homogeneous and heterogeneous drug delivery, *Acta Biotheoretica.* **50**(4), 223–237 (2002).

[5] O. Clatz, M. Sermesant, P.-Y. Bondiau, H. Delingette, S. K. Warfield, G. Malandain, *et al.*, Realistic simulation of the 3-D growth of brain tumors in MR images coupling diffusion with biomechanical deformation, *IEEE Transactions on Medical Imaging.* **24**(10), 1334–1346 (2005).

[6] S. Jbabdi, E. Mandonnet, H. Duffau, L. Capelle, K. R. Swanson, M. Pélégrini-Issac, *et al.*, Simulation of anisotropic growth of low-grade gliomas using diffusion tensor imaging, *Magnetic Resonance in Medicine.* **54**(3), 616–624 (2005).

[7] C. Hogea, C. Davatzikos, and G. Biros, Modeling glioma growth and mass effect in 3D MR images of the brain. In N. Ayache, S. Ourselin, and A. Maeder (eds.), *Medical Image Computing and Computer-Assisted Intervention–MICCAI 2007: 10th International Conference,* Brisbane, Australia, October/November, 2007, Proceedings, Part I (Springer, 2007), pp. 642–650.

[8] K. R. Swanson, R. C. Rostomily, and E. C. Alvord Jr., A mathematical modelling tool for predicting survival of individual patients following resection of glioblastoma: A proof of principle, *British Journal of Cancer.* **98**(1), 113–119 (2008).

[9] P. Macklin, S. McDougall, A. R. A. Anderson, M. A. J. Chaplain, V. Cristini, and J. Lowengrub, Multiscale modelling and nonlinear simulation of vascular tumour growth, *Journal of Mathematical Biology.* **58**, 765–798 (2009).

[10] E. Konukoglu, O. Clatz, B. H. Menze, B. Stieltjes, M.-A. Weber, E. Mandonnet, *et al.*, Image guided personalization of reaction-diffusion type tumor growth models using modified anisotropic

Eikonal equations, *IEEE Transactions on Medical Imaging.* **29**(1), 77–95 (2010).

[11]   E. Konukoglu, O. Clatz, P.-Y. Bondiau, H. Delingette, and N. Ayache, Extrapolating glioma invasion margin in brain magnetic resonance images: Suggesting new irradiation margins, *Medical Image Analysis.* **14**(2), 111–125 (2010).

[12]   R. Rockne, J. K. Rockhill, M. Mrugala, A. M. Spence, I. Kalet, K. Hendrickson, *et al.*, Predicting the efficacy of radiotherapy in individual glioblastoma patients in vivo: A mathematical modeling approach, *Physics in Medicine & Biology.* **55**(12), 3271 (2010).

[13]   S. Gu, G. Chakraborty, K. Champley, A. M. Alessio, J. Claridge, R. Rockne, *et al.*, Applying a patient-specific bio-mathematical model of glioma growth to develop virtual [18f]-FMISO-PET images, *Mathematical Medicine and Biology: A Journal of the IMA.* **29**(1), 31–48 (2012).

[14]   J. Unkelbach, B. H. Menze, E. Konukoglu, F. Dittmann, M. Le, N. Ayache, and H. A. Shih, Radiotherapy planning for glioblastoma based on a tumor growth model: Improving target volume delineation, *Physics in Medicine & Biology.* **59**(3), 747–770 (2014).

[15]   L. Peng, D. Trucu, P. Lin, A. Thompson, and M. A. J. Chaplain, A multiscale mathematical model of tumour invasive growth, *Bulletin of Mathematical Biology.* **79**, 389–429 (2017).

[16]   M. Conti, S. Gatti, and A. Miranville, Mathematical analysis of a model for proliferative-to-invasive transition of hypoxic glioma cells, *Nonlinear Analysis.* **189**, 111572 (2019).

[17]   S. Subramanian, K. Scheufele, M. Mehl, and G. Biros, Where did the tumor start? An inverse solver with sparse localization for tumor growth models, *Inverse Problems.* **36**(4), 045006 (2020).

[18]   D. A. Hormuth, K. A. Al Feghali, A. M. Elliott, T. E. Yankeelov, and C. Chung, Image-based personalization of computational models for predicting response of high-grade glioma to chemoradiation, *Scientific Reports.* **11**(1), 8520 (2021).

[19]   S. Suveges, K. Hossain-Ibrahim, J. D. Steele, R. Eftimie, and D. Trucu, Mathematical modelling of glioblastomas invasion within the brain: A 3D multi-scale moving-boundary approach, *Mathematics.* **9**(18), 2214 (2021).

[20]   A. Agosti, A. G. Lucifero, and S. Luzzi, An image-informed Cahn-Hilliard Keller-Segel multiphase field model for tumor growth with angiogenesis (2022). *Preprint* arXiv:2203.02212.

[21]   J. L. López-Agredo, D. A. Rueda-Gómez, and É. J. Villamizar-Roa, Numerical analysis of a mathematical model describing the evolution of hypoxic glioma cells, *Computers & Mathematics with Applications.* **131**, 138–157 (2023).

[22] J. C. L. Alfonso, K. Talkenberger, M. Seifert, B. Klink, A. Hawkins-Daarud, K. R. Swanson, *et al.*, The biology and mathematical modelling of glioma invasion: A review, *Journal of the Royal Society Interface.* **14**(136), 20170490 (2017).

[23] C. Martens, A. Rovai, D. Bonatto, T. Metens, O. Debeir, C. Decaestecker, *et al.*, Deep learning for reaction-diffusion glioma growth modeling: Towards a fully personalized model? *Cancers.* **14**(10), 2530 (2022).

[24] C. Martens, L. Lebrun, C. Decaestecker, T. Vandamme, Y.-R. Van Eycke, A. Rovai, *et al.*, Initial condition assessment for reaction-diffusion glioma growth models: A translational MRI-histology (in)validation study, *Tomography.* **7**(4), 650–674 (2021).

[25] V. Isakov, *Inverse Problems for Partial Differential Equations*, 3rd edn. (Springer, Cham, 2017).

[26] W. H. L. Pinaya, P.-D. Tudosiu, J. Dafflon, P. F. Da Costa, V. Fernandez, P. Nachev, *et al.*, Brain imaging generation with latent diffusion models. In A. Mukhopadhyay, I. Oksuz, S. Engelhardt, D. Zhu, and Y. Yuan (eds.), *Deep Generative Models: Second MICCAI Workshop, DGM4MICCAI 2022, Held in Conjunction with MICCAI 2022, Singapore, September 22, 2022, Proceedings* (Springer, Cham, 2022), pp. 117–126.

[27] G. Baravdish, B. T. Johansson, O. Svensson, and W. Ssebunjo, Identifying a response parameter in a model of brain tumour evolution under therapy, *IMA Journal of Applied Mathematics* **88**(2), 378–404 (2023).

[28] M. Alwuthaynani, R. Eftimie, and D. Trucu, Reconstruction of mutation laws in heterogeneous tumours with local and nonlocal dynamics (2021). *Preprint* arXiv:2110.13310.

[29] M. Alwuthaynani and D. Trucu, Inverse reconstruction of cell proliferation laws in cancer invasion modelling, *Mathematics in Applied Sciences and Engineering.* **2**(3), 172–193 (2021).

[30] M. Efendiev, *Evolution Equations Arising in the Modelling of Life Sciences*, Vol. 163 (Birkhäuser/Springer Basel AG, Basel, 2013).

[31] G. Nadin and A. I. T. Marrero, On the maximization problem for solutions of reaction–diffusion equations with respect to their initial data, *Mathematical Modelling of Natural Phenomena.* **15**, Paper No. 71 (2020).

[32] R. Jaroudi, G. Baravdish, B. T. Johansson, and F. Åström, Numerical reconstruction of brain tumours, *Inverse Problems in Science and Engineering.* **27**(3), 278–298 (2019).

[33] B. Kaltenbacher, A. Neubauer, and O. Scherzer, *Iterative Regularization Methods for Nonlinear Ill-posed Problems* (Walter de Gruyter GmbH & Co. KG, Berlin, 2008).

[34] Y. Jarny, M. N. Ozisik, and J. P. Bardon, A general optimization method using adjoint equation for solving multidimensional inverse heat conduction, *International Journal of Heat and Mass Transfer.* **34**(11), 2911–2919 (1991).

[35] B. Jin and X. Lu, Numerical identification of a Robin coefficient in parabolic problems, *Mathematics of Computation.* **81**(279), 1369–1398 (2012).

[36] D. N. Hào, P. X. Thanh, and D. Lesnic, Determination of the heat transfer coefficients in transient heat conduction, *Inverse Problems.* **29**(9), 095020 (2013).

[37] K. Cao and D. Lesnic, Reconstruction of the perfusion coefficient from temperature measurements using the conjugate gradient method, *International Journal of Computer Mathematics.* **95**(4), 797–814 (2018).

[38] F. Tröltzsch, *Optimal Control of Partial Differential Equations: Theory, Methods, and Applications*, Vol. 112 (American Mathematical Society, Providence, RI, 2010).

[39] H. T. Nguyen, V. A. Khoa, and V. A. Vo, Analysis of a quasi-reversibility method for a terminal value quasi-linear parabolic problem with measurements, *SIAM Journal on Mathematical Analysis.* **51**(1), 60–85 (2019).

[40] V. A. Khoa, Convergence of a spectral regularization of a time-reversed reaction-diffusion problem with high-order Sobolev-Gevrey smoothness, *Journal of Mathematical Analysis and Applications.* **518**(1), 126666 (2023).

[41] N. H. Tuan, D. Lesnic, and P. T. K. Van, Identification of the initial population of a nonlinear predator-prey system backwards in time, *Journal of Mathematical Analysis and Applications.* **479**(1), 1195–1225 (2019).

[42] G. Leoni, *A First Course in Sobolev Spaces*, 2nd edn. Graduate Studies in Mathematics, Vol. 181 (American Mathematical Society, Providence, RI, 2017).

[43] T. Roubíček, *Nonlinear Partial Differential Equations with Applications*, 2nd edn. (Springer Basel, Basel, 2013).

[44] S. Zheng, *Nonlinear Evolution Equations* (Chapman & Hall/CRC, Boca Raton, FL, 2004).

[45] V. A. Galaktionov and J. L. Vázquez, The problem of blow-up in nonlinear parabolic equations, *Discrete and Continuous Dynamical Systems.* **8**(2), 399–433 (2002).

[46] A. De Pablo, An introduction to the problem of blow-up for semilinear and quasilinear parabolic equations, *MAT Serie A: Conferencias, Seminarios y Trabajos de Matemática.* **12**, 3–28 (2006).

[47] A. Friedman, *Partial Differential Equations of Parabolic Type* (Prentice-Hall, Inc., Englewood Cliffs, NJ, 1964).

[48] J.-L. Lions and B. Malgrange, Sur l'unicité rétrograde dans les problèmes mixtes paraboliques, *Mathematica Scandinavica.* **8**(2), 277–286 (1960).

[49] M. Lees and M. H. Protter, Unique continuation for parabolic differential equations and inequalities, *Duke Mathematical Journal.* **28**(3), 369–382 (1961).

[50] N. T. Long and A. P. N. Dinh, Approximation of a parabolic nonlinear evolution equation backwards in time, *Inverse Problems.* **10**(4), 905–914 (1994).

[51] P. T. Nam, An approximate solution for nonlinear backward parabolic equations, *Journal of Mathematical Analysis and Applications.* **367**(2), 337–349 (2010).

[52] D. N. Hào and N. Van Duc, A non-local boundary value problem method for semi-linear parabolic equations backward in time, *Applicable Analysis.* **94**(3), 446–463 (2015).

[53] N. H. Tuan and D. D. Trong, On a backward parabolic problem with local Lipschitz source, *Journal of Mathematical Analysis and Applications.* **414**(2), 678–692 (2014).

[54] D. N. Hào, N. Van Duc, and N. Van Thang, Backward semi-linear parabolic equations with time-dependent coefficients and local Lipschitz source, *Inverse Problems.* **34**(5), 055010 (2018).

[55] I. Kukavica, Log-log convexity and backward uniqueness, *Proceedings of the American Mathematical Society.* **135**(8), 2415–2421 (2007).

[56] P. Cannarsa and M. Yamamoto, Stability for backward problems in time for degenerate parabolic equations (2023). *Preprint* arXiv:2305.00525.

[57] C. Fabre, J.-P. Puel, and E. Zuazua. On the density of the range of the semigroup for semilinear heat equations. In J. E. Lagnese, D. L. Russell, and L. W. White (eds.), *Control and Optimal Design of Distributed Parameter Systems (Minneapolis, MN, 1992).* The IMA Volumes in Mathematics and its Applications, Vol. 70 (Springer, New York, 1995).

[58] M. H. Protter and H. F. Weinberger, *Maximum Principles in Differential Equations* (Springer-Verlag, New York, 1984). Corrected reprint of the 1967 original.

[59] H. Amann, Compact embeddings of vector-valued Sobolev and Besov spaces, *Glasnik Matematicki Series III.* **35**(**55**)(1), 161–177 (2000).

[60] R. Jaroudi, F. Åström, B. T. Johansson, and G. Baravdish, Numerical simulations in 3-dimensions of reaction–diffusion models for brain tumour growth, *International Journal of Computer Mathematics.* **97**(6), 1151–1169 (2020).

[61] T. Schuster, B. Kaltenbacher, B. Hofmann, and K. S. Kazimierski, *Regularization Methods in Banach Spaces* (Walter de Gruyter GmbH & Co. KG, Berlin, 2012).

[62] E. Casas and F. Tröltzsch, Stability for semilinear parabolic optimal control problems with respect to initial data, *Applied Mathematics & Optimization.* **86**(2), (2022). Paper No. 16.

[63] D. Pighin, Nonuniqueness of minimizers for semilinear optimal control problems, *Journal of the European Mathematical Society (JEMS)* **25**(6), 2127–2162 (2022).

[64] H. Amann, Existence and regularity for semilinear parabolic evolution equations, *The Annali della Scuola Normale Superiore di Pisa, Classe di Scienze (4).* **11**(4), 593–676 (1984).

[65] L. C. Evans, *Partial Differential Equations*, 2nd edn. Graduate Studies in Mathematics, Vol. 19 (American Mathematical Society, Providence, RI, 2010).

[66] J. Nocedal and S. J. Wright, *Numerical Optimization*, 2nd edn. Springer Series in Operations Research and Financial Engineering (Springer, New York, 2006).

[67] J. W. Daniel, The conjugate gradient method for linear and nonlinear operator equations, *SIAM Journal on Numerical Analysis.* **4**(1), 10–26 (1967).

[68] O. Axelsson and A. T. Chronopoulos, On nonlinear generalized conjugate gradient methods, *Numerische Mathematik.* **69**(1), 1–15 (1994).

[69] K. Cao and D. Lesnic, Simultaneous identification and reconstruction of the space-dependent reaction coefficient and source term, *Journal of Inverse and Ill-posed Problems.* **29**(6), 867–894 (2021).

[70] H. W. Engl, M. Hanke, and A. Neubauer, *Regularization of Inverse Problems.* Mathematics and its Applications, Vol. 375 (Kluwer Academic Publishers Group, Dordrecht, 1996).

[71] B. H. Menze, A. Jakab, S. Bauer, J. Kalpathy-Cramer, K. Farahani, J. Kirby, *et al.*, The multimodal brain tumor image segmentation benchmark (BraTS), *IEEE Transactions on Medical Imaging.* **34**(10), 1993–2024 (2015).

[72] S. Bakas, H. Akbari, A. Sotiras, M. Bilello, M. Rozycki, J. Kirby, *et al.*, Advancing the cancer genome atlas glioma MRI collections with expert segmentation labels and radiomic features, *Scientific Data.* **4** (2017).

[73] S. Bakas, M. Reyes, A. Jakab, S. Bauer, M. Rempfler, A. Crimi, *et al.*, Identifying the best machine learning algorithms for brain tumor segmentation, progression assessment, and overall survival prediction in the BraTS challenge (2018). *Preprint* arXiv:1811.02629.

[74] R. Frackowiak, K. Friston, C. Frith, R. Dolan, C. Price, S. Zeki, *et al.*, *Human Brain Function*, 2nd edn. (Academic Press, London, 2004).

[75] Y. Y. Zhang, M. Brady, and S. A. Smith, Segmentation of brain MR images through a hidden Markov random field model and the expectation-maximization algorithm, *IEEE Transactions on Medical Imaging.* **20**(1), 45–57 (2001).

[76] M. Jenkinson, C. F. Beckmann, T. E. Behrens, M. W. Woolrich, and S. M. Smith, FSL, *NeuroImage.* **62**(2), 782–790 (2012).

[77] S. A. Gerschgorin, Über die Abgrenzung der Eigenwerte einer Matrix, *Izvestiya Akademii Nauk SSSR.* **1931**(6), 749–754 (1931).

[78] E. Zeidler, *Nonlinear Functional Analysis and Its Applications. II/B* (Springer-Verlag, New York, 1990).

Epilogue

Raluca Eftimie[*,†,§] **and Dumitru Trucu**[‡]

†*Laboratoire de mathématiques de Besançon,*
Université de Franche-Comté, Besançon, France
‡*Division of Mathematics, School of Science and Engineering,*
University of Dundee, Dundee, UK
§*raluca.eftimie@univ-fcomte.fr*

This volume provides a snapshot of current mathematical modelling approaches in oncology, while focussing one way or another on data: from data-inspired modelling of tumour–immune interactions to data-inspired biomechanical interactions between different tumour cell populations, interactions between different types of therapies for cancers (e.g., chemotherapies and virotherapies), and finally identification of parameters associated with the dynamics of cancer cells using real or synthetic data. Such single-scale or multi-scale data (which might not always be available at this moment) are needed to parametrise the mathematical models, with the ultimate goal of eventually using them as part of personalised anti-cancer treatments. However, even if we are not there yet in terms of the use of the mathematical models for personalised clinical cancer treatment, we can still

---

*The author is also an Honorary Professor at School of Science and Engineering, University of Dundee, Dundee, UK. Email address: r.a.eftimie@dundee.ac.uk.

use these models to explore the basic mechanisms behind the development of cancers and the impact of various anti-cancer therapies. The single-scale and multi-scale mathematical models overviewed here, which described a variety of local and non-local biological interactions occurring across different spatial scales (molecular-level, cell-level, and tissue-level scales), have been used to scrutinise different biological hypotheses and to propose new biological hypotheses for further experimental investigation.

The contributions to this volume were written in 2022 and 2023. We admit that, due to various academic commitments, the volume failed in its vision to showcase a wider range of mathematical models for cancer evolution, e.g., discrete models (agent-based and/or cellular automata) or hybrid models, and rather focussed on continuum models. It also failed to have more expert contributions from clinicians and experimentalists. Also, it failed in having chapters on the promising use of artificial intelligence (AI) on personalised data-driven cancer healthcare: from cancer detection to cancer prognosis and cancer treatment selection. This would have been important since the future of research in mathematical oncology will combine mechanistic modelling with AI approaches to integrate data generated at an even increased rate. The fact that not all generated data are currently useful for the type of mathematical models derived (and many mathematical modellers ask for more specific data to parametrise their models) is also the result of a lack of communication between modellers, experimentalists, and clinicians, each focussing on addressing different questions that they think are important. Nevertheless, the use of AI will also speed-up the integration of these different questions and the development of new mathematical models to take advantage of the currently available data.

Despite all these shortcomings, we hope that the current chapters still provide an overview of some of the current research directions in the vast field of mathematical oncology and further incite the interested readers to develop new modelling approaches and analysis methodologies for these mathematical models.

Finally, we take this opportunity to thank all authors who contributed to this volume and to the publishing team without whom this volume would have not been possible.

Index

www.ingramcontent.com/pod-product-compliance
Lightning Source LLC
Chambersburg PA
CBHW050542190326
41458CB00007B/1885